A Primer of Medicine

A Primer of Medicine

FOURTH EDITION

M. H. Pappworth
M.D., M.R.C.P.

Concerned mainly with
history taking and
eliciting and interpreting
clinical signs

BUTTERWORTHS
London Boston
Sydney Wellington Durban Toronto

THE BUTTERWORTH GROUP

United Kingdom	**Butterworth & Co (Publishers) Ltd** **London:** 88 Kingsway, WC2B 6AB
Australia	**Butterworth Pty Ltd** **Sydney:** 586 Pacific Highway, Chatswood NSW 2067 Also at Melbourne, Adelaide and Perth
Canada	**Butterworth & Co (Canada) Ltd** **Toronto:** 2265 Midland Avenue, Scarborough, Ontario, M1P 4S1
New Zealand	**Butterworths of New Zealand Ltd** **Wellington:** 77–85 Customhouse Quay, 1
South Africa	**Butterworth & Co (South Africa) (Pty) Ltd** **Durban:** 152–154 Gale Street
USA	**Butterworth (Publishers) Inc** **Boston:** 19 Cummings Park, Woburn, Mass. 01801

First published, 1960
Reprinted, 1960, 1961, 1962
Second edition, 1963
Reprinted, 1964, 1967, 1969
Third edition, 1971
Reprinted, 1974, 1975
Fourth edition, 1978

ISBN 0 407 62603 4

© Butterworths and Co (Publishers) Ltd, 1978

British Library Cataloguing in Publication Data

Pappworth, Maurice Henry
  A primer of medicine. – 4th ed.
  1. Diagnosis
  I. Title
  616.07'5   RC71   77–30428

  ISBN 0-407-62603-4

Typeset by Butterworth Litho Preparation Department
Printed by Page Bros (Norwich) Ltd.

This book is dedicated to my daughters,
Joanna, Dinah and Sara.

'Much have I learned from my teachers; more from my colleagues;
and from my students more than from them all.'
Rabbi Judah Ha-Nasi, who lived in the second century CE [AD]
Talmud—Treatise Makkot 10a

In this book there are many quotations from the Talmud which is an
encyclopaedic compendium comprising many large volumes and was
compiled between about 300 BC and 200 CE (AD) and consists of
biblical exegesis, detailed discussion of Jewish law and jurisprudence,
ceremonial and liturgical practices, homiletics, anecdotes and
philosophy.

'Notwithstanding my desire and delight to be the disciple of the
earlier authorities and to maintain their views and to assert them,
I do not consider myself a donkey carrying books. I will explain
their ways and appreciate their value, but when their views are
inconceivable to my thoughts, I will plead in all modesty, but will
judge according to the sight of my own eyes. And when the meaning
is clear I shall flatter none, for the Lord gives wisdom in all times
and in all ages.'
    Rabbi Moshe ben Nachman (1194—1270), generally referred to
as Nachmanides, was a talmudic and biblical scholar and mystic
who lived in Spain.

'Life is short and the Art (of medicine) long, opportunity is fleeting, judgment difficult and experience dangerous. The physician must do the right thing at the right time.' First aphorism of Hippocrates translated by Adams, a nineteenth century Aberdeen doctor and classical scholar.

'It would seem, Adeimantus, that the direction in which education starts a man will determine his future life.' Plato *Republic* iv.

'To study medicine without books is to sail an uncharted sea, whilst to study medicine only from books is not to go to sea at all.'
Sir William Osler (1849–1919), Professor of Medicine, Montreal, Philadelphia, Boston and Oxford.

Preface to the fourth edition

This is primarily a textbook for undergraduates but it is hoped that many postgraduates will also find it useful, and general practitioners who wish either to relearn their medicine or refresh their knowledge may find the information and advice helpful. The book is meant for all doctors however young or old.

In this new edition I have extensively rewritten, rearranged and added to all the chapters and included two new ones.

The power to communicate properly is essential for all students, teachers and physicians and words are the basic element of communication and hence their great importance. However with the prevalence of multiple choice questions and the habit of writing case notes crammed with abbreviations, there is a serious danger of doctors becoming illiterate. I have attempted to counteract this by including a new chapter on Medical Vocabulary. There is also a new chapter dealing with the basic elements of Dermatology, a subject which should be of great importance to all physicians. The chapter on Limbs is an expanded version of the earlier chapter on The Hands.

Preface to the third edition

The whole book has been rewritten and many minor alterations have been made. New chapters have been added on ethical precepts, the arts and science of diagnosis, general appearance, the head and facies, ophthalmology, the neck and the hands.

I have often been advised to include many illustrations such as are present in most textbooks on physical signs. Illustrations add enormously to the cost of a book and I do not consider that they would afford a commensurate aid to the reader. Is a reader really helped by a photograph of a physician doing a rectal examination, eliciting a knee jerk, or percussing a chest?

Preface to the second edition

The first edition of this book has been an enormous success. The many letters of appreciation, helpful suggestions and criticisms from all parts of the world have stimulated me to improve it. I thank the many people who have helped me in this way.

Over five hundred relatively short, but often important, alterations, additions and deletions have been made. Wherever there was any doubt about the clarity of a section it has been rewritten.

Many readers have made suggestions for new sections to be added but I have purposely restricted such additions to a very few. These are on hypertension, cyanosis, cor pulmonale, and the nerve supply of the bladder. This book was never meant to be a comprehensive textbook of medicine or even of physical signs. It is purposely a very personal selection, and I have no desire for the Primer to grow into a large tome. There is not an original idea in the whole of this book and yet I feel that it really is my own child, a personal contribution.

The index is a very important part of any textbook, and I have personally been responsible for the new one.

Contents

1 Ethical Precepts

'Good behaviour is just as important as obedience to the law.'
Talmud Mishna Gadol.

Samuel Johnson (1709–84), the British author and compiler of
the first English dictionary defined ethics as, 'A system of morality'
and quoted Francis Bacon (1561–1626): 'True ethics are but the
handmaid of divinity and religion.'

All great religions have three components, dogma (belief), ritual,
(ceremonial practices), and ethics (conduct in relation to others).
I consider that the ethical aspects are the most important. Logic
and reason should be important guides to right action but they
alone cannot control its quality or value to be a guide to moral
judgments. Personally I am prepared to support wholeheartedly the
controversial dictum of the distinguished lawyer Lord Denning,
who in his Earl Grey Memorial Lecture in Newcastle in 1953 said,
'Without religion there can be no morality and without morality
there can be no law'.

Doctors even more than priests and lawyers have a close relationship with their clients. To be a good doctor one must therefore be a
person of high purpose and moral integrity whose sense of principle
will not be overriden by any lower consideration of expediency or
by the attempts of others to persuade them to any course of action
which conflicts their own ethics or belies their critical judgments.
Medical ethics should never be confined to the narrow meaning of
professional relationships between doctors themselves, which is often
merely a consideration of etiquette.

It is no longer customary for doctors on graduation to be asked
to take the Hippocratic Oath or any such pledge. Much of the
ancient Hippocratic Oath is undoubtedly obsolete but its main
principles are still sound. But today, when medicine is rapidly
becoming dehumanized because of emphasis on laboratory procedures and the domination of many medical schools by research
workers, it is becoming more and more necessary that all doctors
subscribe to, and earnestly and meticulously follow, an agreed ethical
code. Some famous old codes are appended and I have made an
attempt to formulate a set of modern medical ethical principles.

I also believe that para-medical personnel, including nurses and all social workers, should have a recognized and enforced code of conduct.

'I swear by Apollo the physician, by Aesculapius, by Hygiaea, by Panacea and by all the gods and goddesses, calling upon them to witness that, according to my ability and judgment, I will in every particular keep this oath and covenant.

'To regard he who teaches this art equally with my parents. To share my substance, and, if need be, to relieve his necessities and to regard his offspring equally with my brethren and to teach his art, if they should wish to learn it, without fee or stipulation. To impart a knowledge by precept and by lecture and by every other mode of instruction to my sons, to the sons of my teacher and to pupils who are bound by stipulation and by oath according to the law of medicine but to no other.

'I will use that regimen which according to my ability and judgment shall be for the welfare of the sick and I will refrain from that which may be baneful or injurious. If any should ask of me a drug to produce death I will not give it. Nor will I suggest such a counsel. In like manner I will not give a woman a destructive pessary. With purity and holiness will I watch closely my life and my art. I will not cut for stone but give way to those who are practitioners in this work. Into whatever houses I shall enter I shall go to aid the sick, abstaining from every voluntary act of injustice and corruption and from lasciviousness with women or men, free or slaves.

'Whatever in the life of men I shall see or hear in my practice or without my practice which should not be made public, this I will hold in silence, believing that such things should not be spoken. While I keep this my oath inviolate and unbroken may it be granted to me to enjoy life and my art, forever honoured by all men. But should I by transgression violate it, be mine the reverse.' Hippocrates (460–377 BC) lived in the island of Cos. He was a contemporary of the Greek philosophers Plato and Aristotle. His main concern medically was with clinical observations, especially those which were guides to prognosis.

'This is the covenant that Asaph, the son of Barachiah, and Jochanan, the son of Zabda, entered into with their disciples and enjoined them saying,

'Take heed that you will not kill any man with a root decoction. Do not prepare any potion that may cause a woman who has conceived in adultery to miscarry. Do not lust after beautiful women to commit adultery with them. Do not divulge a man's secrets that he has confided unto you. Do not be bribed to do injury and harm and do not harden your heart against the poor and needy, rather have compassion upon them and heal them. Do not follow in the ways of sorcerers to enchant by witchcraft and magic to part a man from his beloved or a woman from the husband of her youth. Do not covet any bribe or reward or assist in sexual misdemeanours. . .

'Do not cause the shedding of blood by essaying any dangerous experiment in the exercise of medical skill. Do not cause a sickness in any man. Do not hasten to maim and do not cut the flesh of man by any instrument or by branding before first observing twice and even thrice and only then giving your counsel. Guard against haughtiness and conceit. Do not bear a grudge against a sick man and beware of revengeful acts.' *The Book of Asaph* – Oxford Hebrew manuscript 2138 translated by S. Muntner. Asaf, known as Asaf HaYehudi (the Jew) and Asaf HaRofe (the Physician) lived in Babylon (modern Iraq) in the sixth century and wrote the first known medical treatise in Hebrew.

A prayer for the young doctor or student:

'Imbue my soul with gentleness and calmness when older colleagues, proud of their age, wish to push me aside or scorn me or teach me disdainfully. May even this be of advantage to me, for they know many things of which I am ignorant.' Maimonides.

A prayer for the older physician:

'Grant me an opportunity to improve and extend my training, since there is no limit to knowledge. Help me to correct and supplement my educational defects as the scope of science and the horizon widens every day. Give me courage to realize my daily mistakes so that tomorrow I shall be able to see and understand in a better light what I could not comprehend in the dim light of yesterday. Bless me with a spirit of devotion and self-sacrifice so that I can treat and heal Thy suffering servants and prevent disease and preserve health to the best of my ability and knowledge.

'Grant that my patients have confidence in me and my art and follow my directions and counsel.

'Oh grant that neither greed for gain nor thirst for fame nor vain ambition may interfere with my work.

'May I see in the afflicted and the suffering only a fellow human being in need.' Maimonides.

Moses ben Maimon (Maimonides), 1135–1204, was a Rabbi, philosopher, biblical and talmudic commentator and physician who practised medicine in Spain and Egypt.

'This is my vow. To perfect my medical art and never to swerve from it so long as God grants me my office, and to oppose all false medicine and teachings. Then to love the sick, each and all of them, more than if my own body were at stake. Not to judge anything superficially but by symptoms and signs. Not to administer any medicine without under-

standing, nor to collect any money without earning it. Not
to guess but to know.' Paracelsus: Philippus Theophrastus
Bombastus von Hohenheim, 1493–1541, a Swiss physician
who took the name Paracelsus by which he is usually known,
was a great opponent of traditionalism and bigotry in medicine.
'You must feel and act as a gentleman . . . But let there be no
misunderstanding as to who is to be regarded as a gentleman.
It is not he who is fashionable in his dress, expensive in his
habits, fond of fine equipages, pushing himself into the society
of those who are above himself in their worldly station, that is
entitled to that appellation. It is he who sympathizes with
others, and is careful not to hurt their feelings even on trifling
occasions; who, in little things as well as great, assumes nothing
which does not belong to him, and yet respects himself; this is
the kind of gentleman which a medical practitioner should
wish to be. Never pretend to know what cannot be known;
make no promises which it is not probable that you will be
able to fulfil.' Sir Benjamin Brodie, 1783–1862, from the
Introductory Discourse in his *Clinical Lectures in Surgery*.
Sir Benjamin Brodie was surgeon to St George's Hospital,
London; he was one of the founder Fellows of the Royal
College of Surgeons of London, and was made in 1858 the
first president of the General Medical Council.

The World Medical Association was founded in 1947 as a direct
consequence of the Nuremberg trials of the infamous Nazi doctors.
In 1948 it issued its own revised version of the Hippocratic Oath,
a compilation called the Geneva Code, which is as follows:

'At the time of being admitted as a member of the medical
profession I solemnly pledge myself to concentrate my life to
the services of humanity. I will give to my teachers the respect
and gratitude which is their due. I will practise my profession
with conscience and dignity. The health of my patients will be
my first consideration. I will respect the secrets which are
confided in me. I will maintain by all the means in my power
the honour and the noble tradition of the medical profession.
My colleagues will be my brothers. I will not permit considerations of religion, nationality, race, party politics or
social standing to intervene between my duty and my patient.
I will maintain the utmost respect for human life from the
time of conception, even under threat, I will not use my
medical knowledge contrary to the laws of humanity. I make
these promises solemnly, freely and upon my honour.'

This Code was later revised as follows:

'Duties of doctors in general
'A doctor must always maintain the highest standards of
professional conduct. A doctor must practise his profession

uninfluenced by motives of profit. The following practices are deemed unethical.

(*a*) Any self-advertisement except such as is expressly authorised by the national code of medical ethics. (*b*) Collaboration in any form of medical activity in which the doctor does not have professional independence. (*c*) Receiving any money in connection with the services rendered to a patient other than proper professional fee, even with the knowledge of the patient.

'Any act or advice which could weaken physical or mental resistance of a human being may be used only in his own interest. A doctor is advised to use great caution in divulging discoveries or new techniques of treatment. A doctor should certify or testify only to that which he has personally verified.'

'Duties of doctors to the sick

'A doctor must always bear in mind the obligation of preserving human life. A doctor owes to his patients complete loyalty and all the resources of his science. Whenever an examination or treatment is beyond his capacity he should summon another doctor who has the necessary ability. A doctor should preserve absolute secrecy about all he knows about his patient because of the confidence entrusted in him.

'A doctor must give emergency care as a humanitarian duty unless he is assured that others are willing and able to give such care.

'Duties of doctors to each other

'A doctor ought to behave to his colleagues as he would have them behave to him. A doctor must not entice patients from his colleagues.'

While recognizing that medical ethics are too complicated to be summarized in a few Olympian phrases, with temerity and due humility I append my own suggested thirteen principles to which all doctors on graduation should agree to conform:

1. I have responsibilities to the medical profession and to the community but the health and welfare of my patients will always be my prime consideration and not what may be for the advancement of science or medical knowledge or what may be for the good of society in general.
2. I will always deal with my patients with sympathy and loving care, regardless of their race, colour, nationality, religion, party politics, or social status.
3. I will not do anything to my patients which I would not readily agree to being done in similar circumstances to myself or my closest relatives.
4. I will never knowingly harm any patient.

5. I will never submit any patient to any operation or investigation without the patient's valid consent. By valid consent is meant consent after full disclosure of what is to be done and mention of all likely discomforts and dangers. The patient, in reference to age and mental state, must be capable of giving consent, and consent must always be obtained with the patient possessing free choice, devoid of all coercion and not engineered by trickery or fraud.

6. I will not abuse or take advantage of the doctor–patient relationship in order to indulge in any sexual activity with a patient.

7. I will take care not to become addicted to alcohol or drugs.

8. I will not advertise or canvass directly or indirectly for patients or entice patients away from any colleagues.

9. I will treat doctors and their wives and husbands and children without any payment in money or kind.

10. I will not take from any patient, or any organization, or the state, any payment for services, including at hospital, which I have not actually performed.

11. I will always behave towards my colleagues – be they my contemporaries, or seniors, or juniors – as I would have them behave towards myself.

12. I will never indulge in dichotomy (fee-splitting).

13. I will never divulge any personal matter which has been confided to me in secret by any of my patients unless I am obliged to do so, in spite of my protests, by order of a judge or statutory obligation. But this obligation to patients does not remove the requirement to assist the law in the detection of crime.

Unfortunately there is a gap which sometimes may be wide between the ideals enunciated in the codes cited above and actual practice. Many acts are done by some doctors in some countries which do not conform with those codes but are not punishable by the laws of their country. But ethical decisions cannot always be left to the conscience of individual doctors. It is arrogant to assume that all doctors' consciences are of a high standard of morality. Moreover there are many doctor–patient relationships of which society as a whole must be the final arbiter.

The Golden Rule as enunciated by Rabbi Hillel (first century BC) should always be every doctor's guide; 'What is hateful to you never do to your fellow man.'

Etienne de Greliet (1773–1855) wrote the following pledge:
'I will pass through this world but once. Any good therefore that I can do, or any kindness which I can show to any human being, let me do it now. Let me not defer it or neglect it for I shall not pass this way again.'

2 Learning and Teaching Clinical Medicine

'And gladly wolde he lerne and gladly teche.' Chaucer (1340–1400), Prologue to *Canterbury Tales.*
Rabbi Ben Zoma said:
'Who is wise? He who learns from all men; as it is said in Psalm 119, verse 99, "From all my teachers I have gotten understanding." ' *Talmud, Sayings of the Fathers*, 4. 1.

Probably in no field of human knowledge is a true start more important and a false one more disastrous than in clinical medicine. The material contained herein is essential for a proper understanding and assessment of any textbook of clinical medicine or specialized monograph.

Many students are surprisingly ignorant of what I consider to be essentials. Although they can prattle of diamond murmurs, clicks, crunches, knocks, ejections, laminar flow, turbulence, vortex shedding and jet impact and aortic run off, they can neither diagnose a common valvular lesion nor discuss logically its differential diagnosis. Others can declaim concerning spike waves on an EEG and yet are unable to enumerate the signs of a posterior column lesion.

The pages which follow are crammed with facts but, although it is fashionable to decry factual knowledge in medicine, it is impossible to be a good clinician without possessing a large store of facts; for example, a doctor cannot safely prescribe drugs without the factual knowledge of their doses and their therapeutic and toxic effects, and he cannot diagnose neurological cases without a deal of factual knowledge about neuroanatomy. Moreover, every fact which is learned becomes a key for other facts. Factual knowledge is not acquired by inspiration, but only by techniques of memorizing and hard work. 'Knowledge is an essential prerequisite to performance' (Rabbi J. H. Hertz, the late British Chief Rabbi).

The phrase 'essential knowledge' is purposely used in preference to the usual 'basic facts'. An oft-repeated advice to students is, 'Master the basic facts of the subject'. Few physicians are in agreement as to which are the basic facts of any branch of medicine. Many consider that the correct way to teach electrocardiography is first to expound at length on electrophysics such as cellular depolarization and repolarization, charge distributions, homogeneous volume conduction and membrane action potentials. A recent textbook written primarily for undergraduates boasts, 'This book emphasizes the concept of vectors using orthogenal lead systems and also stresses the value of the hexiaxial system in analysing frontal plane leads'. All this is completely useless knowledge except for the superspecialist. Any student can become even more than merely competent at electrocardiographic interpretation without such knowledge. Others insist that students must be conversant with the physics of sound and rheology (the science of the flow of liquids and its ultrasonic, thermal and electromagnetic measurement) and wave dynamics, and must know the theories concerning the production of heart and breath sounds before attempting to master the technique of auscultation. Whether or not any of these are 'basic facts' is not worth arguing, but I strongly affirm that they are not essential knowledge for the clinician. We can learn how to drive a car with even more than mere competence without a knowledge of the laws of thermodynamics of the internal combustion engine. Good motor mechanics recognize the cause of an abnormal noise in a car although they probably have no knowledge of physics. A good golf teacher does not insist that his pupil first learns about the laws of dynamics as applied to trajectories. Only the learned ignoramus would teach a child the history of our alphabet before teaching him how to read.

Too many people are over-concerned with the techniques of teaching and pay too little attention to what is taught and by whom. The danger is that today students are often educated to become clever asses. Undoubtedly the greatest of all educational handicaps is poor teaching, and neither the latest audio-visual aids nor drastic revision of the curriculum can overcome such a misfortune. Let teachers stop waffling about learning how to learn and instead imbue their pupils with the realization that hard work is an essential component of learning. A good teacher always acts as a stimulant and never as a narcotic. Enthusiasm, an ability to talk fluently and knowledge of the subject are three essentials of good teaching. Moreover, the teacher must always remember that students are consciously or otherwise imitators of their teachers. This is desirable but places a yoke on the teacher which he must accept gladly, in that he must always be aware of his own eccentricities and slipshod techniques, and that too much exposure of students to these bad examples may have a permanently deleterious effect. Students will never think logically or clearly if their teachers do not do so themselves. The most important pedagogic method is teaching by example.

Some students are difficult to teach because they resent being corrected however politely. Students must learn to value criticism and indications of disapproval. The teacher who overlooks a fault is likely to cause repetition of that fault and commission of others. Students should listen to the advice of Rabbi Eleazer of Worms (twelfth century) who said: 'Cherish not too good an opinion of yourself but lend your ear to remonstrance and reproof.'

My advice to teachers is to guide their pupils without pampering them, and to help them without being meddlesome. The teacher must exhibit a vibrant enthusiasm, a conveying of convictions, a giving of something of himself so that, in the words of Samuel Johnson, 'New things are made familiar and familiar things made new'.

Rabbi Ishmael (*Talmud, Sayings of the Fathers*, chapter 4) said, 'He who learns in order to teach, he will be enabled to learn and to teach but he who learns in order to practice will be enabled to learn, to teach and to practice.' Teachers by carefully preparing their lectures and clinical demonstrations and by expressing their thoughts clearly, by answering questions diligently and with patience, and by taking part in discussions with students, thereby not only improve their students but also improve their own clinical ability and broaden their own mental horizons.

Rabbi Eleazar ben Shomma (*Talmud, Sayings of the Fathers*, chapter 4) advised, 'Let the honour of your students be as dear to you as your own honour.' Students must respect their teachers and the teachers must respect their pupils, being courteous and friendly towards them. But respect for students must never be mere condescension or gratuitous courtesies. If you wish to bring out the best in your students you must not ride roughshod over them and so damage their self-confidence. Neither must you attempt to impress them with your own brilliance compared with their ignorance. Teachers must produce an atmosphere conducive to learning and that depends largely on the force of their personality.

My advice to students is to realize that there are four essential qualities necessary to acquire a worthwhile medical education: (1) intellectual ability, (2) a full stretching of that ability by an indomitable will to overcome all obstacles to learning, (3) a genuine appreciation of the value of education coupled with a desire to be educated, and (4) hard work.

Many students, filled with self pity, complain that they are overwhelmed by the sheer volume of knowledge which is apparently necessary. Whilst I have some sympathy with them I favour the opinion of Dr Burch of New Orleans, 'The idea that there is too much to learn is ridiculous. There is not too much to learn for one who is properly motivated and is healthy in mind and body.' Undergraduate and postgraduate students must realize that their education must be a continuing process and clinical judgment, insight, forbearance and wisdom are all qualities which require for attainment the passage of much time and experience before they even begin to be properly developed.

Socrates (469–399 BC), one of the greatest of all teachers, taught mainly by posing questions, and in his conversations he adopted the pose of a man who himself knows nothing but is asking for information. He declared one of his main aims to be to prick bubbles because amongst others who professed to teach he found pretentiousness, confusion of thought and sheer ignorance. Plato represented Socrates as an intellectual midwife extracting knowledge already existing from those whom he questioned. But I am fully in agreement with the German philosopher Nietzche (1844–1900) who wrote, 'The surest way to corrupt a young man is to teach him to esteem more highly those who think alike than those who think differently'.

I plead for the return to the famous tradition of clinical teaching which was formerly the pride of British medicine, a tradition which insisted that clinical teaching must begin and continue at the bedside, using books, lectures and pictures as mere supplements. Osler's own selected epitaph was, 'He taught medicine in the wards'.

Research and specialization

Two important causes of poor clinical teaching are the domination of the medical schools by research workers and over-specialization by many clinicians. Too often professors of clinical medicine and their assistants are research doctors whose primary and often sole interest is research, and who evince but scant interest in bedside medicine and bedside teaching. The specialist expert is often a person who avoids minor errors in his own speciality which are of little practical importance but makes many major mistakes in other branches of medicine.

'Specialization must be grafted on to a robust stock of general medicine, for like the hybrid rose, it will not thrive on its own roots. The narrow specialist whose field of vision is limited to his own branch of medicine is a menace both to the profession and to the patient; he sees disease through tinted glasses.' Professor Bramwell, 1959, *Clinical Introduction to Heart Disease* (Oxford University Press).

Superspecialization often produces physicians who, though they may be excellent technicians, are incapable of a good doctor–patient relationship and thus are poor clinicians.

The superspecialist or the man who has attained eminence because of a gimmick is very liable to become a pedant who idolatrously worships his subject or gimmick, who exaggerates the importance of his technical jargon and conceptual knowledge, who prides himself on his mastery of the trivia and minutiae of his small subject and who, if perchance he is an examiner, would not hesitate to deem lack of such knowledge a serious fault. His zeal, dogmatism and narrow expertise are often dangerous to students. Such specialists often discuss simple things in a complex and confusing way. Simplification is not always clarification but it very often is. Teachers who do not deign to teach except in extreme depth have a stultifying effect on their pupils. Over fifty years ago Osler wrote,

'The specialist loses all sense of proportion in a maze of minutiae. Everywhere men are in small coteries absorbing subjects of deep interest but of very limited scope or practical application. They quickly lose all sense of proportion and the smaller their field the greater is the tendency to megacephaly.'

Superspecialists become fenced in by their own habits of thought and they look on all other approaches to even their narrow subject as inferior to their own. Each superspecialist possesses only a small fragment of the truth about even his own speciality, but he often believes it to be the whole truth which he carries around in his pocket to bring out and magnify to a gross distortion whenever he teaches, in order to prove to his audience that he has solved all the mysteries of the universe.

Nobody should deny that science is essential for the development of medicine and research is necessary if a university is to flourish. Medical students must have a scientific training, but this itself is not enough. Students must know patients as fellow human beings and they must be familiar with the various types of society in which their patients live. After such long exposure to the outpourings of superspecialists and researchers it is a miracle that any young graduates wish to become general practitioners, and the lost enthusiasm for general practice is wholly deplorable. The aim should be to become genuine bedside doctors and not merely the recipients and sorters of laboratory and X-ray reports. Unfortunately specialization has broken the continuity of clinical teaching, and the general approach and the ability to examine and consider patients as a whole is being ignored.

Reliance on tests

'First, the errors and limitations of these new techniques are not at first appreciated. Often the data yielded by clinical examination are of much greater precision in the identification of disease. Second, a thorough clinical examination, which will only be carried out by doctors who appreciate its worth, is the best method of establishing the spirit of mutual understanding and goodwill which is the core of the doctor–patient relationship. Finally, to rely on data the nature of which you do not understand is the first step to losing intellectual honesty.' Sir George Pickering.

Clinical signs are indeed not infallible, but neither are ECGs, X-rays or biochemical data. A good clinician is always conscious of the fact that laboratory, radiological and even histological reports can be wrong. Neither machines nor those using them are infallible. Moreover, different laboratories, using different techniques, may have different notions as to what constitutes the normal range of many commonly performed estimations, including blood uric acid, cholesterol, prothrombin, many enzymes and even serum calcium.

It is also very important to be always aware that an abnormal laboratory or radiological report, even if true, may be totally irrelevant to the patient's diagnostic problem. For example, a report of a high blood uric acid does not prove that the patient's symptoms are due to gout or even that he has gout, nor does a positive serological latex test indicate that the patient is certainly suffering from rheumatoid arthritis.

'The technically trained physician, as distinguished from the educated physician, may try impulsively, by the unwise and neurotic multiplication of tests and superfluous instrumentations, to achieve the illusion of certainty, and such behaviour may be only a manifestation of another type of superstition, blind faith in the laboratory report. Such a physician, technically overloaded but inadequately educated in the humane sense, is often constrained to maintain a phoney attitude of omniscience.' J. C. Whitehorn, 1961, *New England Journal of Medicine,* **265** (1961) 301. It can be correctly said of clinical investigations that what the fool does in the end the wise physician does in the beginning.

Theories

The clinical teacher and the student must always be concerned primarily with facts and only secondarily, if at all, with theories. They must avoid the frequent habit of first discussing theories which attempt to explain some problem concerning the subject under discussion, instead of first making sure that they are conversant with the accepted facts.

Unfortunately many teachers prefer trotting out the most implausible hypotheses rather than admit ignorance and to stifle commonsense in favour of far fetched theories. 'Profess not knowledge which you do not have' is the advice of Ben Sira (Ecclesiasticus 3:25). The good teacher spends most of his teaching time dealing with what is known for certainty and very little on theories. Students should be taught to recognize theories as speculations and not incontrovertible facts. Students should be taught to observe first and possibly explain later.

Imagination, flair and creative insight are rarely present in medical research today, but are all essential to the formulation of truly new and really important concepts. 'Let us learn to dream and then one day, perhaps, we shall know the truth', was a wise dictum of the chemist Kekule who himself had a stupendous inspiration which led him to formulate his theory concerning the structure of the benzene ring. But no medical teacher should keep on reciting his dreams to his students until the dreams have become reality. In both research and teaching the number of theories expounded is inversely proportional to the number of hard facts.

Whether one accepts the circus theory of causation of atrial fibrillation as a scientific truth or despises such a view as outmoded is of minor importance compared with the clinical ability to recognize and correctly treat atrial fibrillation. No patient has ever suffered because of his doctor's belief or disbelief in the circus theory. But many patients have suffered because atrial fibrillation has been missed or improperly treated. To give another example, it does not help the student to know the view of a leading cardiologist that the bruit of mitral regurgitation is produced by a sudden prolapse of the mural cusps of the valve into the left atrium late in systole, even if this be true.

Disregard of academic waffle is the hallmark of the professional craftsman. We must not let theoreticians bamboozle us with their claims to second sight or their professed ability to unravel all divine mysteries. Blind subservience to any theory which happens to be current is mere foolishness. Byron's riposte, 'I wish he would explain his explanations', is apposite. In clinical medicine what is fobbed off as science is mere speculation, but too many 'scientific' physicians regard speculation and verification as identical.

'So long as men are not trained to withhold judgment in the absence of sound evidence, they will be led astray by cock-sure prophets, and it is likely that their leaders will be either ignorant fanatics or dishonest charlatans. To endure uncertainty is difficult but so are many of the other virtues.' Bertrand Russell.

'Theories are vast soap bubbles with which the grown-up children of learning amuse themselves, whilst the ignorant stand gazing on and dignify these vagaries by the name of science.' Rabbi J. H. Hertz.

A great English social historian, R. H. Tawney, was fond of reminding his students, 'Facts are like swallows pursued by snails, the theories, which never catch them up.'

The student and the teacher must always remember that what is new is not necessarily true and what is true is not necessarily new. The latest theory is not always the best. One should follow the advice of Pope (*Essays in Criticism*, 1711):

'Be not the first by whom the new is tried
Nor yet the last to lay the old aside.'

This advice should also be aptly applied to drug therapy and to surgery. Dean Inge admonished us, 'There are two types of fools; one says "This is old and therefore is good"; the other says "This is new and therefore better".' Indeed, theories like fashions are ever changing, and what is accepted as orthodox today may be deemed absurd tomorrow. Even the very briefest study of the history of science will convince us of the ephemeral nature of many 'scientific' theories and 'established' truths which later are discarded as superstitions or are superseded by yet other theories. The progress of medicine is strewn like a desert track with bleached skeletons, the skeletons of discarded theories which when first propounded appeared to possess eternal life.

'Theories which for many decades have been generally accepted suddenly vanish into the background and are gradually forgotten. After half a century the cycle changes and the old concepts return in the guise of new discoveries. It is necessary to be conversant with these cycles because those who do not remember the past are condemned to repeat it.' Israel Snapper, *Bedside Medicine.*

But old theories are ever being fobbed off as new discoveries. The late Sir Robert Hutchison warned students against 'too much zeal for the new and contempt for what is old; for putting knowledge before wisdom; science before art; and cleverness before common sense.' And he warned teachers:

'Those of us who have the duty of teaching the rising generation of doctors must not inseminate the virgin mind with the tares of our own fads. It is for this reason that it is easily possible for teaching to be too up to date. It is always well before handing the cup of knowledge to the young to wait until the froth has settled.' *British Medical Journal,* **1** (1953) 671.

Cardiologists are often the worst offenders, delighting in bamboozling the young with their theories concerning for example, the aetiology of systematic or pulmonary or renal hypertension; why pain is a feature of pericarditis; why dry pericarditis is frequently present in uraemia; why the first heart sound is loud in mitral stenosis; why atrial fibrillation occurs in thyrotoxicosis; why right bundle branch black is a feature of atrial septal defect; and the mechanism producing pulsus paradoxus. An ability to trot out theories which purport to explain any of these enigmas will not improve ability as a diagnostician.

The student must attempt to discuss the causes of all symptoms and signs in terms of practical clinical medicine and not theories. For example, when considering the causes of increase or decrease of muscle tone the student, as indicated in the neurological chapter, should first consider the anatomical lesions which may be responsible for hypotonicity (posterior column, cerebellar, lower motor neurone extensive sensory root involvement and rarely extra-pyramidal) or for hypertonicity (pyramidal or extrapyramidal). Many would attempt first to discuss the theories as to what constitutes normal muscle tone and what factors operate to keep it normal. Such an approach, though it may sound more scientific, is likely to confuse.

Another example of misguided attempt to explain everything in terms of disordered physiology is when discussing the aetiology of xanthelasma (cholesterol deposits on the eyelids) first to describe the chemistry of cholesterol and its various esters, the different methods of estimating them, theories concerning cholesterol metabolism, and the effects of feeding rabbits with cholesterol and then hanging them upside down, even though the likelihood is that in the patient who is being discussed blood cholesterol is normal. Another example of absurd biochemically orientated teaching is when discussing the causes of pulmonary calcification seen on an X-ray, the teacher first deals with the rival methods of estimating blood calcium and its fractions, and then expounds on calcium metabolism and lists the causes of hypercalcaemia, although all these meanderings are totally irrelevant to the particular patient under review.

The primary task of teaching is explanation and the making of any imparted information meaningful.

3 Medical Vocabulary

A prevalent cause of confusion in clinical medicine is the lack of agreement concerning the exact meaning of even commonly used words and phrases such as apex beat, secondary optic atrophy, exophthalmos, emphysema, osteoporosis and Raynaud's syndrome, and unfortunately quibbling about their definitions has become a fashionable though sterile pastime based neither on science nor on etymological scholarship but on phoney meretricious smatterings of knowledge leading to obfuscation. But agreement is essential if there is to be effective communication, discussion and teaching. If no agreement has been established controversy and confusion arise and the necessity for understanding the different viewpoints.

It is important that no words or terms should be used which cannot be readily defined or are not properly understood. Definitions must be precise and couched in intelligible and logical language devoid of technical or controversial words which themselves require definition and explanation. But on the other hand I deplore the fashionable habit of quibbling about the meaning of such commonly used words as 'bronchitis', 'emphysema' and 'dyspnoea' which lead to long-winded discourses concerning short-winded patients. Words can be used to confuse, to cloak ignorance, to mislead and even to mean the complete opposite of their true meaning. Unfortunately many doctors lack humility and are as illogical as Lewis Carroll's Humpty Dumpty who boasted 'When I say a word it means exactly what I choose it to mean'. Especially medical teachers should oppose any arbitrary extension or alteration of the orthodox and conventional meaning and usage. Admittedly words are not objects handed down unaltered and unalterable from generation to generation, and objections to all neologisms and altered meanings of old words can become pedantry. But one of the horrors described in George Orwell's *1984* was the way in which members of the establishment so twisted and altered accepted meanings as to make it impossible for others to think straight and thereby they lost all hope of revolt against or escape from the dictatorship.

Many medicals have too readily accepted the debased popular usage of medical terms. One of the many examples of this is 'allergy', a term popularly used as a synonym for 'dislike', for example, 'I am allergic to noise'. Neither should 'allergy' be synonymous with 'idiosyncrasy' or 'hypersensitivity' as is often seen in medical literature. The panel of a radio programme, The Brains Trust, which was very popular during the last great war, was asked to explain 'allergy'. The philosopher Professor Joad unhelpfully waffled about its etymology. The biologist Julien Huxley described the production of experimental anaphylaxis (backward reaction) in animals and mentioned the first use of 'allergy' by von Pirquet in 1906. The commonsense Commander Campbell confessed that he had never understood the term but recounted an anecdote which he thought was relevant: when he was a mate on board a ship he was asked to dine with the captain who was baldheaded and Campbell was spellbound to observe that when the captain ate marmalade on his toast steam came out of his head. Triumphantly Campbell proclaimed, 'I think that was allergy' and how right he was. Since then immunologists have invented their own biochemical jargon to define and classify allergies in terms which few doctors and fewer lay people really understand.

A great English wit, Sir Sydney Smith (1771–1845) once heard two garrulous women arguing and yelling at one another from windows on the opposite sides of a street. He commented, 'They will never reach agreement because they are arguing from different premises.' Many physicians when discussing medicine are like those two strident women. For example, they delight in explaining hypothetical differences between terms which are generally considered to be synonymous, such as myxoedema and hypothyroidism, or Addison's Disease and hypoadrenalism. Also in this category are those who insist in a distinction between paresis and paralysis, atonia and hypotonia, anarthria and dysarthria etcetera. Such quibblers do not appreciate that not only to the ancient Greeks but also to our learned immediate forefathers the prefix 'a' or 'an' means 'less' or 'fewer' and not 'total absence'. Patients with achondroplasia have less cartilage than normal but still have a fair amount of that substance in their bones. Moreover such an artificial distinction leads to errors in diagnostic logic because the causes of, for example, a partial paralysis of an upper motor neurone type are exactly the same as the causes of a complete paralysis and the causes of aphasia are the same as the causes of dysphasia. 'Anaemia' does not mean 'without blood' and only a learned ignoramus would talk about 'hypaemias'.

The inventor of the stethoscope, Laennec (1781–1826) wrote with prophetic wisdom, 'Nothing harms medical progress more than the alteration of terms from their customary meaning without sufficient reason and the creation of bad new terms.' Words, like film stars, suffer from an excessive initial success, later losing all sense in a flow of fashionable misuse. A stupid fashion is the replacement of the suffix 'itis' by 'pathy' on the dubious grounds that 'itis' may be derived from the Greek word for 'flame'. Certainly the ancient writers used the suffix 'itis' to indicate 'a lesion of' whatever the cause and in any case their knowledge of pathology was very rudimentary. I see no virtue in replacing 'neuritis' by 'neuropathy', 'retinitis' by 'retinopathy', 'nephritis' by 'nephropathy', 'keratitis' by 'keratopathy', 'arthritis' by 'arthropathy' and 'osteoarthritis' by 'osteoarthrosis', etcetera. The accepted word for inflammation of bone is 'osteomyelitis' and 'osteitis' is a useful word which has been in use for many years to indicate any bone lesion of obscure aetiology, as it was used by Paget himself when he described 'osteitis deformans'. 'Pneumonia' is the accepted word for inflammation of the lung and 'pneumonitis' is a useful word, especially in radiology, to indicate a lung lesion of uncertain aetiology. Some absurdly designate lesions of the choroid 'choroidopathies' and lesions of the macula of the retina 'maculopathies' although neither of these words are euphonious. Bursitis is rarely inflammatory but should we talk about 'bursopathies'? Is it incorrect now to talk of 'alcoholic gastritis' or 'uraemic pericarditis' or 'periostitis' due to sarcoma of bone?

Neologisms

Undergraduates and postgraduates alike suffer from those whose answer to my problem is the invention of new words and terms whenever ideas fail them. Admittedly, when we have a conception for which no name exists, or invent a new drug, or (which is extremely rare) discover a genuinely new syndrome or disease, we are forced to invent new words and terms. But, with very few exceptions, neologisms far from helping merely add to the confusion. As the German author Goethe (1749–1832) wrote, 'When true concepts fail an idle word steps in to take their place'. Baron Corvisart's aphorism written in 1797 is still apt, 'The physician should be very conservative with regard to innovation and he should accept new words only when the need for them is clearly proved'. Alexander Pope in his *Essay on Criticism* (1771) wrote,

'Words are like leaves, and when they most abound
  Much fruit of sense is rarely found.'

The extent of the problem can be gauged from the fact that the latest edition of a standard medical dictionary contains 7,199 words not in the previous edition. Many clinicians delight in using neologisms, labouring under the delusion that they are making an important contribution to the advancement of medical knowledge. Many have been misguided into using those neologisms erroneously believing that their frequent repetition is the hallmark of 'advanced medicine'. The American humorist Ogden Nash wrote in 1962,

'Coin brassy words at will, debase the coinage,
We're in an if you cannot lick them join age.
A slovenliness provides its own excuse age,
Where usage overnight condones misusage.
Farewell, farewell to my beloved language,
Once English now a vile orangatanguage.'

The following are a few of the very many neologisms to which I object. Drugs acting on the heart have been classified into inotropic, chronotropic, bathotropic and dronotropic. Extrasystoles have been subdivided into ectopics, escape, beats and parasystolic beats. Even neurology has succumbed as witnessed by 'asterixis' (flapping tremor), 'akathisia' (restlessness), 'polypia' (monocular diplopia), 'prosopagnosia' (inability to recognize familiar faces), 'pallaesthesia' (vibration sense), 'cephalgia' (headache), 'ageusia' (loss of taste) and 'cerebral dysrhythmia' (epilepsy).

Other neologisms are 'haematochezia' (blood per rectum), 'algodystrophy' (traumatic rarification of spine), 'thelarche' (premature breast development), 'mucoid dysporia' (fibrocystic pancreatitis), 'balanoprosthitis' (indicating that infection of the glans penis often spreads to the prepuce), 'balanochlamyditis' (lesion of clitoris), 'claudicant' (person with intermittent claudication), 'testees' (candidates doing multiple choice examinations), 'virgynatism' (sexual desire between husband and wife) and 'matutolagnia' (lust felt in the morning). The last two words are examples of psychiatric neologisms. Amongst physicians, psychiatrists are undoubtedly the worst offenders rivalling even sociologists.

Some misguided doctors boasting of their linguistic ability justify their introduction of yet more neologisms on the ground of etymological purity, pointing out that many medical words are bastards derived from two different languages, for example, 'idioventricular' (Greek and Latin). 'kernicterus' (German and Greek), 'chancroid' (French and Greek) etcetera. But many of such words have been in use for many generations and we should not agree to their alteration merely to pacify pedants.

Personally I hate most of all the ugly compound words which are besmirching medical literature such as 'hyperelectrolyteaemia', 'corticonigropallidothalamic', 'neurodermatoangiomysositis', 'polydysspondylisia', 'dolichostenomelia', 'autopagnosia', and 'cardiotachometry'.

Also very disturbing is the proliferation of terms for the identical syndrome or disease. There are at least twenty synonyms for 'myelofibrosis', twelve for 'chronic infective hepatitis', six for 'periarteritis nodosa' and five for 'Stevens—Johnson syndrome' and at least ten for the condition intermediate between 'angina' and a definite 'coronary thrombosis'.

Jargon

The use of some technical jargon is inevitable but should be kept to a minimum. The blind faith of the power of jargon to transmute the base metal of superstition into the pure gold of genuine science is acknowledgement of a belief in magic and witchcraft. Jargon often accentuates mental confusion because it often attempts to conceal confusion by rendering every technical subject into a great mystery which can be understood only by the initiated. It also accentuates the fragmentation of knowledge and thereby prevents a true appreciation and understanding of technical subjects outside a small sphere, thus creating an iron curtain which prevents roaming into adjacent fields of knowledge. Jargon is often used to demonstrate that when its users talk about commonplace matters they do so in a superior manner and not as others do. So they abuse and pollute the language. The torrent of medical jargon poured out creates a tropical jungle defying penetration except by the most intrepid of explorers. Sir George Pickering (*Lancet,* 1961) asked the rhetorical question, 'Why do doctors like to use strange words which others do not understand?' His own answer was, 'I am quite sure that usually it is nothing more than a bad habit which many acquire unwittingly. But the underlying basis is more than that. Its purpose is to advance the standing of the users; its method is deception of others and ultimately self deception.'

Dr Jacobides in a letter to *The Lancet* said 'Specialization tends to take the form of a closed cult and all new members have to go through a period of initiation in which the apocryphal words of the cult must be mastered for clearly such words have a magical value because they signify the concentrated wisdom of the "speciality" and become irresistible in their perpetual use, dominating the predisposed members of the cult, and, in moments of mystical ecstasy may lead to full blown neologisms should the right mutations take place.'

Many medicals are prepared to listen to and to read jargon even if it be mere gibberish, gobbledegook, codswallop and mental garbage, without admitting that they do not understand it. Some are so uncritical that they seem to believe that unintelligibility is evidence of profundity simply because it is beyond their understanding, and so assume that it must be important. They are as foolish as the Molière character who proclaimed proudly, 'That must be wonderful because I do not understand it at all'! We should all follow Schopenhauer's advice, 'Say extraordinary things by using ordinary words'. Lucidity, simplicity and euphony should always be the prime aims. The *Oxford Dictionary* defines jargon as 'a noise like the twittering of birds'.

Dr W. B. Bean amusingly wrote, 'The pseudo-prestige of long and difficult words transcends the useful scientific terms and they are diffused widely through medical papers. Simple things are made complicated and the complex is made incomprehensible. Chaos reigns. The so-called medical literature is stuffed to bursting point with junk written in a hop-scotch style characterized by a Brownian movement of uncontrolled parts of speech which settle in restless unintelligibility.'

As described in chapter 2, modern cardiology is crammed with obscure jargon. According to Boswell's biography, Johnson, the great lexicographer, 'was much offended at the general licence, by no means modestly taken in his time, not only to coin new words but to use many words in senses quite different from established meanings, and those very fantastical'. An objectionable but now popular term is 'cardio-vascular accident' and doubly so when it is abbreviated to 'CVA'. The term 'accident' in this context is certainly not orthodox. Those who are ignorant of neurology smugly and glibly proclaim that the explanation of almost every positive neurological sign is 'a CVA' but when questioned are unable to state the precise nature of the vascular lesion or, and more important, which vessel is involved.

Probably the most abused word in medicine today is 'parameter'. This is actually a mathematical term which very few doctors really understand. A standard textbook of mathematics defines it: 'In conic sections it is an indication of the third proportional to any given diameter and its conjugate. In statistics it is a quantity which determines the distribution of a random variable which can be estimated from simple data as the co-ordinate of a locus.' I am not proud of the fact but admit that I have not got a clue as to the meaning of the above definition. But our medical smart Alecks pompously use this word as a synonym for values, variables, factors, tests, results, measurements etcetera. I am in full agreement with an editorial in the *Journal of the American Medical Association* which proclaimed, 'The doctors who write about parameters ought to have their heads examined in both the antero-posterior and transverse diameters'.

Abbreviations

A few abbreviations such as CSF are unequivocal and useful but many doctors talk in a muddy mixture of jargon and abbreviations. The worst example I have ever seen was a case sheet which contained the following:

    ♂57 CC(PTA) SOB PI & FH nil. Exam. CCF JVP+ Oedema 2+
    CVS AF AR MS & MR (MS dom) PR 80 BP 130/80
    AS K° S° L° CNS PERLA MW° SD° RN P↓↓

With mock seriousness I remonstrated with the perpetrator saying that it was monstrous to describe a patient as the 'son of a bitch'.

Does PI mean present or past illnesses; MS mitral stenosis or multiple sclerosis; GU gastric ulcer or genito-urinary? Many do not appreciate that there is no uniformity with regard to abbreviations and different teaching hospitals have their own preferences.

Romance descriptions

The use of romantic descriptions are best avoided altogether. They often are unfamiliar or outdated terms such as 'hardbake' to describe splenic involvement with lymphadenoma; or they are borrowed from the language of a different sensory impression, for example, describing a bruit as 'diamond'; or they are far-fetched, for example, 'swan-neck deformity' or 'rugger jersey spine' or 'buffalo obesity'.

Medicine is a cliché-ridden subject and probably will always be so, but you should be aware of those clichés which when correctly used have a very special and limited connotation indicative of a certain final diagnosis which does not allow for any manoeuvrability which is often so essential, as exemplified by the alternative approach stating that X is probably due to 'this' but is possibly due to 'that' or 'the other'. Examples are 'sabre tibia', a term correctly used indicating a definite syphilitic aetiology, or 'tufting of phalanges' which implies acromegaly, or 'pin-point pupils' which means literally the size of the point of a pin and indicates either pontine haemorrhage or opium poisoning as the cause.

Every physician should develop an accuracy of description and this is especially essential when using such significant terms as 'root pain', 'lightning pains', 'intermittent claudication' and 'tophi' − all terms which demand an accuracy of usage and description readily recognized by every cognizant physician. Such manifestations cannot be assessed mathematically, but their correct description constitutes a discipline as scientific and as valuable as any laboratory investigation. Moreover accuracy of description is essential for meaningful communication between doctors themselves. Unfortunately medical literature is crammed with fashionable words such as 'stress' and 'strain' which are incapable of precise definition but convey a spurious notion of complete understanding.

Etymology

Teachers and examiners are too often overconcerned with niceties of etymology rather than the correct use of words. It does not help to know that 'comedone' derives from a word meaning glutton; 'lupus' a wolf; 'alopecia' a fox; 'cretin' a Christian; 'sarcoid' fleshy;

'herpes' to creep; 'eczema' to boil out (presumably, the humors); 'atheroma' porridge; 'cirrhosis' tawny; 'cancer' a crab; 'jejunum' hungry; that the 'pituitary' was so named under the erroneous belief that it produced nasal secretion; and 'syphilis' was the name of a youth in a poem written by Fracastorius in 1530. It is usually those who have but little Latin knowledge and even less Greek who are most vociferous with such information. Common usage determines the meaning of words and that consideration should outweigh any etymological considerations.

Eponyms

With regard to eponyms – the naming of things including syndromes, signs and diseases after people – it is fitting and proper to pay tribute to the really great and revere their memory, but many of those who have been honoured in medicine by an eponym have had greatness thrust upon them, often by ignorant writers, rather than having achieved distinction by either genius or true originality. One of the worst examples of this is the undeserved elevation of Reiter to fame: in 1916 he wrote a bad paper describing a single patient who had urethritis, conjunctivitis and arthritis, in whose blood he claimed spirochaetes were found. Later he wrote another paper about the same one patient but mentioned the additional symptom of diarrhoea and forgot the spirochaetes. This bears no relation to the symptoms often referred to as Reiter's syndrome or even disease.

Ecclesiastes reminds us 'There is nothing new under the sun'. Indeed when attempting to be original it is advisable not to read too much lest you be disillusioned to find that it has all been described before. Medicine throughout the ages has rarely been advanced by some brilliant completely original discovery of any single man but has been a gradual development, a superimposition and integration of many minor contributions of others. This truth is often forgotten by those who delight in pettifogging arguments concerning priorities of descriptions, and the use of rival eponyms fans this noisy pastime.

The use of eponyms also sometimes engenders brayings as to what Dr X actually did describe. That the report was originally published in an obscure journal impossible to obtain, or that the person who is laying down the law concerning this has no knowledge of the language in which the original article was written, does not deter them. Probably there is more misinformation on this score than concerning any other branch of medicine. Examples of this are the syndromes usually attributed to Behçet, Simmonds and Libman and Sachs.

B

Another fruitless argument arising from the use of eponyms is how many features are essential before the title is used. If Dr A described four features, are the presence of only two or three sufficient? Furthermore, if Dr B wrote of some condition about which our ideas have since then profoundly changed should we still talk of the B syndrome although we are describing something only remotely resembling that which B himself described?

Statistics

Clinicians whatever the depth and breadth of their mathematical knowledge must always exhibit a healthy scepticism concerning statistics and not be mesmerized by those who appear to have mastered this difficult and highly specialized branch of mathematics. Statistics can never be a genuine substitute for medical knowledge but should be regarded as no more than a minor, even though sometimes important, aspect of the whole spectrum of medicine. Medical statistics are like bikinis, concealing what is vital and revealing much that is occasionally interesting.

Many symptoms and signs such as pain and anxiety cannot be measured in terms of numbers. At best we can express their degree by an attempted accuracy of verbal description. Often words such as 'slight', 'moderate', or 'marked' are the most accurate possible in the circumstances. It is not scientific to describe one systolic bruit as grade 2 and another as grade 3 or to categorize leg oedema numerically. There is a commonly held fallacy that what cannot be measured cannot be understood or even known. Many clinicians use statistics in a way reminiscent of a drunken man clinging to a lamp-post for support and not for illumination.

Quoting percentages often gives an illusion of accuracy and a false accolade of exactitude. The statement that some symptom or complication occurs in 13.5 per cent of cases of a particular disease is an unwarranted accuracy. Phrases such as 'the majority' or 'a large number' or 'a few' are nearly always as precise as is justifiable. There is no such thing as either a 'never' or 'an always' in clinical medicine; 'never' means 'hardly ever' and 'always' means 'nearly always'.

Statistics become very absurd when used by those who want to demonstrate that something is a truth when its reality is dubious. Statistics often distort vision, especially when they claim to measure such things as growth rate or intelligence, ignoring the immeasurable aspects even when those are very important features. Statistics are frequently used in clinical medicine to conceal inadequate data or to mould data into a preconceived mould, often in an attempt to hide bad planning of an experiment. Dr Bean of Iowa has written: 'The mathematical manipulation of data cannot create significance out of artefact.' The physicist Professor Dingle wrote: 'It is a delusion that any idea which lends itself to mathematical development is thereby justified as true. . . No intelligent person would underestimate the importance of mathematics or question its importance but it cannot bring truth to an error. If it is applied to truth it will produce truth and if applied to error it will produce error.'

A patient's trust in his physician is never based on a controlled study of the doctor's therapeutic successes and failures.

4 The Art and Science of Diagnosis

Foundations of diagnosis

Diagnosis is a creative art belonging to the realm of discovery. It is detective work with logic as its basis. Logic in this context means the principles relating to correct reasoning and the drawing of the proper inferences from unequivocal premises which have been garnered from a good history and the skilful elucidation, assessment and interpretation of positive and negative physical signs. The skills of history-taking and clinical examination can be mastered only at the expense of much time and patience.

Clinical medicine is essentially a technical skill, and its techniques can be demonstrated and taught properly only by those who themselves genuinely practice those skills. Such methods are the foundation of clinical medicine and without them it is meaningless. Students must not be misled into regarding the elucidation of physical signs as a phoney and spurious pastime unworthy of their intellects, but, by their teachers' example, they should come to regard this skill as honest and intellectually rewarding. Today, unfortunately, physical signs are often denigrated as things of but little import in medicine, especially by those who do not themselves know how to elicit and interpret such signs correctly.

Lack of method in arriving at a diagnosis is often due to a basic misconception as to the meaning of diagnosis. Diagnosis must always be considered in stages, and in the great majority of cases the stage 1 diagnosis should be an anatomical one, stage 2 the general pathology and stage 3 the special pathology. To state that a patient has a cerebellar lesion is a diagnosis — only a stage 1 diagnosis, it is true, but nonetheless a diagnosis. Moreover, it may be that the stage 1 diagnosis is the only one which can be made with certainty, and that the other two stages must be considered in terms of probabilities and later possibilities, always discussing the most likely diagnosis first and leaving remote possibilities till last. Be like a good electrician who regards his first job to be the location of a fault and not speculation about its cause.

Any diagnosis must be based on three firm foundations: history, physical signs and necessary investigations, all interpreted in the light of a wealth of factual knowledge and clinical experience. Diagnosis must not be 'wrung from speculations and subtleties but common sense and observation', as Sir Thomas Browne (1605–82) advised in his *Religio Medici.* Diagnostic talent can never be developed by reliance on lucky guesses. Guesswork in clinical medicine can easily become a pernicious habit spasm, which if performed often degenerates into an incurable disease rendering the doctor incapable of ever becoming a proficient clinician. Intuition, if by that is meant an immediate apprehension without apparent reasoning, must never be relied upon as a diagnostic method, even though it may have the apparent virtue of speed. The late Lord Samuel advised, 'We must never put our trust in intuitions unless they are supported by reason' (*In Search of Reality*). Experience itself is of course useless unless we have the inherent capacity for learning from experience, and that is intelligence. However brilliant the teacher, he cannot give you that which Nature failed to do.

Watch the expert neurologist and observe how he pays great attention to the details of his techniques, and contrast his methods with the slipshod, misleading and inadequate performance of many other doctors when examining the nervous system. Surely, if such attention to details is necessary for the expert before he is willing to arrive at his conclusions, it is even more necessary for the inexpert. 'Trifles make perfection and perfection is no trifle', was Michelangelo's motto. Also, it is important to realize that the absence of any physical sign may be just as significant as its presence, and slight deviations from the normal may be as significant as grosser changes, provided, of course, that the observer is certain that the deviation is really present. Neglect of minor abnormalities and focusing of attention only on grosser changes is a common cause of diagnostic error. Be mindful of the advice of the American author J. R. Lowell (1819–91): 'It is not the finding of a thing but the making of something of it afterwards that is of consequence.'

Touch, hearing and, above all, sight are the cornerstones of physical examination. Every medical student should take for his own the motto of Leonardo: *Sapere vedere,* learn to see things. Indeed, the most important instrument for any doctor is a pair of observant eyes used like a wide-angle lens, simultaneously seeing many things in sharp focus. However the distinction should be made between what we really see and what we intellectually infer, because seeing is a complex process of interaction and integration, and it is often the power of expectation rather than the power of conceptual knowledge which moulds what we claim to have seen. To many doctors 'believing is seeing'; radiologists especially sometimes allow themselves to be duped by that delusion. Undoubtedly imagination often plays a prominent part in visual interpretation. Erroneously some even deny that skill plays a leading role in visual perception and interpretation, regarding such ability as little more than a registering of sensory data on the retina acting like a photographic film.

> 'We learn a lot about training the eye to see but this phraseology can be misleading if it hides the fact that what we can learn is not to see but to discriminate. . . . Perception may be regarded as primarily the modification of an anticipation. It is always an active process conditioned by our expectation and adapted to the situation. Instead of talking about seeing and knowing we might do a little better by talking about seeing and noticing. We notice only when we look for something and we look when our attention is aroused by some disequilibrium, a difference between our expectation and the incoming messages.' E. H. Gombrich, *Art and Illusion.*

Unfortunately the student may have defective acuity of any of his special senses, but even this handicap may in large measure be overcome by diligent practice. Our powers of observation can be developed and considerably improved by non-medical activities, including the recognition of flowers, trees, plants, birds, paintings and music. By such exercises the accuracy of our auditory and visual sensations can be repeatedly tested and improved. May the application of the advice given in this book be the mordant which will fix things in your memory.

> 'Medicine is to be learned only by experience; it is not an inheritance; it cannot be revealed. Learn to see, learn to hear, learn to feel, learn to smell, and to know that by practice alone you can become expert. Medicine is learnt by the bedside and not in the classroom. Let not your conceptions of the manifestations of disease come from words heard in the lecture room or read in a book. See and then reason and compare and control. But see first.' Sir William Osler.

ABSENCE OF SIGNS

Absence of any physical sign may be just as important as a positive finding. For example, lack of wasting of the tibialis anticus and peronei would rule out a lower motor neurone lesion of these muscles as a cause of foot drop of more than a few weeks' duration. Certain (if this is possible) absence of a blowing diastolic bruit rules out aortic regurgitation even though the patient has a collapsing pulse. On the other hand, absence of any physical sign usually found in a particular condition often does not rule out the diagnosis, but it should always make us reconsider our tentative diagnosis and think of alternatives.

One must never be over-impressed by the exceptional case in whom somebody has diagnosed X disease even in the absence of a physical sign considered essential. For example, it might be true that an untreated patient has Addison's disease of the suprarenals even in the absence of any pigmentation or hypotension, but it must be realized that such a contingency is extremely unlikely. The making of such a diagnosis in the absence of what are generally considered to be essential findings, whatever may be the results of biochemical investigations, will probably prove to be wrong and, what is even worse, lead to grave therapeutic errors.

EQUIVOCAL FINDINGS

It is only experience and continuing self-criticism that will guide the clinician as to when he should take cognizance of and when he should ignore an equivocal finding. But here also the patient's symptoms must always be related to such findings. For example, an equivocal plantar reflex must never be lightly disregarded in a patient complaining of difficulty in walking, but it may well be of no significance in a patient who is completely free from any symptoms referable to the nervous system.

As a general rule, when in doubt as to whether or not any finding is really present it is much wiser to ignore it rather than to base a diagnosis upon such a shaky foundation. Do not suffer from *folie de doute*, and when uncertain do not repeat a procedure again and again, because with each performance you are likely only to further confuse and not enlighten yourself. For example, it is easy for some to delude themselves into a wrong diagnosis by repeated percussion of the same area of the chest, or by repeatedly stroking the sole of the feet to 'make sure' whether a plantar response is flexor or extensor (often done in spite of the patient's obvious discomfort and even protests). The same applies to cardiac auscultation, for repeated and prolonged listening may cause increasing uncertainty and even auditory hallucinations. With regard to any physical sign considered to be positive or negative, the clinician must make up his mind quickly and decisively. Repeated performance usually indicates lack of self-confidence. One of the three maxims of the Great Assembly of Rabbis was 'Be deliberate in judgment' (*Talmud, Sayings of the Fathers*, 1, 1).

IRRELEVANT SIGNS

Another important realization is that positive signs or investigations may be irrelevant to the patient's symptoms. Extreme examples are that a hallux valgus would not explain dyspnoea, or bleeding haemorrhoids dysphagia. Less obvious instances are that osteoarthritis of the spine, demonstrated radiologically, may not be the cause of the patient's backache; that a palpable lower pole of the right kidney may not indicate the cause of urinary symptoms; or that either gallstones or hiatus hernia, diagnosed radiologically, may not provide the correct explanation of abdominal symptoms.

COMPLETENESS OF EXAMINATION

Examination of patients must always be thorough but never be pushed to absurdity, for example doing a rectal examination in a patient whose sole complaint is a sore throat. A spurious completeness of examination is equally often otiose, is often impracticable and may be absurd. For example, a commonly enacted crime, made all the more heinous when done in front of students, is the brief flashing of a light in front of a patient's eyes and the scratching of his feet, followed by the proclamation, verbally or in writing, that the patient's nervous system is normal. Better not to examine the nervous system at all than make such a puerile gesture to a supposed completeness or thoroughness.

RARE DISEASES

The adage, 'The commonest things are the commonest', is wholly true in clinical medicine. He who frequently diagnoses rare diseases frequently makes diagnostic errors. A rare disease should be seriously considered only when the pattern of symptoms, signs and investigations does not fit into that of any common disease, always taking into account the great variations which may occur in the course of all common diseases. It is essential in this context to know the various patterns seen during the progress of different diseases and how the clinical features may be modified by treatment, all of which can be summarized by the important phrase 'the natural history of disease'. A correct prognosis is likely only if the physician is familiar with the natural history of the disease from which the patient suffers, and this entails not only knowing the various modes of presentation, the various possible patterns of its development and its likely response to any particular therapy, but also what Osler referred to as 'the kind of patient the disease has'.

THE SEARCH FOR A SINGLE DIAGNOSIS

It is very important to attempt to make a single diagnosis which will explain all the symptoms and all the signs. But the physician must not be a slave to this concept. Many patients, especially the elderly, have more than one disease, so one should not attempt invariably to drag all symptoms and signs under a single diagnostic umbrella when they obviously cannot be covered thereby.

DIAGNOSTIC PROOF VERSUS PROBABILITY

It must be accepted that the making of a diagnosis is nearly always an estimation of probabilities and only occasionally the assertion of certainties. Moreover any commitment to a supposed certain diagnosis should always be subject to revision if new information comes to light.

Exact proof of many minor ailments and many chronic diseases is either not possible or attempts to establish such proof may not be justifiable because of the hazards involved in the necessary investigations. A diagnosis of coronary thrombosis can be made without resource to coronary angiography, and a diagnosis of disseminated sclerosis or Parkinsonism should be made without attempting histological proof during life. Many diagnoses must be considered acceptable even in the absence of so-called proof. It is the over-zealous attempts by some 'scientific' doctors to establish 'final proof' that have been a contributory factor leading to the sorry dehumanization of clinical medicine.

It is a truism that accurate diagnosis should precede treatment but clinical medicine is full of situations where to push a diagnosis to its ultimate finality, though perhaps intellectually satisfying, may expose the patient to risks without altering his management at all. Those who seek for certainty and perfection are just as likely as those medieval churchmen who, pursuing the millennium, caused hell on earth.

On the other hand, each clinician must repeatedly reformulate his accepted criteria for diagnosis of many diseases, always distinguishing between the certain, the probable and the possible diagnosis. What, for example are your criteria for diagnosing rheumatoid arthritis, gout, emphysema, chronic pancreatitis, or a lumbar disc protrusion? There must be clear and critical thinking on such issues. Moreover, in many endocrine diseases and in some types of arthritis – to name but two of many possible examples – an important question to ask oneself is whether or not to accept the findings of some clinical pathologist when one's own clinical criteria are absent. I remain very sceptical of, for example, a diagnosis of rheumatoid arthritis in the absence of any history of swelling of joints but based on positive serological tests, or a diagnosis of gout in the absence of any history of joint pains, including of the hallux, and based solely on a reputedly high serum uric acid. And I strongly deprecate the fashionable habit of regarding a biochemical finding such as hypokalaemia as a clinical diagnosis or diagnosing an excess of growth hormone when acromegaly is meant.

THE IMPORTANCE OF DIFFERENCES

Too often similarities between various conditions are stressed. This in part arises from an uncritical enthusiasm for compiling long lists of causes of various symptoms or signs. Much more important than emphasizing similarities is the stressing of differences. 'Wherefore is this disease different from all other diseases?' is a way of thinking which should be ingrained. It is an approach to clinical medicine which is of great value but rarely taught.

For example, ptosis may be due to a third nerve lesion, a sympathetic paralysis or a lesion of the levator palpebrae superioris muscle itself. Any of these lesions may cause ptosis, and this they all have in common. But at least equally important is the knowledge that in each cases the ptosis will have its own special features (*see* Chapter 16). Another example is consideration of bowing of the tibia. Syphilis, rickets and Paget's disease all have this sign in common, but what is very important is to be able to describe how the bowing itself and associated findings differ in each of these conditions.

DISCUSSION FROM GENERAL TO PARTICULAR

It is often wrongly insisted that it is wrong to generalize. But in fact generalizations are a useful and convenient method of indicating, for example, some special feature of a disease. If any danger exists in generalizations it is due to applying the general rule without listing the exceptions. Diagnostic discussions should always be approached from the general to the particular. For example, the suggestion that a patient has a blood disease such as acute leukemia rather than particularizing that the diagnosis is probably acute leukemia. This order of discussion allows us to consider later other probabilities and then possibilities within the group of blood diseases. Or, to give another example, rather than suggesting that a patient's bilateral facial weakness is probably due to myasthenia gravis, it is usually better to consider that the finding is probably due to a muscle disease such as myasthenia gravis, or to dystrophia myotonica or facio-scapular myopathy.

Diagnostic pitfalls

THE SIN OF GREED

Beware of the sin of diagnostic greed. Overwhelming evidence is not essential for correct diagnosis, and the absence of some expected symptom or sign often does not invalidate an otherwise reasonable diagnosis. For example, a posterior column lesion may be present even if joint and vibration sense are intact, or a patient may have mitral stenosis even if there be no opening snap. Before making any diagnosis, the physician must always be self-critical and ask himself what points are against such a conclusion. If there are such symptoms or signs, then he must think of some more acceptable alternative, some condition which has fewer points against it, sticking to the original diagnosis only if no better alternative can be thought of.

The evidence for any diagnosis is often not clear-cut, but all diagnoses at whatever stage should always be considered by a careful weighing up of all the pros and cons. For example, a patient may have an upper motor neurone lesion of his lower limbs and a lower motor neurone lesion of his upper limbs, and motor neurone disease may be considered to be the correct diagnosis. But supposing the history of limb weakness was of over ten years' duration and the arm reflexes were absent, it should then be appreciated that these are two important points against that diagnosis, although not excluding it, and an alternative diagnosis such as syphilitic amyotrophy might be considered and might actually be the correct diagnosis, even though the pupils were normal. This is another example of avoidance of the sin of diagnostic greed.

PRESUMED DIAGNOSIS OF OTHERS

Never accept another doctor's actual or presumed diagnosis or what a patient may tell you was the opinion of another doctor without careful scrutiny of the evidence, especially the basis on which it was made or presumed to have been made, and the status and, if known, the clinical ability of that doctor and the likely accuracy of the ancillary aids at his disposal.

THE CRIME OF PROCRUSTES

The crime of procrustes is prevalent in clinical medicine. According to a Greek legend, the robber Procrustes often feigned hospitality to strangers and then tied them to his bed; if they were too long for the bed he amputated their limbs, and if they were too short he stretched them. There is a Talmudic story recounting that the inhabitants of Sodom and Gomorrah also perpetrated this crime.

In clinical medicine the crime of Procrustes is committed by those who make a diagnosis without good evidence, often after a snap decision, and then make the physical signs fit in with the erroneous diagnosis, perhaps, as explained previously, imagining that he has actually seen something which he expected to find. Never let it be forgotten that even experienced doctors may suffer from illusions and hallucinations when examining patients. Such a doctor always finds what he expects to find and always fails to find any signs which he has decided beforehand will not be present, even though in actual fact they are. For example, the clinician may diagnose aortic regurgitation correctly but then delude himself into believing that the pulse is collapsing when in fact it is not. Or he may correctly recognize a collapsing pulse and, because he automatically assumes that the patient has aortic regurgitation, delude himself that he can hear the appropriate bruit, even though no such bruit is present and the collapsing pulse is due to some other cause.

Or else he may on seeing a patient with a hemiplegic gait, due actually to unilateral Parkinsonism, immediately decide that the patient has an upper motor neurone hemiplegia and then persuade himself that the plantar reflex on that side is extensor. It is often advisable that initial impressions be left fluid, open to correction and possibly not recorded.

To give a more complex example, the clinician may elicit a difference of percussion note between the two sides of a chest and draw the wrong conclusion as to which side is abnormal; thus misguided, he may diagnose an upper lobe fibrosis and then proceed to support this illusion and aggravate his initial mistake by wrongly convincing himself that the trachea is deviated because this supports his diagnosis. Imagine his chagrin when he finds that the X-ray shows a pneumothorax on the opposite side!

Another common cause of the Procrustean crime is observer bias based on advance information obtained from investigations. It has unfortunately become an increasingly common practice for some clinicians always to look at the results of investigations before they examine the patient. This practice must inevitably lead to the denigration of the techniques of eliciting physical signs and must have a profoundly bad influence on students. Such clinicians always blame the inaccuracy of the physical signs, but the real fault is in their own shortcomings, their failure to master the methods of physical examination. Such procedures lead to the perpetration of Procrustean crimes such as the supposed hearing of a fourth heart sound or a wide splitting of the second sound merely because the phonocardiogram is reputed to show this. The crime of Procrustes is perpetrated far more often in clinical medicine than is generally realized or admitted, and in no branch of medicine is this better exemplified than in cardiac auscultation.

Clinical judgment

Without a good deal of medical knowledge and experience, nobody can become a good clinician. On the other hand, it is possible to know a good deal of medicine and yet be a poor clinician. Logic is of prime importance in diagnosis, but beyond logic there is undoubtedly an important phenomenon called clinical judgment. This is difficult and perhaps impossible to define. It is certainly not guesswork and not some mystique. It depends on an amalgam of knowledge, experience, and a constant awareness of the spectra of the natural history of many diseases. In addition it depends on the physician's understanding and appreciation of his patients as individual sick human beings. It includes the ability to distinguish the essential from the non-essential and it can be taught only by the example set by teachers.

A. R. Feinstein, in his brilliant book, which all doctors should read, *Clinical Judgment* (Baltimore: Williams & Wilkins, 1967), describes the physician who possesses clinical judgment as follows:

'He knows the many clinical distinctions that tell him when death is imminent or hope abundant; when to treat and when to wait; when to sedate with drugs and when to sedate with words; when to stop treatment, change or add; when to treat aggressively for cure, palliatively for relief and consolingly for comfort. The physician knows that these therapeutic decisions may depend on such distinctively bedside observations as the strength of the patient's handgrip; the posture of his body, the noise in his chest, the smell of his breath, the sweat of his brow, the grimace on his face, the quiver in his voice and the anguish of his family. The physician knows that the therapeutic decision may depend on such distinctly clinical nuances as a particular continuation of symptoms and signs, whether the patient complains of certain symptoms or tolerates them quietly, whether the disease was found before or after symptoms developed, whether the symptoms were of short duration or long, and whether the symptoms had preceded one another or followed. The good clinician knows all these things and many more distinctly clinical features that are his harbingers of prognosis and determinants of therapy. But he cannot express these specifically or consistently.'

The late Professor J. A. Ryle of Guy's and Cambridge, himself a fine teacher and clinician in an address to the Medical Society of London in 1939 said of clinical judgment which he called 'clinical sense'.

'This attribute is not something which is innate or intuitive but a complex faculty built upon prolonged training and exercise of the special senses together with a sound knowledge of pathological possibilities. Observational ability, the observational habit, observational accuracy and a retentive memory for observed phenomena, together with an aptitude for the sifting and correlation of experience, these are the main ingredients. What is wrong with medical education is that while multiplying diagnostic aids and instilling more basic science than our fathers had it fails in its cultivation of judgment and the faculty of perception from which judgment derives.'

With the growing emphasis on technological development in medicine and the use of ever more complex instruments, all of which have the effect of keeping doctors away from patients, there is an ever-increasing loss of this power of clinical judgment which primarily depends on the greatest instrument known to man, the human brain. To quote Feinstein again:

'The art of clinical examination comes from attitudes and qualities that are neither obtained nor easily detected by scientific procedures: the physician's awareness of people and human needs; his ability to temper the rational aspects of his work with a tolerant acceptance of the irrationalities of mankind; his perception of faith, hope and charity, love and other elements of the human spirit and human emotions. These properties of care and compassion, although sometimes dismissed as merely "bedside manners", are the fundamental and most important tool of any clinician. With them he can often give healing and comfort where science fails or does not exist. Without this his science is unsatisfactory no matter how excellent.'

Instrumental and laboratory investigations can never be a good or even adequate substitute for clinical judgment. Indeed, when the latter is at variance with the results of any investigation, it is always better to repeat the test than to discard or alter one's clinical judgment. A grain of clinical judgment is worth a ton of biochemical results.

'Medical practice is not knitting and weaving and the labour of hands, but it must be inspired with soul and filled with understanding and equipped with the gift of keen observation. These faculties combined with accurate scientific knowledge are the indispensable requisites for proficient medical practice.'

So wrote the great Maimonides eight hundred years ago.

Allied to clinical judgment and sometimes a part of it is imperturbability in the face of surprising and unforeseen happenings and emergencies. Osler in *Aequanimitas* wrote in 1904:

'Imperturbability means coolness and presence of mind under all circumstances, calmness amid storm, clearness of judgment in moments of great peril, immobility, impassiveness, or, to use an old and expressive word, phlegm. It is the quality most appreciated by the laity, though often misunderstood by them; and the physician who has the misfortune to be without it, who betrays indecision and worry, and who shows that he is flustered and flurried in ordinary emergencies, loses rapidly the confidence of his patients.'

Criticism and self-criticism

An enquiring and self-critical mind is a requisite of the good clinician. 'The greatest of all faults is to be conscious of none' (Carlyle). A well-developed critical faculty should teach us to disregard theories lacking in real proof and instead to follow the Rabbinic advice, 'Teach thy tongue to say, I do not know, lest you are led into falsehood' (*Talmud Berachot* 4a).

Teaching hospitals should be centres for the fostering of criticism, including self-criticism, because only by this means can continuing improvement in clinical ability be achieved. Too much agreement with authority and the development of the 'yes-man' may result in preferment, but will eventually lead to an organization in which the bland lead the bland, and mental constipation will prevail. Neither the student nor the teacher should waste time in noisy discussion of the undiscussable. Which came first, the hen or the egg? This is a type of question very popular in many medical schools. For example, do the skin changes precede or follow the vascular disturbance of sclerodactyly? Another type of futile question is why any particular disease has a predilection for one specific part of the body — for example, why poliomyelitis attacks the anterior horn cells, and syphilis spares the cerebellum? Why are subungual haemorrhages linear and longitudinal in bacterial endocarditis but transverse in trichiniasis? Why are the bone lesions of myelomatosis usually round and well-defined? Why are gout, thrombo-angiitis and intestinal lipodystrophy predominantly diseases of men, and lupus erythematosus and lipodystrophia progressiva predominant in women? There are hundreds of such unanswerable questions which are too frequently discussed at boring length. Moreover, teachers especially must always rethink things and avoid believing in some fantasy merely because it has been oft repeated by them to students. The truly religious man does not claim to be endowed with any knowledge which he does not possess, and no teacher should attempt to impress his students with smatterings of dubious validity poured forth as though he were the confidant of the Almighty and not merely an observer of His mighty acts and mysterious ways.

'To discuss endlessly what silly people mean when they say silly things may be amusing but can hardly be important. Does the full moon look as large as half-a-crown or a soup plate?' Bertrand Russell.

Every doctor should at least once attend a court of law during an important criminal trial and listen carefully to a skilled cross-examination. Throughout his career the doctor should always, when making his diagnostic and therapeutic judgments, imagine himself being cross-examined by a brilliant lawyer and having to justify those decisions. May the voice of the questioning and demanding lawyer, call it conscience or reasoning faculty if you so prefer, be always with you throughout your medical activities, whatever they may be.

'Within the sum total of these diseases there is one which is widespread, and from which men rarely escape. This disease varies in degree in different men, just as all bodily diseases vary. I refer to this, that every person thinks that his mind is clearer, cleverer and more learned than it actually is. I have found that this disease has attacked many an intelligent person who is well versed in physical science, or mechanical

art or one of the positive sciences. But they express themselves not only upon the sciences with which they are familiar,
but also upon other sciences about which they know nothing.
If they are applauded and heeded, so does the disease become
aggravated.'

This was a warning given by Maimonides, twelfth century Rabbi
and physician, to his pupils. A good student, graduate or undergraduate, should always ask himself whether he really understands
the subject under discussion and, if not, must seek out somebody
who, or a textbook which, will enlighten him. Above all, he must
never be afraid to ask for guidance from even the most senior of
doctors, and every teacher should welcome such inquiries.

'The bashful cannot learn' (*Talmud, Sayings of the Fathers* 2.6).
The fear of being embarrassed should never outweigh the desire for
information. If you do not ask for an explanation of your difficulty
in understanding a problem you will never learn.

Abuse of investigations

A pernicious habit has become commonplace of routinely ordering a
large number of investigations which are often demanded as though
ordering goods wholesale, or as though behaving like an uncritical
shopper in a supermarket who, allured by the machinations of the hidden persuaders and the sight of a plethora of possible purchases, buys
indiscriminately. Unfortunately many students are initiated into the
bad practice of ordering multiple routine tests at an early stage of
their career and later find it very difficult to discard the habit.
Routine investigations have become with some doctors an obsessional
routine often designed to protect themselves from the uncomfortable
and possibly disturbing admission that they have not got the foggiest
notion as to what is the matter with a patient.

Anybody who orders any investigation must be prepared to
justify it in front of critical colleagues, both senior and junior.
What are the investigations which are essential and which can be
readily justified in any particular case? Clinical judgment and not
routine procedure should always be the main guide. The craze for
lists of so-called routine investigations which are ordered automatically is the antithesis of good medical practice. A patient with
high fever, purpura and shock requires neither detailed investigation
of his platelets nor biochemical tests of suprarenal function. Indeed,
if his life is to be saved, antibiotic therapy must be instituted immediately even before the results of blood culture are known.

Too often tests are ordered to gain time in an apparently difficult
case, or in an attempt to impress people, or as a futile indulgence in

the often sterile pastime of accumulating yet more statistics. There is also a peculiar group of doctors who attempt to justify even their most esoteric activities — such as renal angiography in all patients with hypertension, or combined right-sided and left-sided cardiac catheterization, a battery of enzyme estimations and coronary angiography on all patients with acute myocardial infarction — by claiming that they would be liable to be sued for negligence if they failed to attack their patients in such ways. In addition there are those clinicians, generally of poor calibre, who attempt to justify the extent of their investigations on the grounds of thoroughness. There is undoubtedly such a thing in clinical medicine as being too thorough. In this category could be mentioned esoteric histology using the latest electron microscopes on pieces of viscera, yielding results which very rarely influence the treatment of any individual patient. The cult of the attempted complete investigation of all symptoms, the creed that even if a patient will not himself directly benefit in any way, and that it is unscientific not to order all possible tests which are available, must be strongly condemned. We should never forget that the results of any test cannot be more than one item in the total balancing of findings when formulating a diagnosis. The search for so called accuracy and finality of diagnosis may be dicing with danger. Such clinicians often justify their attacks on patients by the phrase, 'It would be interesting to know' — but whether it would be of any benefit to the patient is not even considered. Doctors used to regard investigations as a means of confirming or refuting diagnostic probability which was considered likely after careful history-taking and examination, but nowadays many regard investigations as an essential prerequisite even before considering a provisional diagnosis. Worst of all is the routine initial ordering of a large barrage of investigations without considering their order of importance, and without first waiting for the results of a few key tests before demanding others.

Another frequent reason for doing many investigations is ostensibly to reassure the patient that he has not got any organic disease. This is often an admission of a poor doctor–patient relationship, and such acts may produce or aggravate rather than cure anxiety, often fortifying the patient's denial or lack of acceptance that his symptoms are entirely psychogenic. Tests can and often do aggravate pre-existing symptoms and frequently produce new symptoms.

There are other uncritical clinicians who always arrange for the investigations of most recent introduction, however complicated or hazardous they may be and however unprepared the laboratory or X-ray department is to undertake the new procedure. They know full well that there is but an infinitesimal chance of any such tests yielding any useful information, but they justify these antics by the phrase, 'Just in case it might show something'. Such clinicians, if further challenged, maintain that they cannot afford the risk of blighting their reputations by missing anything. An example of this is the submission of patients with a typical history of migraine for many years, who have no positive physical signs, to ventriculography and/or cerebral angiography. Another example is the routine estimation of growth hormone, follicular stimulating hormone, luteinising hormone, X-rays of spine, skull, hands and heel and ventriculography on all patients with acromegaly. Indeed many doctors order investigations for no better reason than that they are the latest. If they read in a medical journal that it has recently been discovered that rheumatoid arthritis may be associated with a raised blood caviare or rhubarb, or that it causes a subtle change in the mitochondria of the Kupfer cells of the liver, they automatically thereafter demand for all their patients with rheumatoid arthritis, however certain be that diagnosis, that they have blood rhubarb or caviare estimations and liver punctures. This uncritical application of the latest research findings to clinical medicine is the bane of many hospitals and a consequent exposing of patients to the diabolical machinations of these meddlesome medical muddlers.

Many investigations are often repeated a number of times because the results are equivocal or unexpected or the bewildered physician is playing for time, feigning an active intervention when masterly inactivity would show better clinical judgment. Routine quantitative bacteriological investigations on sputum and urine specimens, with the pathologist's frequent report of a moderate growth of three or four different organisms and the sensitivity tests on each organism to a wide variety of therapeutic agents, are commonly a waste of time, effort and money, too often yielding results which the wise physician ignores. A further instance is the repeated estimation of different steroids in urine, giving results which are liable to be inaccurate or useless. If clinically there is diagnostic doubt in many common endocrine diseases, then biochemical tests – even if reliable, which they often are not – nearly always give equivocal results. The same applies to routine folic acid, B_{12} and iron estimations in the sera of all anaemic patients. The vast majority of iron deficiency anaemias in women can be diagnosed correctly without serum iron or iron binding capacity measurements. Indeed, if the anaemia is not hypochromic then those results are likely to add to diagnostic confusion, and if the anaemia is hyperchronic the same applies to folate and B_{12} estimations. Furthermore many seriously ill patients have a low serum folate but this is not the cause of their illness and even massive folate therapy by all possible routes will not help the patient. Investigations should never be used to confirm what is not in doubt.

A fundamental rule when ordering investigations is that there must be a start with the simplest tests and a gradual progression to the more and more complex. By simple as opposed to complex, I refer not only to the comparative difficulty of the techniques themselves but also to the amount of discomfort and inconvenience that may be caused to the patient and the possible hazards.

The technically trained physician as distinct from the properly educated physician tries impulsively by an unwise and neurotic multiplicity of tests to achieve a delusion of certainty. Such behaviour may also be a manifestation of another superstition, a blind faith in laboratory and X-ray reports. A good physician is always aware that laboratory results may be wrong and X-rays may be misinterpreted. Neither the latest machines nor those using them are infallible and many laboratory procedures have a degree of specificity and sensitivity causing falsely positive and falsely negative results.

Investigations are commonly done under the guise of routine when what in fact is performed is some experimental work, some research project. Medical research must go on, but only after due safeguards are strictly observed. These problems have been discussed fully in my book *Human Guinea Pigs* (Routledge & Kegan Paul, 1967; Boston, Beacon Press, 1968).

There are two main issues concerning experiments on humans: (1) Valid consent; (2) Do ends justify means? By valid consent is meant consent after full disclosure of the whole of the proposed procedure and not merely part of it; and full explanation of the purpose of the experiment including any possible relationship, or lack of it, to the patient himself; and the probable duration of the experiment. Consent must be freely given, devoid of any coercion, and never engineered by trickery or fraud. All known risks, hazards and discomforts must be given honestly and never ignored or minimized. The patient in regard to age and mental state must legally be capable of giving valid consent. In my opinion dying patients and those suffering from any disease with a grave prognosis should never be submitted to any experiment that is not primarily and unequivocally intended to relieve their own suffering. It is never a physician's prerogative to take advantage of a presumed hopeless prognosis, even if that be certain. He must be aware of the tempting sophistry that the 'hopeless' are expendable and therefore especially suitable for experimentation. Utter hopelessness from whatever cause should demand complete protection and even those deemed to be a burden on society and recalcitrant to the social purpose have rights equal to those of any experimental physician.

Do ends, however noble, always justify means, however distasteful? Is it ever justifiable to do wrong in order that good may possibly come of it? I think not. No doctor is ever justified in placing science or the public welfare first and obligations to his patients second. The experimental physician is not the acknowledged agent of society or of the selfish interests of either co-sufferers or future sufferers from the particular disease being investigated. It is always wrong and never right to make the misfortunes of people a convenience for furthering alien aims. Any claim to act for the good of society should be regarded with extreme distaste and even alarm as there is a real danger that such proclaimed altruism may be a high-flown expression to cloak outrageous acts. Nobody has the right to select martyrs for society.

Some investigators become accustomed to deceit and manipulation of others and this breeds contempt for others which is fanned by the physicians' boast of possible benefits to mankind that may accrue from their work. These are prating coxcombs. Listen to the plea of Sir Robert Hutchison, 'From making the cure and investigation of a disease more grievous than the endurance thereof, good Lord deliver us'.

A physician's duty to his patients has been brilliantly epitomized as follows:

Guerir quelquefois — to cure occasionally
Soulager souvent — to relieve often
Consoler toujours — to comfort always

This statement of intent is often attributed to Dr E. L. Trudeau and is actually carved on his monument in Sarane Lake, New York, but it is an old saying dating back at least 400 years. To this advice I personally add, *Mais nuire jamais* — but never harm. May it always be your proud motto.

Fashions in aetiology

Aetiology is a word which is often misused, thereby creating confusion. There are still many diseases of which the aetiology is obscure, and some of them cannot even be fitted into the conventional general pathological groupings, namely congenital, inflammatory, toxic, traumatic, neoplastic, degenerative and metabolic.

The term reticulosis was introduced in 1910 to describe a group of conditions of unknown aetiology characterized by a systematized hyperplasia of the reticulo-endothelial system. By 'systematized' is meant that in any individual patient, identical histological features are found in all affected sites. To diagnose a reticulosis is to to give an anatomical-cum-cytological description but not an aetiology.

Another nosological term is collagen diseases, a group of conditions of unknown aetiology in which the essential similarity is that of the histology, which is a fibrinoid necrosis of collagen tissues. The warning of Klemperer, who first used the term in 1941, is still very apt:

'In spite of the impatience of clinical investigators and the peculiar worship of diagnostic terms which has led to an exaggerated popularity of the diagnosis "collagen disease", there is a danger that it may become a catch-all term for maladies with puzzling clinical and anatomical features.'

Because certain diseases have a common histopathology, this does not mean that they have an aetiology or anything else in common. The two most popular terms at present in discussions on aetiology are (1) genetically determined and (2) auto-immune. There is a great danger that either of these phrases will be regarded by the uncritical as a complete solution of all diagnostic problems. Declaim, with no real knowledge but with mock seriousness, that some condition is genetically determined as an autosomal recessive with poor penetrance, and you are likely to be immediately hailed as a genetic expert.

The great German pathologist Virchow* over fifty years ago wrote:

'If one surveys the almost immeasurable number of diseases which have been held to be hereditary, it seems obvious that the habit of some doctors of recognizing the hereditary character of certain diseases has changed almost according to fashion. An inclination in this direction has always existed and the acceptance of heredity as the cause protects against further mental efforts concerning the aetiology of the condition.'

Virchow pointed out that tuberculosis, scabies and leprosy were all considered to be genetically determined until their real causes were found.

The term idiopathic, although it was originally used to indicate a disease arising of itself, nowadays is understood to mean of unknown cause. Terms such as 'primary' and 'essential' should be regarded as synonyms. There is no justification for the neologisms 'cryptogenic' or 'agnogenic', which latter term sounds as if it indicated a relationship to lambs.

---

*Rudolf L. K. Virchow (1821–1902)

5 History Taking

History taking is a major diagnostic procedure usually no less important than physical examination or investigation, and should be considered as an essential complement to these other techniques and never a completely separate discipline. The greater the skill of the interviewer the more reliable and the more extensive will be the facts on which he later will formulate a diagnosis. Unfortunately many students are never taught properly how to interview patients and never to appreciate the true value of good history-taking, and so never bother to practise and thereby acquire this difficult yet rewarding art. In medical education history-taking should be, but rarely is, a basic element and major discipline and its teaching and genuine supervision should extend throughout the student's undergraduate and immediate postgraduate life and not be confined, as it often is, to a brief period at the commencement of clinical studies. In some organic conditions, such as angina and peptic ulcer, the history is often more important than the physical signs or even investigations. The symptoms of more than half the patients seen by the average general practitioner are primarily psychogenic and history-taking is the chief diagnostic weapon in these cases, especially if the physician regards, as he should, psychological ilness as a positive diagnosis and not merely the exclusion of the organic.

I strongly deprecate the common practice of recording histories on standard printed sheets which are ticked or crossed on the appropriate lines or demand monosyllabic or extremely brief replies. History recording should never be a stereotyped performance but should be evolved like a well written narrative with a literary form and style. Patients will usually answer all questions properly if properly presented at the proper time. The students must be taught and thereby gradually learn how to develop a history in logical sequence, and to appreciate how, as experience increases, the patient's primary symptoms will automatically demand the appropriate follow-up questions. A cardiologist does not need a printed sheet to remind him that a patient with dyspnoea must also be asked about swelling of the legs, or a neurologist that the patient with vertigo must be asked concerning tinnitus and deafness. It is amazing how often in teaching hospitals the consultants themselves use such printed forms, especially in out-patient clinics. Series of pre-arranged printed questions with a predetermined sequence cannot cater for all possible contingencies or all possible combinations of symptoms, and can never assess the reliability of answers or evaluate important emotional factors.

The instant a patient enters the room and while obtaining the history the examiner must keep his eyes wide open, carefully observing the patient, because he may notice many things, for example pallor, swelling in the neck or tremor, gait and cyanosis or jaundice, and also observing the patient's general demeanour, his facial reactions to questions and his alertness, all of which may give him important guides to subsequent questions. In other words, the physician should seek out physical signs even whilst obtaining a clinical history.

Doctor–patient relationship

The doctor's general appearance, especially with regard to tidiness, cleanliness and being reasonably well groomed and conventionally dressed are matters which must not be ignored, because neglect of them may at least initially detract from a patient's belief in a doctor's ability.

To obtain a good history it is essential to be on good terms with the patient. The introductory remarks are of vital importance because they often determine the doctor–patient relationship. A good understanding with a patient depends on an ability to communicate skilfully; such an ability is rarely a natural gift and is not awarded as a bonus on medical qualification but has to be gradually developed.

A good doctor–patient relationship depends in large measure on mutual trust and respect, is in large measure emotionally determined and not dependent on logical considerations, and is enhanced by symbolic values attached to small acts and inconsequential behaviour. We must attempt to make the patient appreciate that we recognize him as an individual and our approach must be kind and sympathetic, not arrogant and blown out with the air of feigned superiority or ultra-sophistication. It is only by adopting a friendly, warm, gracious and good-mannered attitude that we will obtain the confidence of many patients, and complete confidence is essential for good histories. The doctor must try to ward off any possible hostility which he may feel towards a patient because of his personality, irritating mannerisms, or psychological defences. Hostility breeds aggression which will be counter productive. If we are courteous to patients any problem of communication will probably disappear. 'Politeness does not consist merely in gesture or words which may be hypocritical and deceptive but in being courteously disposed towards people' (André Maurois). Humility and a genuine interest in all people are two necessary ingredients of the good physician. Humility is the surest shield against intellectual arrogance but it must be genuine and not a mere pretence or fatuous self delusion, and must not only be felt but also demonstrated.

Another essential quality is that of being a good listener, allowing the patient to talk freely and in simple language and yet skilfully guiding him away from irrelevancies and towards a logical continuity of his story. But the wording of questions must never be such as to suggest that a particular answer is required. Most patients are anxious to talk and one must give them the opportunity. An impatient doctor can never be a good doctor. Listening is an art which not only enables a physician to obtain facts but also to gain insight into the patient's personality and emotional reactions.

No one can ever share completely the feelings of another, but the mere effort to do so brings the doctor closer to the patient. This ability is in itself an expertise just as important as the correct elucidation of physical signs. Interest in a patient's disease should never rule out a passionate regard for his suffering. An anonymous author wrote, 'The milk of human kindness has been curdled by molecular biology and the robot generation of milli-equivalent practitioners'. The physician's rapport with his patient determines not only the amount of significant information he obtains but also its quality.

Empathy is the ability to feel what another is feeling, an appreciative perception and understanding without necessarily sharing a patient's emotional reactions. But the physician must preserve a degree of detachment, otherwise his own objectivity will be destroyed and his clinical judgment will become biased and faulty. Empathy is not identical with sympathy. In sympathy the doctor may suffer with his patient but in empathy, although he knows and appreciates how the patient feels, he himself does not necessarily have the same emotions and may even believe them to be false or wrongheaded. Empathy is not concerned with advice, criticism or reassurance.

Non-verbal communication

The first communication a patient has with his doctor is often non-verbal and the degree of emotional warmth displayed thereby may profoundly affect subsequent rapport. Facial expression, nods, gestures, grunts or groans are usually under control but conscious control is often far from complete. If the doctor genuinely feels an emotion then the desirable facial expression comes of its own accord. Control of non-verbal expressions may be very difficult if the physician is tired or in a hurry or is consulted by somebody whom he does not wish to see. But however difficult the physician feels he should act friendly towards his patients from the first instant of their meeting and this attitude should continue throughout the interview.

The physician should never by facial expression, gesture or spoken aside betray boredom, anger, surprise or disgust, or directly or by innuendo pass moral judgment on anything a patient may say about himself. At appropriate times laugh with patients, but this must always be engendered by genuine emotion and never be counterfeit, and you must never give an impression that you are laughing at a patient.

It may surprise some to know that an impassive poker face, sometimes deliberately adopted, may provoke uncertainty in a patient with resultant anxiety. Such passivity may be wrongly interpreted as evidence of boredom or lack of interest or feeling or understanding or that the doctor is holding back something.

By non-verbal communications the doctor also expresses his own self-confidence and assuredness. All of this is often ridiculed and dismissed as 'bedside manner', but in reality is an effective help in treating patients. But faced with a blatant over-confidence or an attempt to convey a veneer of omnipotence and supreme prestige, a discerning patient, irritated by the incongruity of the physician's pompous pose and arrogance, will be alienated.

Periods of silence may indicate serious reflection and thought on the part of the physician and may impress the patient, but sudden silences are more likely to produce anxiety not only in the patient but also in the doctor himself, especially if he is inexperienced. The pause may be because the patient is attempting to recall something which he considers is important and he then may be helped by the physician's assurance that accuracy of detail, for example of a date, is not important. On the other hand the patient may be hesitating about giving some information and then the doctor should by a nod or by leaning forward in his chair or by alteration of facial expression, or a simple phrase (or preferably a single word) indicate to the patient that he is listening attentively and wishes the patient to continue. If the patient's manner indicates distress then a few words of encouragement such as, 'Please go on' or 'Yes, I understand' or 'I appreciate that it is difficult but try and tell me'. However the commonest cause of silence is poor interviewing technique including hesitation as to what further questions to ask, or tactless remarks, or frequent interruptions or signs of lack of concentration on the part of the physician. Moreover it is during such periods of silence that the patient is likely to concentrate on the physician's facial expressions and gestures which themselves might indicate boredom or continuing interest.

The physician must never attempt to relieve any tension caused by silence by inane, facetious or irrelevant remarks. On the other hand silences may have a calming effect relieving any anxiety and producing a desirable measure of serenity.

The classical dictum, 'Know thyself' is an essential prerequisite and the physician must always be aware of his own mannerisms which may detract from obtaining a satisfactory history. The physician should ask himself how he would feel if when he was telling somebody something important that person was constantly gazing at the ceiling or at his shoes or repeatedly tapping his pencil against some furniture or doodling or scribbling notes furiously.

Eliciting the symptoms

After noting the patients full name, address and age, the first essential is to learn from him what initially motivated him to seek medical advice, and thus to know exactly what his complaints are. It is often the emotional disquiet produced by symptoms rather than the symptoms themselves which make a patient seek medical advice. For each individual symptom, roughly the date and more precisely the mode of onset, whether it came on with dramatic suddenness, reaching its maximum within minutes or about one hour; fairly suddenly reaching its maximum in one or a few days; or more gradually. How it has subsequently progressed is important, whether it has gradually or suddenly got worse or better and whether there have been remissions and exacerbations, and, if so, on average for how long and what direct and indirect factors are held responsible for them. All possible factors, including past treatment, aggravating and relieving each symptom must be carefully gone into. With any pain its site, radiation, character (including severity), duration, aggravating and relieving factors, frequency and periodicity must always be elucidated. Enquiry should be made concerning other symptoms associated with or coincidental to or produced by the primary symptom. The patient should be asked concerning any therapy he may have received for each individual symptom and its effect on each symptom. Of course, the questions which the examiner asks are influenced by the symptoms, but he must not allow the patient to skip from one to another before he has given a full account of each individual symptom in turn.

ANGINA

To illustrate the importance of history let us consider angina. Phobias, neurosis or any disease of the chest wall or spine or of the diaphragm or of any thoracic or abdominal viscus may cause chest pain simulating angina. But the features which distinguish angina from all other pains must be emphasized rather than any similarities, and if those distinctive features are absent then some other cause of the pain should be sought.

Angina starts in the sternal area and although it may radiate widely it never starts in another site and radiates to the sternum. Angina may radiate to the left mammary or inframammary area, or to the left shoulder and down the arm. Rarely it radiates to the right and sometimes to the neck or epigastrium but again it must be emphasized that it does not radiate in the reverse direction towards the sternum. Radiation is not essential and when the pain is of atypical distribution angina is not likely.

Angina is described as a feeling of constriction, of being squeezed, or of a pressure and is only rarely described as a sharp or stabbing pain. It is brought on by exertion or marked emotional disturbance and its severity gradually increases as the activity is continued but it never starts very abruptly (except when infarction occurs) or immediately the exertion begins and it does not wax or wane in intensity during the exertion but gradually increases in severity, finally forcing the patient to stop which always causes a gradual but complete disappearance of the pain. The severity of the exertion or emotional upset which produces the pain is far more important diagnostically than the exact nature of the precipitating factor, and if a patient complains of chest pain when doing some particular exertion but does not experience the same pain when doing some different but equally strenuous activity then the patient has not got angina. I have seen several patients who have been wrongly labelled as angina who were able to demonstrate to me their ability to do strenuous floor exercises for about ten minutes without causing pain, thus proving that they did not have angina.

Angina never starts while a patient is at complete rest and rarely lasts for more than five minutes and if for over ten minutes either the diagnosis is wrong or the patient has a myocardial infarction. Rapid and complete relief in less than five minutes on sucking a glyceryl trinitrate or equivalent tablet is an important feature of angina, but many who have not got angina also claim such relief but usually not so dramatic and they may even become habituated to those tablets, insisting on their efficacy. In such cases a trial with a placebo should always be instituted and it will be found that patients with cardiac neurosis or with organic lesions of other viscera will be equally improved. It is true that angina is very occasionally atypical, but then an alternative diagnosis should always be seriously considered. I have known patients with chest pain which was definitely not angina who have been deliberately frightened by their physicians attaching the angina label to them in order to persuade them to alter their habits and to drink or smoke or work less or lose weight. This is shocking medicine. Fear of impending death is often not a feature of angina and when present with chest pain is not pathognomonic.

Angina has been discussed in detail because with this condition clinical examination is often completely normal as are also investigations, including ECG before and after a standard exercise, enzyme estimations and even coronary angiography which means that a careful history is all important and decisive in many patients with chest pain. A distinguished cardiologist has written: 'Any capable physician can determine the presence or absence of angina effectively and reliably at the bedside without any fancy or diagnostic gadgets or cost, pain, suffering, or apprehension to the patient.'

In their monumental tome on *Heart Disease* E. N. Silber and L. N. Katz* have stated: 'More erroneous diagnosis of heart disease is made by a hasty superficial interpretation of the patient's symptoms than by either lack of knowledge or failure to elicit or properly interpret physical signs.'

Leading questions

The patient must be free to talk about the things he personally feels are important but the quasi-legal notion that doctors should never ask leading questions is bad advice; but such queries must be as few as possible and be used only to help the patient formulate his story in a logical pattern. There must always be a subtle guiding of the conversation along the channels most likely to be profitable. Wisdom borne largely of experience will help in the decision when and if to curb a loquacious patient or the person who goes into unnecessarily elaborate details and guide him back to the important issues. The physician should never passively listen to volumes of irrelevancies, but on the other hand he must not behave as though he were a lawyer grilling a recalcitrant prisoner.

If the patient is of poor intelligence and unable to explain himself properly it is essential to ask direct and leading questions, guiding the conversation so as to obtain as clear answers as possible.

Some leading questions which provoke the patient to give one type of answer rather than another, or a definite instead of a vague reply, though intruding some bias, may yield important information quickly. This technique can be especially useful in testing the reliability of answers to various interrelated questions — for example, concerning headache, by the loaded final question, 'Would you then agree that your headaches come on only when you are emotionally upset?'

When he has apparently completed the voluntary history, the examiner must always ask leading questions, for instance concerning appetite, bowels, micturition and weight, if these have not previously been mentioned. In other patients other leading questions are necessary, such as asking in a neurological case whether there is disturbance of vision or attacks of loss of consciousness, or asking

*E. N. Silber and L. N. Katz, *Heart Disease,* Collier-Macmillan, 1975.

a patient with dyspnoea whether he has pain on exertion. Good instruction and experience should teach the student the essential questions for each system.

If a patient is of poor intelligence and unable to explain himself properly, or is garrulously bubbling over with irrelevant details, then it is essential to ask direct and even leading questions, subtly guiding his conversation so as to obtain as clear answers as possible.

Misunderstandings

Whilst appreciating that a patient's history may be unreliable do not too readily dismiss his account as it may be the best source of information concerning his condition and may turn out to be correct even if it sounds preposterous. Do not reject anything the patient says because it sounds implausible or because you cannot explain its significance. Similarly do not dismiss any symptom as psychogenic because you cannot explain its significance.

Never accuse a patient of misleading you unless you are absolutely certain that it is not you who have misled him. The patient must be asked to explain exactly what he means by any words or phrases which are obscure or mean different things to different people, such as weakness, tiredness, rheumatism etcetera. The physician must not put his own interpretation on such words, but must be very patient when listening to attempted explanations and realize that even the most intelligent person has difficulty in describing, for example, the character of pain or any very transient phenomenon such as dizziness.

The examiner must always beware of automatically translating symptoms expressed by the patient in lay terminology into technical terms. This may result in many false equations and false premises. For example, if the patient complains of unsteadiness when walking, do not automatically assume that he is ataxic; or if he complains of light-headedness, that he has vertigo.

Especially, do not jump too hastily to the decision that a particular system is involved and that therefore your questions must revolve round this. For example, shortness of breath on exertion does not necessarily imply cardiac involvement, nor difficulty in walking, neurological disease.

Always be sure that the patient really understands your questions. Many patients give misleading replies rather than admit to incomprehension. Constant interruption by the doctor often makes the patient suspect that he is being regarded as unintelligent, and he is then liable to give misleading information. Neither should the physician use technical words and phrases even of the simplest type, such as heartburn or palpitations, without explaining to the patient exactly what is meant by such terms. There is nothing of importance in clinical medicine which cannot be explained to, or enquired about by, ordinary people using ordinary words. To be precise and at the same time to be colloquial may be difficult sometimes but is never impossible. It should also be appreciated that patients often express their emotional problems in a variety of ways and frequently the presenting symptom is only an excuse in an effort, which is often subconscious, towards making it easier to discuss those emotional problems. Frequently such patients use the language of physical symptoms and not commonly used psychiatric terms. For example, 'palpitation' may refer to an awareness of the heartbeat, or it may imply a very rapid heart or even a slow pounding beat. Especially when the clinician has a prejudice in favour of some particular diagnosis, he may wrongly accuse the patient of poor observation or of a misleading description of his symptoms when the truth is that the symptoms have been correctly stated but are atypical. In such circumstances the clinician may upset the patient and make him give answers which approximate more to those which the doctor expects but which are actually incorrect.

Psychiatric aspects of history

Physical diseases especially of the brain, kidneys and liver may cause and even start with mental disturbance and mental disease may present with a symptom such as dyspnoea which is usually associated with organic disease. A large percentage of patients complaining of headache, weakness of limbs or abdominal pain have no organic disease and a large number of those with organic disease have some purely emotional reaction (psychogenic overlay) to their physical illness. A history obtained by every physician even though he is not a psychiatrist must include questions on which to base an assessment of mental state and intelligence, noting the facility with which questions are answered, the ability to recall past events and the degree of mental alertness exhibited. Moreover it is only by history-taking that delusions, hallucinations and the grosser forms of mental disturbance may sometimes be recognized if no other witness is present. Every physician should learn how to identify and assess personality defects, obsessions, phobias, paranoia, depression and hysteria. Many symptoms are caused by psychological defects and the sufferer's inability to cope adequately with the varying circumstances and problems which are a normal part of living. Also patients have different emotional reactions to an organic disease which they have. Such understanding on the part of the physician will help him to explain to the patient whatever is thought essential for him to know and understand about his illness and such understanding must be the basis of effective reassurance. The good physician realizes that the unfounded fears of only a few are resolved by such trite expressions as, 'Do not worry', or 'Everything will be fine', or 'Pull yourself together', unless accompanied by further explanations and reasons which the physician hopes will be accepted by the patient as to why those fears are groundless. Reassurance, if it is to be effective, depends on an excellent doctor—patient relationship. The bald statement, 'There is nothing organically wrong with you' is also unlikely to be convincing as it makes no attempt to explain the symptoms which initially brought the patient to the doctor. Sometimes the best approach for the physician is to admit ignorance but explain that many patients do have symptoms for which no valid answer can be found and then explain that one of the main duties of a physician is to differentiate serious from non-serious symptoms; the latter, whatever academic explanations may be given, are merely a nuisance, either major or minor, and not indicative of any serious disease, such as cancer or heart disease. The language used by the physician must always be simple and show due consideration. To give answers obscured by technical jargon will only increase anxiety. It is also important, especially in patients who have some organic disease, that any reassurance is not given with strings attached, for example, 'You can live a normal life but do not drive your car when alone', or 'You will be fine provided you do not have another attack'.

Attentive listening to a patient's recital of his woes is often more help to him than the employment of a vast armentarium of laboratory and radiological tests in an attempt to assure the patient that he has not got any organic disease, and the doctor that he has not missed anything important. Most patients go to their doctor in the hope that he will understand not only their disease but also their personality. Being treated with respect by a prestigious person, a doctor, in itself often boosts a patient's self-esteem. Allowing the uninhibited expression of the patient's current emotional problems and helping him to form his own solutions without the physician delving too deeply into the past is the essence of good psychotherapy. Psychiatrists are not the only ones capable of dealing with emotional problems of others, and anyway a doctor cannot send all his patients to psychiatrists.

Lack of knowledge of the bloated voluminous jargon of psychiatry should not deter the ordinary physician. Indeed any attempt to help a patient by giving him explanations of his symptoms in technical jargon, even if those terms are properly understood by the physician himself, is valueless, as are grotesque theories which purport to explain to patients the basis of their emotional problems, such as the dogmas of psychoanalysis concerning penis envy, the oedipus complex and the subconscious wish to castrate a parent.

General remarks

In every case the patient's occupation should be asked, and it may be important in an appropriate case to enquire about its exact details. The consumption of alcohol and tobacco is often important, and every patient must be asked what medicines he is taking, including hypnotics, because so much illness today is produced by the indiscriminate and careless use of drugs.

Family history and previous illnesses must always be gone into, either briefly or in detail according to the likely diagnosis, but the answers must be kept relevant, otherwise a great deal of time and emotional energy will be expended unnecessarily. If previous illnesses and family history are dealt with before the details of the present complaint have been elaborated, this may cause a lessening of a good doctor–patient relationship. The patient's mind is fully occupied with his own present troubles and too detailed an enquiry about his own or his family's past illnesses are likely to be regarded as irrelevant or even irritating. For example, if the patient is complaining of recent shortness of breath and the doctor goes into long-forgotten particulars of some exanthem of childhood or the details of his father's last long illness due to cancer before completing the information concerning the patient's immediate symptoms, the patient may wrongly consider that the doctor is uninterested in his real complaint and may regard him as eccentric or incompetent. History-taking like physical examination can be too thorough, more detailed than the occasion demands.

Three important areas of experience, work, friendships and sex life should always be asked about, diplomatically. With regard to employment, the number of jobs the patient has had since he left school and his relationships with his employers and fellow-workers are often much more important than the technical details of his occupation. With the craze for super-specialization, inquiries about a patient's sex life are considered to be the prerogative of priests, psychiatrists and social workers. But just as the general physician must be prepared to examine the various orifices of the body, so must he also be prepared to inquire about the sexual life of his patients. Such personal matters, when dealt with in a tactful manner, should be considered no more an intrusion into a patient's privacy than the physical examination of some part of his or her body which is normally clothed. At the same time the physician must guard against those few patients who obtain an erotic satisfaction from recounting and being questioned about their sexual experiences. Likewise the physician must himself beware of any voyeuristic tendencies of his own which may induce him into asking greater details than are either necessary or judicious.

Again it must be emphasized that history-taking and clinical examination are complementary and not two completely different approaches and it may be essential during or after the physical examination to obtain further details of the clinical history. Often the sudden change from the armchair interview to the greater intimacy of the examination couch stimulates the patient to mention spontaneously problems not previously aired or accept such questions being asked without them causing any embarrassment. This is especially true of sexual matters. Too early probing may produce defence reactions with resultant evasiveness, vagueness or even amnesia because the patient wonders why the doctor wants to know such intimate details, especially if they seem to be irrelevant to the main complaint. Uncovering of the body often makes uncovering of the mind much easier.

Every patient should be questioned about his own views and fears concerning the cause of his symptoms and must also be asked what he considers is the matter with himself and his ideas about his diagnosis and if he has fears that he has some particular condition such as cancer or heart disease.

It is usually true that if after a well taken history the physician has no reasonable idea of the diagnosis then it is unlikely that he will be much wiser after full physical examination. In fact a good history often gives valuable clues as to the correct assessment of physical signs discovered later. An accurate history does however depend on the patient's memory and veracity and either may be defective, and in such cases if the physical findings conflict with the history then the former is likely to be the better guide to a correct diagnosis.

If after completing the history and physical examination you consider that further investigations are necessary, then the reasons for them and their nature must be explained to the patient in language which he can understand. Other than in exceptional circumstances, the patient should be told your provisional or considered diagnosis and have the rationale of your proposed treatment explained to him and he should be asked if he has any further questions and if he is satisfied with the explanations which have been given to him. All these explanations in themselves constitute a most important therapeutic weapon. It must never be forgotten that the psyche and the soma are two interrelated and inseparable aspects of every patient's personal identity.

C

6 Fever

Taking the temperature

There are some rules about taking temperatures which, although elementary, must be observed scrupulously. The thermometer must be aseptic, having been washed before putting away and, whenever possible, being kept in an antiseptic solution. One must first make sure that the mercury column has been shaken down to below 98°F (36.5°C). In the conscious adult it is not important whether the temperature is recorded in the mouth or the axilla, although it is often ½ to 1 degree Fahrenheit higher in the mouth. In an infant or child it should be recorded in the groin with the hip fully flexed, or in the rectum. In drowsy, stuporose, semi-comatose or comatose patients it must always be taken in the rectum, using a special thermometer which can record below 95°F (35°C), or the important and serious condition of hypothermia may be missed. The thermometer must always be kept in position for one minute at the very least, even if the instrument is labelled 'half minute'. The normal temperature is generally presumed to be 98.4°F (37°C) but may vary between 97°F and 99°F. There is normally a diurnal variation of about 1.5°F with the highest temperature in the late afternoon and the lowest in the early hours of the morning.

The temperature record is an important physical sign in every patient and, except in ephemeral fevers lasting only a day or two, an explanation for a raised temperature must always be sought.

The temperature chart

The type of fever may be a great help in diagnosis. Often, however, the classical terms given to the different categories of fever — remittent, intermittent, continued and undulant — are incorrectly used.

REMITTENT PYREXIA

A remittent pyrexia is one in which the difference between the maximum and minimum temperatures (usually the evening and morning temperature respectively) is more than 1.5°F (1°C), the temperature being raised throughout the whole or almost the whole of the day. Most fevers are of this type.

INTERMITTENT PYREXIA

An intermittent pyrexia is one in which there are paroxysms of fever, usually high, which last for only a comparatively short period of the day and are often accompanied by a rigor. A rigor is characterized by marked shivering, the patient feeling very cold. This occurs in the period immediately prior to the actual rise of temperature and is due to a marked generalized reflex vasoconstriction in order to conserve body heat. The rapidly rising temperature is accompanied by profuse sweating associated with generalized vasodilatation.

The temperature chart therefore shows high peaks, with subsidence to the normal line or below. The paroxysms may occur daily or every third or fourth day — these being called quotidian, tertian and quartan fevers respectively. Malaria, pyaemias, acute pyelitis, intermittent biliary obstruction due to stone or neoplasm, and septicaemias commonly give rise to this type of fever.

CONTINUED PYREXIA

A continued pyrexia is one in which the temperature remains high throughout the day, with a difference between the maximum and minimum temperatures of less than 1.5°F (1°C). In Britain there are only three common causes of a prolonged continued pyrexia — the enteric group of infections, miliary tuberculosis and infective endocarditis. Very rarely a virus pneumonia may cause such a fever. Miliary tuberculosis is often very difficult to diagnose clinically, for there is usually an absence of physical signs in the lungs and there may be no meningeal signs. A slight cyanosis is often present in these cases and should arouse suspicion.

UNDULANT PYREXIA

An undulant pyrexia (sometimes called 'relapsing') is one in which periods of continued fever alternate with completely afebrile periods. The brucellosis group of infections and lymphadenoma are the two commonest causes of this type of fever, but the relapsing fevers and spirochaetal infections conveyed by bites or scratches of various animals — especially rats, cats, ferrets and humans — are of this type.

Brucellosis may be present without the typical undulant type of fever. The occasional, although rare, occurrence of an undulant fever (Pel–Ebstein fever)* in lymphadenoma is of great importance because it may be the presenting manifestation, especially in those cases which do not exhibit palpable lymph nodes or splenomegaly, any enlarged nodes being confined to the chest or abdomen.

There are various relapsing fevers, each due to a distinctive organism such as *Borellia duttonii* and each peculiar to a localized part of the world. In all the relapsing fevers a short febrile period of 4–10 days, starting and ending abruptly, is followed by an apyrexial period of 1–2 weeks and later by a further paroxysm of fever, the number of relapses being up to about ten. It is extremely unlikely that any of these relapsing fevers will be encountered in Britain unless the patient has very recently arrived from a region where it is endemic.

With bite and scratch fevers, between one and two weeks after the initial wound a relapsing type of fever develops, and paroxysms of pyrexia alternating with apyrexial periods may go for many weeks. A diagnostic difficulty is that the wound may have healed and the initial incident be forgotten before the fever starts. There is often enlargement of the lymph nodes draining the area, and there may be a morbilliform eruption which may wax and wane with each bout of fever.

It is sometimes stated that untreated infective endocarditis may cause an undulant fever, but this is not true. If the charts are studied carefully, it will be seen that there are no truly apyrexial periods, although the fever may spontaneously abate to near normal for a few days.

Marked sweating with fever is a feature of tuberculosis (especially pulmonary), brucellosis and rheumatic fever. Prolonged fever with widespread pruritus without any other skin involvement is suggestive of lymphadenoma. High fever and purpura should always suggest a septicaemia or primary blood disease such as leukaemia.

Pulse rate in fevers

The pulse rate in relation to the temperature is a point always worthy of consideration. For every degree centigrade (1.5°F) elevation of temperature above normal, there is usually an increase of eight beats per minute in the pulse rate. In typhoid fever, brucellosis, psittacosis, virus pneumonia and meningitis, the pulse rate is slower than would be predicted from the temperature chart. In polyarteritis and rheumatic fever the tachycardia is often very marked although the temperature may be only slightly raised.

*P. K. Pel (1852–1919), Dutch physician and Wilhelm Ebstein (1836–1912), German physician.

Respiratory rate in fevers

A marked increase in the respiratory rate/pulse rate ratio in a patient with fever suggests a pulmonary infection even though there are only equivocal or no positive signs in the chest. However, pneumonias, especially virus, do not always cause an increase in the respiratory rate, and such an increase may be due to conditions other than pneumonia.

Fever of uncertain origin

The task of diagnosis in a patient with pyrexia of uncertain origin demands a close alliance between clinician and pathologist — an alliance based on a full understanding of each other's powers and limitations. On the one hand, the clinician must have a sound knowledge of the tests which he asks the pathologist to carry out; on the other hand, the pathologist must not be used merely as a sort of penny-in-the-slot machine to deliver an answer of 'yes' or 'no' to such questions as, 'Has this patient systemic lupus erythematosus?'

Ephemeral fevers lasting for less than ten days, to which so frequently no accurate diagnostic label can be assigned, and which are often due to virus infections and for which the term febricula is sometimes used, are outside the scope of this discussion, as are also the common exanthems.

HISTORY

A careful history of the illness, especially of its onset, is of the first importance, for example in typhoid fever the onset is usually very gradual, but sometimes the classical ingravescent fever with gastrointestinal symptoms does not occur and the presenting symptoms may be bronchial. Particular attention must be paid to any symptom which cannot be attributed to the pyrexia *per se* such as cough, dyspnoea, dysuria, localized pain or diarrhoea, because such a symptom will give an obvious lead to the anatomical site of the disease. Symptoms such as headache, anorexia, lassitude, sweating which is not very marked and loss of weight have no diagnostic or localizing value, being common to all feverish patients.

Previous illnesses may afford a clue to the present condition, which may be a relapse, a complication or a sequel of either a recent or a long-standing disease. Has the patient been abroad, particularly in the period directly preceding the illness? If so, the type of fever common in the foreign parts visited must be kept in mind. Are other members of the family or fellow workers similarly affected?

If the latter, Weil's disease should be considered as an industrial hazard; in Britain minor epidemics have been reported among sewer labourers, coal miners, bargemen, fish workers and tripe makers, and it is important to realize that more than half the cases are not jaundiced. Usually the disease has an abrupt febrile onset followed by marked prostration, muscular pains, evidence of nephritis without oedema, frequently meningismus and marked injection of the episcleral vessels of the conjunctivae and haemorrhages from various sites, most commonly the nose.

It is always very important to know the details of any drugs which the patient has had recently because they may have modified the more usual course of the disease and rendered it atypical, or the drug itself may be the direct cause of the fever. This is especially so with antibiotics, sulpha compounds, iodides, antithyroid drugs and the anti-convulsants, including the barbiturates.

EXAMINATION

Complete and careful examination of all systems is essential and should always be carried out scrupulously before any investigations are ordered. Moreover any initial examination with completely negative findings must not be presumed to be a constant feature, and a detailed clinical examination should be carried out fairly often, as new signs such as rashes, heart bruits, or lymph node enlargement may develop after the first examination.

Enlarged lymph nodes demand examination of the area of lymphatic drainage. A generalized lymphadenopathy may be due to a generalized infection such as glandular fever, tuberculosis, secondary syphilis, or sarcoidosis; or a primary blood disease such as leukaemia; or a reticulosis such as lymphadenoma. In all these conditions splenomegaly may also be present. The presence of splenomegaly as an isolated finding is rarely helpful but does exclude cancer as the likely cause. In acute infections the spleen is never huge but it often is in chronic protozoal infestations and with a reticulosis such as lymphadenoma, and with some of the primary blood diseases, especially leukaemias. In any of these conditions causing splenomegaly pyrexia may be the presenting feature. Enlargement of any other abdominal viscus may indicate the cause of pyrexia. Examination of the chest must be meticulous because a pulmonary condition may be the cause of an obscure pyrexia even in the absence of cough or sputum.

The presence of a systolic or diastolic bruit should arouse suspicion of the possibility of an infective endocarditis and the less dramatic manifestations such as occur in the skin or purpura in mouth or conjunctiva or microscopic haematuria should be sought.

Meningitis is the only neurological condition which is likely to present as a pyrexia of over ten days' duration. Nuchal rigidity,

especially if associated with severe headache and photophobia, demands lumbar puncture to exclude meningitis. Choroiditis and high fever suggests miliary tuberculosis and pyrexia and retinal haemorrhages suggest septicaemias (including infective endocarditis) leukaemia or systemic lupus.
Lesions of the nails especially clubbing, spontaneous haemorrhages or white bands, all of which are described in a later chapter, may help in elucidating the cause of an obscure fever.

INVESTIGATIONS OF PYREXIA

It is outside the scope of this book to detail the investigations which should be done in a patient with fever of unknown cause, especially if there are no positive physicial signs, or to detail the interpretation of the results. Certainly, X-ray of the chest, blood culture, and a full blood count and differential white cell count are the tests which are most often helpful. With regard to the white cell count, a leucopenia suggests typhoid, miliary tuberculosis, systemic lupus, brucellosis, agranulocytosis (often due to drugs), aleukemic leukemia or a chronic virus infection. Leucocytosis with lymphocytosis suggests glandular fever (which clinically is often atypical and the Paul–Bunnell test may be negative) or lymphatic leukemia. Leucocytosis with eosinophilia suggests polyarteritis nodosa or trichiniasis. Other helminth infestations cause eosinophilia but are very unlikely to cause a prolonged fever. The frequency and diagnosis value of eosinophilia in the diagnosis of lymphadenoma has been grossly exaggerated. A raised sedimentation rate is of no value in this problem unless it is extremely high which would suggest myelomatosis. Some general rules must be stressed.

1. All investigations must follow a logical sequence which may be determined by the slightest clue from symptoms or signs. A barrage of laboratory and radiological tests should be held in abeyance until the system suggested by even a minor symptom or sign has first been investigated. Blunderbus investigations are rarely helpful but are costly and may be very unpleasant.
2. Investigations should never be done as though buying goods wholesale or in a supermarket. The simplest tests, meaning those likely to cause the least discomfort and inconvenience to the patient, must be carried out first.
3. Hazardous investigations are never justifiable in such a patient. Remember that patients who are very ill but have had a persistently high fever for even months have ultimately made a complete and spontaneous recovery without the supposed benefit of a diagnostic label.
4. If investigations have been unhelpful, nothing is to be gained by the automatic repetition of tests done previously.

5. Until the correct diagnosis is definitely established, no prognosis should be given, even though the pyrexia has persisted for a long time and constitutional manifestations are marked.

6. A grave condition such as lymphadenoma, even if strongly suspected, should never be diagnosed as definite unless there is irrefutable proof.

7. It may be tempting to regard any undiagnosed pyrexia as due to tuberculosis, or a collagen disease, or a 'hidden' cancer. However, tuberculosis is rarely the cause of an unexplained and long continued fever, and it is just as blameworthy to label and treat a patient as tuberculous when this is not true as to fail to diagnose the disease when it is present. To suggest a diagnosis of some collagen disease without supporting evidence is the refuge of the diagnostically destitute, because in this group of conditions it is rare to get prolonged fever without focal symptoms or signs. (A possible exception is sarcoidosis localized to the intra-thoracic lymph nodes.) Many patients with cancer have fever, often due to infection of a nearby organ, but with the exception of renal cancer it is unusual for any cancer to present without any focal symptoms or signs.

8. Most patients with obscure pyrexia have not got any rare disease but have some unusual form of a fairly common condition.

9. There is no justification for administering antibiotics or sulpha drugs unless the patient is so ill that delay cannot be justified. To give antibiotics merely because the patient demands them, or because the physician is afraid that if he keeps to simple symptomatic remedies like aspirin the patient will seek advice elsewhere, is extremely bad medicine. Antibiotic therapy, especially when a combination of them is used, often obscures the clinical picture without serving any useful purpose. However in cases of suspected malaria, amoebiasis or septicaemia in patients who are very ill and getting worse then a therapeutic trial of an appropriate drug may be justifiable.

10. One should beware of a snap diagnosis because this is likely to lead to Procrustean errors, and one should be prepared to retain the label 'obscure' or 'uncertain' until the evidence is really sound.

11. If a patient develops fever after surgery it is nearly always related to the surgical procedure in spite of denials by the surgeon.

12. It is sometimes considered that some obscure interference with the hypothalamic control of the heat-regulating mechanism may cause a persistent pyrexia, but this diagnosis should not be seriously entertained. There are indeed a few

cases in which the most diligent search fails to reveal the cause of a fever which has lasted many months or even years, but this must not be considered an adequate excuse for attaching a spurious diagnostic label to such a patient. In nearly all these cases of very long-lasting pyrexia, the fever is of low grade and ultimately abates spontaneously.

13. It should always be suspected that the patient has been faking the temperature if in an adult it is over 105°F (temperatures even above this are fairly common in infants and children), if his appetite and general nutrition remain good in spite of the persistent pyrexia, if variations in the pulse rate are not commensurate with the alterations in temperature, if the temperature lacks the normal diurnal variation, or if with any sudden lowering of the fever there is no sweating. In cases where such faking is suspected, the temperature must be recorded rectally and a trusted nurse must supervise its taking. Well-known methods of faking a temperature are (*a*) holding the thermometer near a light bulb, radiator or hot water bottle, or lighted matches or cigarette lighter, (*b*) vigorous rubbing of the thermometer with fingers or tongue, or bed sheets, and (*c*) shaking the thermometer held upside down.

7 General Appearance

Nutrition

Normal people differ considerably in body build from the two extremes of the tall and thin (the asthenic) to the short and stocky (the hyperasthenic), with the majority not conforming precisely to either pattern but representing one of the myriad of possible intermediate body configurations. The association of body build with specific disease predilection — for example, the asthenic to pulmonary tuberculosis and duodenal ulcer, and the hyperasthenic to gastric ulcer and coronary thrombosis — is a reputed statistical correlation but probably has no clinical application to the particular patient who is being examined.

The general nutrition of every patient must be assessed, whether or not the person is obviously excessively fat or abnormally thin. The patient should be weighed. Minor deviations from figures obtained from published tables are of no clinical significance.

Obesity is sometimes defined as a body weight over 20 per cent above the ideal given in standard tables. Some dispute that figure and others quibble as to whether obesity and overweight are synonymous. An alternative method of assessment of obesity is by taking various measurements and comparing them with standards, allowing for differences due to sex, age and body build. The measurements usually recorded are the maximum circumference of the chest (including breasts), of the abdomen, of the pelvis (including the buttocks). Often our experienced eyes give just as meaningful and good an assessment. Moreover, fat distribution is often not generalized.

Obesity in Cushing's* syndrome, whatever its cause, involves especially the trunk, neck and face with relative sparing of the limbs. In other obese patients the fat is evenly distributed over the face, limbs and trunk, but occasionally the excess fat is almost entirely on the buttocks and thighs (steatopygia). The vast majority of cases of obesity are due to an excess of food intake over body requirements. Many patients who deny that they over-eat will accept this pedantic phraseology if it is explained to them in simple terms, possibly using the petrol requirements of a car as an analogy. Over-

*Harvey Williams Cushing (1869–1939), a pioneer American neurosurgeon.

eating may have a psychogenic basis. Obesity is only rarely truly genetically determined and when all members of a family are fat this is very likely to be due to their identical eating habits. Comparatively few cases of obesity are due to endocrine disorders such as myxoedema, Cushing's syndrome, Fröhlich's* syndrome or primary gonadal disease. Moreover, all these conditions can nearly always be readily diagnosed or excluded on clinical examination without resource to biochemical or other investigations.

Multiple lipomas are lobulated swellings, all feeling alike, with no involvement of the overlying skin or other dermatological accompaniment. The lobulation can be readily felt if the swelling is compressed between a finger and the thumb of the hand and then palpated with the fingers of the other hand. Although it may be difficult to demonstrate that the skin immediately over a subcutaneous swelling can be moved independently of the mass, but if when the edge of the lump is pressed by the end of the finger it is felt to slip away from beneath the finger, this indicates that the swelling is subcutaneous. Lipomas are usually seen on the limbs rather than the trunk and should not be mistaken for neurofibromas. Very rarely they are painful.

Grossly poor nutrition from whatever cause results in emaciation and a generalized loss of fat, which in severe cases contrasts vividly with the marked abdominal prominence that sometimes occurs due to intestinal distension and hypotonicity of the abdominal muscles. Normal skin exhibits a turgor demonstrable by momentarily picking up a fold of skin between finger and thumb and then quickly releasing it; the normal skin drops back immediately to its resting place, but dehydrated skin remains raised in a pinched condition for some seconds or even minutes. Turgor is best evaluated where there are no loose skin folds such as below the clavicles. With marked dehydration, the Hippocratic facies (described later) may develop.

Height

Height depends upon a mixture of genetic, environmental, nutritional and endocrine factors.

*Alfred Fröhlich (1871–1953) worked for a short time with Starling in Liverpool and on returning to Vienna in 1901 he published his paper, 'Dystrophia adiposa genitalis', acknowledging his indebtness to Trousseau for the title, in which he described a single case due to a craniopharyngoma which was removed successfully via the nose. He later became successively professor of pharmacology and professor of toxicology in Vienna but had to flee the country in 1939. He settled in Cincinnati, USA.

GIGANTISM

Gigantism is a marked increase of height well above the average. It is due to either a hyperplasia of the eosinophilic cells of the pituitary or a gonadal hypoplasia occurring before union of the epiphyses of the long bones. The pituitary hyperplasia may later develop into an adenoma with resultant acromegaly.

DWARFISM

Dwarfism is smallness of stature but its precise definition is arbitrary and I think that the term should be used only when the stunting of growth is marked. Those physicians who indulge in a supposedly more scientific definition describe dwarfism as a height below the third percentile for his or her community in accordance with standard tables. If, for example, the mean average height of the British adult male aged over twenty is 5 feet 8 inches, then a man below about 5 feet 6½ inches in height would be considered by these mathematical enthusiasts to be a dwarf — a viewpoint which I, probably because of my own shortness of stature, consider to be untenable. It must be appreciated that undoubtedly there is a wide variation in the rate of growth of normal healthy infants and children, and bone age as shown radiologically is more closely correlated with maturity than is the chronological age. With dwarfism due to thyroid deficiency the bone age is grossly retarded but when it is due primarily to lack of growth hormone it is only marginally affected.

The causes of dwarfism are:

1. Bone or joint disease, especially rickets, achondroplasia, tuberculosis of the spine and Still's* disease.
2. Any severe chronic disease occurring during the growth period. This includes a large number of conditions in which the three essential factors — severity, chronicity and onset in childhood — are present. For convenience these may be classified anatomically as follows:
   (*a*) Cardiovascular diseases, especially cyanosed congenital heart conditions such as the tetralogy of Fallot.†
   (*b*) Respiratory disease such as extensive bronchiectasis. Note that pulmonary tuberculosis in childhood is rarely both severe and chronic in the same patient.
   (*c*) Abdominal disorders such as coeliac disease and allied conditions and renal disease (renal rickets).
   (*d*) Neurological lesions which cause a spastic paraplegia, with lack of growth of the limbs, due to cortical cerebral involvement in early life — for example, cerebral palsy,

*George Frederic Still (1868–1941), a London physician.
†Etienne–Louis Arthur Fallot (1850–1911), a French physician.

congenital hydrocephalus or craniostenosis. Bilateral extensive lower motor neurone lesions of the lower limbs, due for example to poliomyelitis, occurring in childhood may also result in dwarfing, but this is much less common.

(e) Chronic infection such as malaria, schistosomiasis or ankylostomiasis, especially if accompanied by malnutrition. This is an especially potent cause of dwarfism in the underdeveloped areas of the world.

3. Endocrine diseases affecting the pituitary, thyroid or gonads, or prolonged steroid therapy in childhood. With precocious puberty the children are often initially tall but later because of premature fusion of ephyses growth ceases early.

Infantilism

Infantilism is a retention in adult life of the sexual characteristics of childhood. Some physicians add to this definition the presence of childhood mental and physical features. But 'mental' is the wrong word if it implies poor intelligence, and if by it is meant the emotional make-up of a child, the problem is that this phrase is incapable of exact or acceptable definition. To imply that infantilism must always be accompanied by the physical characteristics of childhood indicates that dwarfism is a necessary finding, and this creates the difficulty of attempting to define dwarfism in mathematically precise terms. It also raises the question whether or not eunuchoidism, producing as it does poor sexual development, should be included as a cause of infantilism, because of such patients being usually tall. By my definition, eunuchoidism is included as a cause because dwarfism is not considered to be an essential feature.

The causes of infantilism are:

1. All the groups of chronic diseases listed above under the causes of dwarfism, provided they are very severe and occur before puberty has been reached.
2. Endocrine diseases. An important feature of pituitary infantilism is that although the person is small, he or she is perfectly proportioned; this is assessed in adults by measuring (a) the outstretched span, which should equal the height, and (b) the distances from scalp to pubis and from pubis to ground, which should be equal. In eunuchoidism the arms and the legs are abnormally long compared with the trunk. This is also a feature of dwarfism due to spinal disease, especially tuberculosis. In hypothyroidism starting in infancy or early childhood the ratio of limbs to trunk is diminished.

3. Chronic and malnutrition.
4. Chromosome abnormalities such as Turner syndrome (described later).

Three important diagnostic principles are:

1. Never diagnose infantilism in a young person unless you know the exact age; in other words, unless you know that the patient has passed the age when puberty should normally have occurred. For example, it is absurd to diagnose infantilism in a boy of ten because his genitalia are considered to be small. Furthermore, in fat males the genitalia nearly always appear to be comparatively small because they are embedded in fat.
2. The presence or absence of infantilism can often be readily diagnosed at a glance by looking for secondary sexual characteristics such as facial hair in the male and breast development in the female.
3. Marked dwarfism unaccompanied by infantilism is likely to be due to bone disease.

8 The Head and Facies

The head

The posterior fontanelle normally closes at about six weeks. The anterior fontanelle starts to diminish in size after the first year and should be completely closed by about sixteen months. Delayed closure of the fontanelles occurs in rickets, cretinism and congenital hydrocephalus. Normally the fontanelles bulge while any infant is crying, but persistent marked bulging indicates raised intracranial pressure. Conversely, the fontanelles become depressed as the result of the presence of dehydration. The skull sutures are normally closed by about six months.

SHAPE

The shape of the head varies enormously in normal people, depending mainly on genetic factors. Many normal people have hatchet-shaped, elongated heads (dolichocephaly), while others have broad almost cubical or spherical heads (brachycephaly). It is only grossly abnormal shapes, noticeable at a glance, which are pathological.

This pathological group is collectively called the craniostenoses, craniosynostoses or stenocephalies, these terms being synonyms. The condition is characterized by a very peculiarly shaped head due to premature synostosis (fibrous union) of some of the skull bones occurring in intra-uterine life or soon after birth. The group is sometimes subdivided according to the shape of the skull which depends on which of the many sutures, especially the major four, are involved. Hence such terms as oxycephaly (with a very high receding forehead); acrocephaly (a marked sloping of the occiput and frontal bones so that the skull is pointed); turricephaly (the frontal and occipital bones being extremely high and more or less vertical so that the skull has a tower shape); scaphocephaly (the crown being abnormally flat or even concave); and plagiocephaly (gross asymmetry of the two sides of the skull, including the facial bones). Any craniostenosis may be associated with any or all of the following additional features: low intelligence; epilepsy; upper motor neurone lesions of any number of limbs; exophthalmos; primary optic atrophy; strabismus (usually of the concomitant type) X-ray changes in the skull, showing the abnormal shape and a gross exaggeration of the normal pattern (described as a beaten copper or silver appearance) which is not in these patients due to raised intracranial tension, the mechanism of its production being obscure.

SIZE

The maximum circumference of the head at birth is about 13 in. (33.5 cm); by the age of one year it is 18 in. (45 cm); at seven years of age it is 20 in. (50 cm), and in adults it varies between the narrow limits of 21½ in. (53.75 cm) and 23 in. (57.5 cm). Prior to the age of two, the maximum skull circumference is roughly equal to the circumference of the thorax. These figures indicate that although there is a wide variation in the shape of normal heads, there is comparatively little variation in their size. Enlargement of the head may be due to any swelling involving the scalp, such as a sebaceous cyst, or to any localized or generalized enlargement of the skull bones.

It is usually easy to decide whether or not any swelling of the head involves the skull. A swelling involving the skull may be a secondary neoplasm from a primary growth in the lung, breast, kidney or thyroid, or rarely from some other site; a primary neoplasm such as an osteoma or a meningioma which has eroded the skull; a reticulosis such as myeloma or lymphadenoma or a lipoidosis; a chronic inflammatory swelling secondary to a chronic osteomyelitis, especially syphilitic; or an acute inflammatory swelling, a subperiosteal abscess, secondary to an acute osteomyelitis complicating a compound fracture or sinusitis. The inflammatory causes are rare nowadays.

The two commonest causes of generalized skull enlargement are congenital hydrocephalus and Paget's disease.* The latter is seen only in those aged over forty, but it must not be forgotten that congenital hydrocephalics may survive to beyond this age. Whereas the skull of the hydrocephalic is always smoothly and symmetrically enlarged, the skull in Paget's disease is often irregular, a fact which is better appreciated by palpation. In many dwarfs, especially achondroplasiacs, the head appears to be abnormally large, but this is in relation to height and is not an actual enlargement.

OTHER OBSERVATIONS

Rachitics are often brachycephalic and may exhibit craniotabes, an abnormal thinness of the skull, especially the occipital bone, which can be appreciated, especially in younger children, by digital pressure,

---

*Sir James Paget (1814–1899), London surgeon, wrote his treatise in *Trans. Med. Chir. Soc. London* in 1877.

which gives the impression that the bones can be indented. Rickets may also cause a localized prominence of the frontal and parietal bones. In congenital syphilis there may be a similar prominence of the frontal and rarely of the occipital bones which is often referred to as bossing.

A rare phenomenon is head nodding synchronous with the heartbeat, seen rarely in patients with severe aortic regurgitation. Other involuntary movements of the head, and percussion and auscultation of the skull, are discussed in Chapter 16 on neurology as is also the value of percussion and auscultation of the skull.

Head and body hair

Premature greying, or the presence of whitish-grey tufts in otherwise normal hair, is nearly always genetically determined and of no genuine diagnostic significance although it may occur in a large number of patients with pernicious anaemia and sometimes it occurs after a severe acute illness or a marked emotional disturbance, but in other cases it may suggest premature ageing. In kwashiorkor the normally dark hair of the head in those affected becomes depigmented, often with reddish streaks.

LOSS OF HAIR

Alopecia, which is a loss of scalp hair, is generally partial and rarely complete. It may have the following causes:

1. A local scalp infection (which in children is often fungal) or part of some more widespread skin disease such as seborrhoea, psoriasis, lupus erythematosus or erysipelas.
2. Acute infection such as secondary syphilis, pneumonia or typhoid may be followed by alopecia.
3. Irradiation or burns of the scalp.
4. Drug therapy, especially with the cytoxic drugs and with heparin and thallium (which is sometimes given orally in the treatment of fungous infections of the scalp).
5. It may be genetically determined, and then on the scalp is usually frontal or tonsoral, or it may be part of a generalized paucity of hair.
6. It may be due to myxoedema or uncontrolled diabetes mellitus. In myxoedema the loss of hair is occasionally generalized but is more often confined to the scalp and the eyebrows (especially their outer third) and the remaining hair is coarse and very dry. In Simmonds' syndrome (panhypopituitrism) there is a generalized loss of body hair, especially pubic and axillary. This condition is nearly always due to a vascular lesion of the main pituitary artery following pregnancy.

7. Loss of hair may be due to liver disease especially of an alcoholic aetiology. It is then usually mainly of body hair and associated with concomitant gonadal atrophy.
8. Alopecia, especially frontal, is common in those with dystrophia myotonica (myotonia atrophica).
9. Alopecia areata is a condition characterized by patchy baldness of unknown aetiology. The lesions are well defined, of various sizes and shapes, and the affected skin is smooth and not ulcerated or scarred.

In anorexia nervosa the body hair is greatly diminished but the face becomes covered with lanugo hair resembling the fine, soft, silky, very fair hair present on a normal foetus which disappears soon after birth. Lanugo hair is sometimes seen over the back, shoulders and limbs of infants and children with hypothyroidism.

HIRSUTISM

Hirsutism is a male texture and distribution of hair occurring in females. Differences in the amount, distribution and texture of hair are often genetically determined, for example, Chinese men and women have normally very sparse facial and body (especially pubic) hair.

Chinese normally have little body hair, and male American Indians do not have beards. Many normal women have a hairy upper lip and hairy limbs, and this will be more obvious in brunettes. Such hirsutism is usually genetic and often racial. Sometimes a transitory hirsutism occurs during pregnancy and disappears after parturition. But in women, other than a few wisps, in the following sites is always abnormal: the chin, the region of the external auditory meatus of the ear, the chest, the abdomen extending much above the pubic bone, and over the knuckles.

Hirsutism is but one aspect of virilization (signs of masculinity in a female). Hirsutism in an obese female, especially when associated with amenorrhoea, strongly suggests Cushing syndrome due to any of its several causes. Virilism without obesity is most often due to a neoplasm of the suprarenal cortex. The Stein–Levanthal syndrome is characterized by hirsutism and amenorrhoea or oligomenorrhoea starting about a decade after a normal menarche (puberty) and causing sterility and is due supposedly to follicular ovarian cysts. Some experts deny that there is such an entity and certainly removal of the cysts does not cure the condition.

The facies

An awesome thought is that there are probably no two people, apart from identical twins, in the whole world who are exactly alike as regards facial appearance. Greek philosophers, physiognomists, phrenologists, criminologists, artists and writers have all endeavoured to describe and define the facial features which are unique to every individual, and each of these groups of observers has claimed, with far more romance than science, an ability to relate those special facial features to both character and intelligence. Many stress the importance of the eyes in this connection, but what they are observing and attempting to define and describe are not the eyes themselves but the facial musculature around the eyes.

The facial muscles are an important guide to the patient's emotional feelings and should always be noted and taken into account. For example, the facies may indicate undue anxiety or depression, and even if the patient does not verbally describe such feelings, the good physician will diplomatically veer his questions towards elucidation of the source of that anxiety or depression.

Neurological lesions which affect the face, producing ptosis, squints, paralysis of the facial muscles and involuntary movements of the head, tongue, lips or facial muscles are described in Chapter 16.

The facial appearance may arouse in the wide-awake physician an immediate strong suspicion of endocrine disease, especially of Cushing's syndrome, myxoedema, thyrotoxicosis or acromegaly. Indeed, in these diseases the facies is often the most important single diagnostic feature. In acromegaly all the parts of the face which are normally prominent, both bony and soft tissues, are enlarged. The mandible often projects much further forward than the maxilla (prognathism).

In myxoedema, in contrast with acromegaly, only the soft tissues are affected, giving rise to bloated and coarse features. The skin is dry and thickened, and there is usually bagginess under the eyes. The hair of the scalp and outer part of the eyebrows is thinned. Myxoedematous patients are nearly always pale due to anaemia and this contrasts with a waxy yellowish or reddish colour of the cheeks, giving a 'strawberries and cream' complexion.

In Cushing's syndrome, obesity of the face and neck is always present and the facies is plethoric due to a secondary polycythaemia. In women there is frequently a masculine distribution of hair. In thyrotoxicosis the resultant exophthalmos and lid retraction (*see* Chapter 10) often produce a virtually pathognomic appearance. Oedema of the face may be due to any form of nephritis, myx- oedema, angioneurotic oedema, superior vena caval obstruction, erysipelas, trichiniasis or cellulitis of the face. The degree of oedema in any of these conditions may vary from a slight puffiness below the eyes to a marked swelling involving the greater part, but especially the upper half, of the face. Slight puffiness below the eyes may be seen in normal people, especially after late nights and during men- struation, but beware of such a facile explanation of any infra- orbital oedema until all the other causes have been carefully considered.

In any severely dehydrated patient the hollow cheeks and sunken eyeballs (enophthalmos) will be evident. Hippocrates described the facies in such patients, especially when death is imminent, as follows: 'The sharp nose, hollowed eyes, collapsed temples, the ears cold and contracted and their lobes turned out, the skin about the forehead distended and parched, the colour of the whole face being greenish, blackish, livid or lead-coloured.' The classical causes of the Hippocratic facies are the later stages of typhoid fever and advanced peritonitis.

MONGOLISM

The diagnosis of mongolism can be readily made from the face alone. All mongols look like members of the same family because they all have the same facial appearance, and it is that and not features which may be present elsewhere which is diagnostic. Their palpebral fissures are small and narrow and their closely set eyes are slanted. They are invariably brachycephalic and their hair is always scanty and straight, never curly. Their eyes often show epicanthic folds in the region of the inner canthus and a strabismus, which is usually concomitant, is common as is also bilateral ptosis with overaction of the frontalis. The mouth is often kept permanently wide open showing a fissured tongue. The ears are often abnormal in shape and size. It is the sum total of all these features which gives a pathognomonic facial appearance.

It has become fashionable to refer to mongolism as Down syndrome but this is another example of a bad eponym. Langon-Down in *The London Hospital Report,* **3** (1866), 259 wrote a paper entitled, 'Observations on the ethnic classification of idiots' in which he pointed out that although mongolism occurs in all racial groups it is far commoner in Europeans and this results in 'degeneration' (his word). Down believed that the European represents the apex of evolution and mongolism a reversion to an Asiatic type. I advocate the retention of the old term 'mongolism' even though these patients have only a superficial resemblance to certain Mongolian races (especially the Kalmucks). It is now known to be due to a chromosome abnormality, usually trisomy 21.

TRIANGULAR FACIES

There are three causes of a triangular-shaped face, namely congenital hydrocephalus, Paget's disease and achondroplasia. In congenital hydrocephalus the calvarium is enlarged but the facial bones are normal. In Paget's disease the calvarium is enlarged, often irregularly, the forehead often appearing to be unduly prominent, but the facial bones are not involved except in the rare variant called leontiasis ossea which produces bony nodules over the face and hard palate. The so-called leonine facies of leprosy can be distinguished because in the latter the nodules are in the skin and subcutaneous tissues and do not involve bone. In achondroplasia the triangular facies is produced by the lack of proper development of the facial bones with a normal head circumference, the face resembling that of a pug dog because of the depressed bridge of the nose and the squashed-in appearance of the whole face. Many dwarfs are wrongly diagnosed as achondroplasiacs, a mistake which would never occur if it was remembered that the outstanding feature differentiating achondroplasia from all other forms of dwarfism is the striking facial appearance which is always present.

The nose in diagnosis

In acromegaly and in myxoedema the soft tissues of the nose are enlarged, adding to the unprepossessing but distinctive appearance. Achondroplasia causes a depressed bridge of the nose due to poor development of the nasal bones. A similar appearance is seen in congenital syphilis, but in this condition it is a direct consequence of the snuffles (infection of the nasal mucosa) which occurs soon after birth and results in destruction of the nasal cartilage. Tertiary syphilis may produce the same end result, which is then often complicated by destruction of a large part of the nasal septum. Tuberculosis, in the form of lupus vulgaris, may also destroy the nasal septum, but this is then always secondary to the skin lesion with its marked ulceration and subsequent scarring. In similar ways both tuberculosis and syphilis may destroy part of the hard palate. Yaws may simulate syphilis, and leprosy tuberculosis. Rarer causes of destruction of the nasal septum are epithelioma spreading from the nearby skin and Wegener syndrome characterized by granulomatous lesions of the nasal mucosa which may cause destruction of the nasal cartilages and also by severe intractable rhinitis and sinusitis, granulomatous pulmonary lesions and severe chronic glomerulonephritis. Wegener, a German, described the condition in 1936. Industrial chrome poisoning may also cause destruction of the nasal septum.

Hypertelorism is a condition characterized by overgrowth of the lesser wings of the sphenoid which can be recognized on a lateral skull X-ray. It results in a very wide separation of the orbits, an extremely broad base of the nose and often bilateral exophthalmos. It is a congenital anomaly which is often accompanied by other congenital abnormalities, especially of the skull and teeth.

Many skin lesions commonly affect the nose and cheeks and these are described in a later chapter.

The ear in diagnosis

The external ear (auricle or pinna) rarely helps in diagnosis. Congenital abnormalities of the ears are fairly common; the ears may be
very large or very small or absent, they may be grossly asymmetrical
or of a peculiar shape, or there may be accessory auricles, usually in
the region of the tragus. Any such congenital abnormality may occur
in an otherwise healthy person, but in such an individual the finding
of some additional abnormality, for example in the heart, would
indicate that the heart lesion is congenital.

In any patient, other than a pre-menopausal woman, with arthritis
the ears should be carefully scrutinized for tophi, which are deposits
of urates and pathognomonic of gout. The skin over the cartilage of
the ears is thin and so ulceration of tophi in this site is an early
feature, but the whitish nature of the deposit may be visible even
before actual ulceration occurs. Deposits of calcium pyrophosphate
as occurs in the condition of chondro-calcinosis may be present in
the ear, simulating tophi. Darwin's tubercle, the skin over which is
always normal, is situated on the upper part of the straighter margin
of the helix, is a normal finding and must not be mistaken for a
tophus. The ears exhibit a bluish discoloration in patients with
moderate or severe cyanosis. In ochronosis associated with either
carbolic acid poisoning or alkaptonuria, the ear cartilates are bluish-
black.

Sturge–Weber syndrome

This is a condition characterized by a cutaneous facial angioma
which is often confined to one side of the face but may be bilateral
and may extend on to the neck and trunk. It is often associated with
a large and discoloured lower lip due to a cavernous angioma. It
may be associated with mental disturbance, epilepsy, an upper
motor neurone lesion of any number of limbs often with lack of
growth and buphthalmos (congenital glaucoma). An X-ray of the
skull always shows horizontal bands of calcification which are
almost invariably unilateral and confined to the posterior half of
the skull.

The salivary glands

PAROTID SWELLING

A parotid swelling is situated mainly in front of the tragus of the
pinna and may extend upwards towards the zygoma and downwards and slightly backwards towards the sternomastoid, obliterating

the depression normally visible below and in front of the lobule of the ear. An important differentiation from a pre-auricular adentis, is that the latter never obliterates that depression. An attempt should be made to differentiate between enlargement involving the whole of the parotid and a swelling confined only to a part of it because the latter is nearly always due to a neoplasm of the gland. Parotid neoplasms often cause a lower motor neurone facial palsy. Enlargement of the submandibular salivary glands produces a swelling beneath and in front of the angle of the jaw. Because the gland has two portions, the cervical and the buccal (which lies above the mylohyoid muscle), examination of the gland must be a bimanual procedure, with one hand palpating the neck in the region of the angle of the jaw and a gloved finger feeling the floor of the mouth and demonstrating contiguous and joined buccal and cervical swellings. This is an essential procedure to differentiate enlargement of the submandibular salivary gland from enlarged submandibular lymph nodes.

Parotid swelling may be due to an acute inflammatory lesion, most commonly mumps, and is then nearly always bilateral. Parotid enlargement may occur in debilitated patients, especially those with bad oral hygiene, and in semi-comatose or comatose patients. Suppuration, usually unilateral, often develops in such circumstances. Syphilis, tuberculosis and sarcoidosis may cause unilateral or bilateral parotid enlargement. Diabetics and alcoholics are prone to develop a parotitis. The gland may also be involved in lymphadenoma and leukaemia. Unilateral parotid enlargement may be due to a mixed cell tumour, and in such cases a lower motor neurone facial palsy is a frequent complication. Blockage of the parotid duct by a calculus with consequent glandular enlargement is rare, but this is the commonest cause of a unilateral submandibular salivary gland enlargement. Any salivary gland enlargement due to calculus is often intermittent and may be seen to get appreciably larger if the patient sucks some strongly flavoured substance such as a lemon. Mixed cell tumours of the submandibular salivary gland are very rare.

In any patient with a salivary gland enlargement, the openings of the parotid ducts, which are small papillae situated opposite the crown of the second upper molars, and the openings of the submandibular salivary gland ducts in the floor of the mouth must always be examined. This is particularly informative if the lesion is unilateral, when the difference between the orifices on the two sides may be readily visible. With suppurative parotitis, pus may be expressed from the orifice.

Mikulicz's* syndrome is a condition characterized by enlargement, usually bilateral, of the salivary and lacrimal glands. The parotid enlargement may be associated with a lower motor neurone

Johann von Mikulicz-Radecki (1850–1905), Breslau surgeon.

facial palsy. The common causes of this condition are sarcoidosis, syphilis, tuberculosis, lymphadenoma and leukaemia. Acute inflammatory lesions such as mumps and glandular fever very rarely cause this syndrome. The uveo-parotid syndrome is a condition characterized by bilateral parotid swelling together with iridocyclitis and often choroiditis. The causes of this syndrome are the same as those of Mikulicz's syndrome, but it is important to realize that anatomically these are two different syndromes.

Sjögren, a Swedish ophthalmologist, in 1933 described a syndrome the essence of which is an abnormal dryness of the mucous membranes. This causes xerophthalmia (dryness of eye) with resultant keratoconjunctivitis sicca, and because of the shedding of the epithelium from the conjunctiva and cornea there may be a blockage of the lacrimal ducts and the production of a dacryo-adenitis (*see* Chapter 9). The abnormal dryness of the mouth (xerostoma) may similarly cause salivary duct obstruction, with resultant salivary gland enlargement. This syndrome is probably never a clinical entity, but it is seen in patients with vitamin A deficiency, rheumatoid arthritis and systemic lupus erythematosus. It may also be accompanied by splenomegaly, hepatomegaly, Raynaud's syndrome, fever, bilateral pulmonary fibrosis and serological abnormalities including hyperglobulinaemia.

9 Ophthalmology for the Physician

In any eye lesion whether it be ulceration, abnormal opacification, haemorrhage, dilated blood vessels or any other finding, the first task is to localize the abnormality, that is to determine which anatomical structure or structures are involved.

The eyelid

The recognition and causes of ptosis are discussed in Chapter 16.

RETRACTION OF UPPER LIDS

This is usually considered to be due to a spasm of the levator palpebrae superioris, but overaction of the smooth muscle of Müller may play a part. Upper lid retraction may be readily visible when the patient is looking straight ahead because it causes a staring appearance with a widened palpebral fissure (the breadth of the transverse diameter between the upper and lower lids) and visible sclerotic above the margin of the iris. With ectropion (*see* below) or when the eyeball is pushed forward by a retro-orbital mass of any kind, the sclerotic may be visible below the inferior margin of the iris.

Lid retraction may be demonstrated by any of the following techniques:

1. If the patient is asked to follow the examiner's finger held at least ten inches away and moved very slowly (this is important) in a vertical plane starting above the patient's head, which is kept horizontal by the examiner's other hand, then it will be noticed that the upper lid does not keep pace with the level of the moving finger. For example, when the finger is 45 degrees above, or at, or 45 degrees below the horizontal, the upper eyelid will normally be in the same horizontal plane, but in the presence of lid retraction the eyelid will be above this, hence the term lid lag. Again, it is important to emphasize that this phenomenon can be observed only if the finger is moved very slowly.

2. The patient is asked to look into the distance and then quickly at the examiner's finger, which is suddenly placed a little above the horizontal plane and a few inches away from the patient's eyes. With lid retraction, instead of the upper lid lowering a little as part of the normal accommodation-convergence reflex it will be seen to elevate transiently.

3. The accommodation-convergence reflex is demonstrated by bringing the finger in a horizontal plane gradually towards the patient's eyes. This produces three distinct components occurring in the following chronological order: lowering of the upper eyelids, diminution in size of the pupils, and convergence of the eyeballs. Lid retraction causes interference with the first component of this reflex.

These associated eye signs of lid retraction are important because they are often early manifestation of thyrotoxicosis, occurring before the exophthalmos is demonstrable.

BLEPHARITIS

Blepharitis is an inflammation (usually staphylococcal) of the lid margin which leads to reddening, thickening, crusting and depilation. It is often accompanied by conjunctivitis. The cause may be obscure, but possible aetiological factors are cosmetics, measles, acne rosacea and allergic conditions. The condition is common in the elderly and in patients with seborrhoea or rosacea.

ECTROPION

Ectropion is retraction (eversion) of the lower lid. Especially in elderly people, it is often secondary to a chronic blepharitis with resultant cicatrization of the lid. It may be a feature of any long-standing lower motor neurone facial palsy.

HORDEOLUM

A hordeolum (sty) is a tender red pimple-like swelling with a yellow summit, involving the lid margin, and is associated with infection around the eyelash insertion.

CHALAZION

A chalazion is a chronic granuloma of the meibomian (sebaceous) glands and is easier to see from the skin than from the conjunctival surface of the lid. The conjunctiva locally in relation to the swelling is usually deep red. The swelling feels like a bead in the lid.

OEDEMA OF LIDS

Oedema of the eyelids, especially the lower, may be a feature of congestive cardiac failure, renal disease and myxoedema. Oedema localized to the upper eyelids may be due to cavernous sinus lesions, local infection, eczema or angioneurotic oedema (often due to cosmetics). The significance of infra-orbital swelling is discussed elsewhere.

XANTHELASMA

Xanthomas are deposits of cholesterol or cholesterol esters in tissues and, when they occur in the eyelids, are known as xanthelasma. Like xanthomatous deposits in the skin and subcutaneous tissues elsewhere, they may be secondary to the known causes of a hypercholesterolaemia which has been present for at least a few months, namely diabetes mellitus, chronic obstructive jaundice, nephrosis and myxoedema. These four conditions can be easily recognized and excluded, the last three often by a glance at the patient's face. The vast majority of patients with xanthomas in whom these conditions have been excluded have a normal blood cholesterol and the cause of the xanthomas is obscure; only a very small percentage have a hypercholesterolaemia, which may be genetically determined.

Lacrimal gland enlargement (dacryo-adenitis)

The normal lacrimal gland occupies a fossa situated on the medial aspect of the zygomatic process, which is in the upper lateral quadrant of the bony orbit. The gland is not normally visible or palpable, but when it enlarges it produces a swelling in the outer half of the upper eyelid. Bilateral dacryo-adenitis may be due to sarcoidosis, tuberculosis, syphilis, lymphadenoma or leukaemia, and is a rare complication of mumps and glandular fever. Its association with salivary gland enlargement and Sjögren's syndrome is discussed in Chapter 8.

Enophthalmos

Enophthalmos is a sunken appearance of the eyeball. It may be a feature of a normal facies, and is then always bilateral and usually racial. Bilateral enophthalmos may be seen in a patient with marked dehydration. Unilateral enophthalmos is a described sign of a cervical sympathetic paralysis but is rarely demonstrable. An artificial eye is usually more sunken than a normal eye.

Exophthalmos

Prominence of the eyes may be seen in normal people (especially in those who have prominent supra-orbital ridges) and in Negroes, and is a common appearance in patients with a very high degree of myopia. In buphthalmos (ox eye), which is associated with congenital glaucoma, the eyes are often prominent.

A significant undue prominence of the eye is called exophthalmos or proptosis. Some clinicians use the former term only when prominence is accompanied by lid retraction, and others use the term proptosis only when the prominence is unilateral, but I do not favour these distinctions. Exophthalmos is usually readily recognizable, but if there is any doubt when looking at the patient from the front, it is often possible to resolve that doubt by examining him in profile. A further test is that a ruler or card placed on the supra-orbital ridge and the malar bone will not touch the eyeball unless the latter is abnormally protruded. Minor degrees of exophthalmos are sometimes recognizable by standing, without leaning forward, behind the seated patient, holding his head between your palms and slowly tilting his head backwards while you yourself look almost vertically downwards. Normally you will first see the patient's supra-orbital ridges and then, as his head is gradually tilted backwards, his malar prominences, but without seeing his eyes between these two bony landmarks unless exophthalmos is present. An exophthalmometer is an instrument for measuring accurately the degree of forward protrusion, but such a critical assessment is rarely required except to assess the value of any new therapy.

Bilateral exophthalmos may be due to the following causes:
1. Thyrotoxicosis. It is then usually associated with lid retraction.
2. Exophthalmic ophthalmoplegia (malignant exophthalmos), which is often regarded as a variety of thyrotoxicosis. This is seen in middle-aged, often male patients, and the exophthalmos is always out of all proportion to any other manifestations of thyrotoxicosis; indeed, the exophthalmos may gradually increase in spite of the patient having been rendered myxoedematous by medical or surgical treatment. This means that exophthalmic ophthalmoplegia occurs in euthyroid, myxoedematous or thyrotoxic patients.
3. Cavernous sinus lesions. In such cases the exophthalmos, which may initially be unilateral, is associated with chemosis and ophthalmoplegia.
4. Hand—Schüller—Christian* syndrome. This is a condition characterized by deposits, usually of cholesterol esters, in the skull, producing bilateral exophthalmos and diabetes insipidus.

*Alfred Hand (1868–1949) an American physician, H. A. Christian (1876–1951) an American paediatrician, and Arthur Schüller (1874–) a Viennese neurologist. These authors wrote their accounts independently in 1893, 1920 and 1926 respectively, each adding new concepts.

5. Craniostenosis (*see* previous chapter).
6. Hypertelorism (*see* previous chapter).
7. It is a rare accompaniment of three common conditions, namely internal hydrocephalus, superior vena caval obstruction and emphysema.
8. Lesions behind the eye such as secondary neoplasm (classically due to primary suprarenal tumour), deposits of lymphadenoma or leukaemia may cause bilateral exophthalmos, but in these conditions the exophthalmos often remains unilateral. Any retro-orbital swelling due to a primary neoplasm, such as an osteoma, meningioma of the sphenoidal ridge or dermoid, aneurysm, cellulitis or haemorrhage (spontaneous or traumatic) may cause exophthalmos, but in these disorders it will be unilateral. Obviously any bilateral exophthalmos may be preceded by unilateral involvement. Asymmetry of a bilateral exophthalmos is of no diagnostic significance apart from the fact that when the difference between the two eyes is gross, the lesion may be mistaken for a strictly unilateral one. Lesions behind the eye often cause displacement of the eye with resultant strabismus.

Pulsating exophthalmos is due to an arterio-venous aneurysm, usually between the internal carotid and the cavernous sinus, and is most often the result of trauma. In addition to the exophthalmos, the condition causes conjunctival injection, and the angular vein and its branches can be felt to pulsate synchronously with the carotid pulse. A rumbling bruit may be heard over the orbit, and the exophthalmos can be diminished by pressure over the carotid. Ophthalmoscopy may show grossly distended retinal veins and there may be papilloedema.

A lower motor neurone facial palsy which causes widening of the palpebral fissure due to the weakness of the orbicularis palpebrarum may give a false resemblance to exophthalmos. In a patient with unilateral enophthalmos the normal eye may incorrectly be regarded as exophthalmic.

Conjunctival lesions

The normal conjunctiva is glistening, smooth and translucent, the normal white of the eye being due to sclera. Pengueculi are fatty deposits on the conjunctiva which are always near the limbus and of no significance.

In all patients the tarsal conjunctiva of the lower lid must be examined for pallor, cyanosis, icterus and plethora. Conjunctival haemorrhages may be due to an injury of the eye itself or to a fracture of the anterior fossa of the skull. Spontaneous conjunctival haemorrhages are common in infective endocarditis (they are then often petechial), Weil's* disease and trichiniasis. They may occur, but are not common, in any primary blood disease associated with a bleeding tendency. They may complicate pertussis. Often no cause is found.

Conjunctivitis is characterized by injection of the conjunctival vessels, sometimes by small haemorrhages and very rarely by ulceration (phlyctenules). Conjunctivitis unless due to foreign body or blocked tear duct is nearly always bilateral. Common causes are localized infection, foreign bodies, including irritation by contact lenses, allergic conditions and repeated undue exposure to bright light. Systemic diseases which may involve the conjunctiva are sarcoidosis (the lesions may then be nodular); tuberculosis, which typically causes chronic indolent ulcers; measles; Weil's disease; rickettsial infections, especially typhus, non-specific urethritis, and gonorrhoea (which has been spread from the urethra by the patient's fingers, when the disease is usually purulent and affects the tarsal as well as the bulbar conjunctiva, producing marked swelling of the lids). Trachoma (due to chlanydia trachomatis, which although some experts do not regard it as a true virus, is often referred to as the tric virus) is endemic in many tropical and subtropical countries, is localized to the eye and causes a progressive hypertrophy of the conjunctiva, spreading on to the cornea and causing blindness.

The Stevens–Johnson† syndrome is a condition characterized by severe conjunctivitis, urethritis, bullous lesions of the skin and mucous membranes, and occasionally an erythematous macular rash. Behçet, a Turkish dermatologist, in 1937 described a triad characterized by recurrent conjunctivitis (and sometimes iritis) and recurrent painful superficial ulcers of the mouth and genitalia which heal spontaneously after a few days. The condition is most often seen in young women, and the ulcers often have a definite time relationship to menstruation.

Oedema of the bulbar conjunctiva is called chemosis and may be (1) caused by severe infection, either localized to the conjunctiva or involving other eye structures; (2) due to interference with the conjunctival blood supply, for instance by a retro-orbital swelling of any kind or a cavernous sinus thrombosis, in which case chemosis is an early sign; (3) a complication of any marked exophthalmos, especially if it is associated with exophthalmoplegia; (4) rarely part of a generalized oedema, for example due to renal disease. The conjunctiva of the lower lid should always be inspected for pallor and the bulbar conjunctiva for icterus or marked injection as occurs with polycythaemia.

---

*Adolf Weil (1848–1916), a German physician.

†Albert Stevens (1884–1945) and F. C. Johnson (1894–1934) were American pediatricians.

The sclera

The sclerotics normally have a slight bluish tint in infancy, but a pronounced blueness is a feature of fragilitas ossium and is a very rare finding in rheumatoid arthritis and iron deficiency anaemia. The sclerotics are affected by jaundice but not by cyanosis. In phenylketonuria and also in alkaptonuria, there are often diffuse or localized areas of blackish pigmentation of the sclerotics. In alkaptonuria the pigmented area is usually semilunar in shape and situated roughly midway between the margin of the cornea and the inner and outer canthus. Involvement of the sclera may be seen in rheumatoid arthritis, in sarcoidosis, polyarteritis and temporal arteritis and in the first two conditions the lesions may be nodular, and sometimes with scleral oedema. Episcleritis is a lesion confined to the superficial layers of the sclera and it does not occur as a complication of any systemic disease and its cause is rarely ascertainable.

The cornea

In daylight the cornea is best examined by asking the patient to look towards a window and observing the image of the window in his cornea, or by moving a small light moving obliquely over the corneal surface. There should be no distortion or loss of clearness of that image. Small lesions of the cornea may not be visible except by fluorscein staining.

Keratitis means any lesion of the cornea, but some limit this term to inflammatory lesions. In acute or subacute keratitis there is injection of the corneal vessels, but in view of the fact that the cornea is a comparatively avascular structure this injection is usually confined to the corneal margin or circumcorneal vessels, and is only slight, producing what is often referred to as a salmon pink colour compared with the much brighter redness of conjunctival lesions. In severe cases ulceration occurs. With chronic keratitis, which is nearly always the result of previous subacute infection, the important finding is a clouding of the cornea, which loses its normal transparency and becomes opaque. The lesion may be confined to a small segment of the cornea. An important cause of bilateral keratitis is congenital syphilis, and because it involves the deeper layers of the cornea is labelled as an interstitial keratitis. The line of junction where the transparent cornea fuses with the sclera and conjunctiva is called the limbus.

In any lesion of the sensory part of the trigeminal nerve, but especially in lesions of the Gasserian ganglion (herpes zoster), a neurokeratitis may develop which is secondary to loss of corneal sensation, and resultant desquamation of the epithelium may render the cornea opaque. In herpes zoster ophthalmica, vesicles on the cornea are a rare additional hazard.

Vitamin A deficiency and also Sjögren's* syndrome may be associated with xerophthalmia (an abnormal dryness of the eye), and this may lead to keratitis and sometimes even to a complete disorganization and softening of the cornea (keratomalacia). Bitot's† spots are small triangular white foamy patches on the cornea; these are sometimes incorrectly regarded as a manifestation of vitamin A deficiency, but they are of no significance. In hepato-lenticular degeneration (Wilson's disease) brownish rings, due to deposition of copper granules, may be seen at the margin of the cornea (Kayser—Fleischer rings).‡

An arcus senilis consists of white rings, caused by intracellular and extracellular fat deposits, one to two millimetres wide and forming a partial or complete circle around the cornea just medial to the limbus, but separated from the sclera by a very narrow clear zone which is sharply defined on its peripheral side. The condition does not interfere with vision. It is seen in a large number of normal elderly people, but its presence in younger age groups is suggestive of premature ageing.

In any condition causing persistent hypercalcaemia there may be white or greyish-white dots, bands or flecks of opacification in the cornea which are usually confined to the nasal or temporal margin. In sarcoidosis this may be an early sign. In Fanconi's⊕ syndrome, an inherited defect of renal tubule absorption together with inherited defects of protein and amino acid metabolism, there is not only an excretion of cystine in the urine but also an accumulation of this substance in the tissues, and it may be deposited in the cornea. In gargoylism, intense clouding of the periphery of the cornea is common.

The uveal tract

The uveal tract consists of the iris and the ciliary body, which are anterior, and the choroid, which is posterior, and all these structures are normally pigmented. Each of them may be involved singly, but more often in combination. Choroiditis is described in more detail in Chapter 16.

---

*H. S. C. Sjögren (1899–   ), a Swedish ophthalmologist.
†Pierre Bitot (1822–88), a French surgeon.
‡S. A. Kinnear Wilson (1877–1937), a London neurologist. Bernhard Kayser (1869–1954), a German ophthalmologist, described the condition in 1902; Bruin Fleischer (1874–   ), a German ophthalmologist, described the same condition in 1903.
⊕Guido Fanconi (1892–   ), a Swiss paediatrician.

An acute iritis is characterized by dilatation of the blood vessels. It may become chronic, and an important result is then the development of adhesions between the iris and the lens (posterior synechiae) or between iris and cornea (anterior synechiae). With any iritis the delicate pattern of the iris, instead of being clear and sharply defined, becomes blurred and indistinct (muddy) and its colour alters – a fact which is especially noticeable in the blue-eyed. In severe cases white spots (keratitis precipitation) form in the centre of the pupil. Haziness of the iris must not be mistaken for keratitis. Any iritis affects the pupil: this is often small (unless it has been treated with mydriatics); it is irregular in at least a small part of its margin, and there is interference with its reaction both to light and to accommodation. The synechiae are best seen by focal illumination.

In many parts of the tropics a common cause of uveitis is the filarial worm, onchocerca.

Generalized diseases associated with iritis are syphilis, sarcoidosis, tuberculosis, ankylosing spondylitis, non-specific urethritis, rheumatoid arthritis and related conditions, toxoplasmosis and ulcerative colitis. In most of these conditions the iritis is usually a complication of a severe conjunctivitis which is the primary lesion. Uveitis affecting any or all parts of the tract occurs in the uveo-parotid syndrome. Both in diabetes and in gout there is an increased liability to infection of any part of the eye, and rarely this may involve the iris. However, the cause of an iritis is often unknown. In mongols the periphery of the iris is sometimes speckled with greyish-white spots arranged in concentric rings around the pupil but they are not pathagnomonic. A congenital defect of any part of the eye is known as a coloboma and the commonest site is the iris when it is usually inferior, whereas a similar appearance is caused by a surgical iridectomy but is then usually superiorly situated.

The lens

Cataract is opacification of the lens. This can more readily be seen by inserting a +10 or stronger lens in the ophthalmoscope. Lens opacities can be seen without instrumental aid only if large. When seen by oblique illumination, cataracts are greyish-white or yellowish, but as seen with an ophthalmoscope they are blackish. A large percentage of elderly people develop cataracts, fortunately often small, and probably they represent part of the ageing process. Diabetes is a common cause of cataracts in the elderly. Congenital cataracts are usually lamellar and anterior capsular and are generally due to malnutrition during intra-uterine life or early infancy. An associated defect of the tooth enamel is often a clue to this aetiology. Maternal rubella during early infancy is an important cause of

D

cataracts. Other causes of cataract are local injury, drugs (including steroids) and galactosaemia. Cataracts due to rickets, myotonia atrophica or hypoparathyroidism may develop at an early age but do not cause symptoms until adult life. In myotonia atrophica the cataracts are multiple, small and peripheral.

Congenital subluxation of the lens is a feature of Marfan's syndrome and may also be found in homocystinuria (in which other features of Marfan's syndrome may occur). It gives rise to an easily visible tremulousness of the iris.

The vitreous

Haemorrhages into the vitreous may occur with local injury, blood diseases, diabetes and hypertension. Large haemorrhages in the retina if there is a defect in the hyaloid membrane may spread into the vitreous. Recurrent spontaneous haemorrhages into vitreous of unknown aetiology do occur.

10 The Neck

Whenever possible the neck should be examined in a good light striking the neck obliquely and the patient sitting upright.

Congenital lesions

An abnormally short neck is a fairly common congenital abnormality, but it cannot be correlated with any one specific type of the many cranio-vertebral anomalies. Klippel and Feil in 1912* described a syndrome characterized by a congenital abnormality of the cervical spine and rarely also of the upper dorsal spine, some vertebrae being fused or of an abnormal shape. This syndrome produces a very short neck with limitation of its movements and often an abnormal tilting of the head. Rarely it may be associated with compression of the spinal cord and, even more rarely, with a foramen magnum syndrome (identical with that seen in the Arnold–Chiari† deformity) characterized by bilateral lower motor neurone lesions of the last four cranial nerves and upper motor neurone lesions of all four limbs.

Webbing of the neck is due to either a fan-like fold of skin extending from shoulder to neck or an abnormal splaying out of the trapezius, and is a congenital anomaly. It may form part of Turner's‡ syndrome, a condition seen in females which is characterized by webbing of the neck, infantilism and dwarfism and is due to absence of one of the X sex chromosomes. Other congenital abnormalities added since the original description are often present involving the external genitalia; the limbs (arachnodactyly, polydactyly or cubitus valgus); the heart (usually an anomaly of the aorta); or the chest (abnormally broad in comparison with the patient's height, with the nipples very wide apart).

*Maurice Klippel (1858–1942) and André Feil (1884–   ), French neurologists.
†Julius Arnold (1835–1915) and Hans Chiari (1851–1916), German pathologists, described the condition in 1891.
‡H. H. Turner (1892–   ), an American endocrinologist, described the condition in 1938.

Swellings

The following remarks, although dealing specifically with swellings of the neck, are equally applicable to any swelling wherever found in whatever part of the body. The discovery of a swelling is one of the commonest and one of the most important signs in clinical medicine. A swelling having been found, it is imperative that a logical technique be used both in eliciting the details of the swelling and later in discussion of its likely cause. Wild guessing must be scrupulously avoided.

The first stage diagnosis must always be the determination with as great an accuracy as possible of the anatomy of the swelling – that is, which tissue it involves. Only after having determined this should the clinician proceed to the second stage diagnosis, which is the general pathology (inflammatory, neoplastic, etcetera). The special features which must be elicited in the case of any swelling are:

1. Its size.
2. Its shape.
3. Involvement of the overlying skin by any acute inflammatory process; by a sinus (common in tuberculosis and actinomycosis); by peau d'orange (a wrinkling and pitting of the skin making it look like a Jaffa orange, indicating lymphatic obstruction); or by collateral veins or telangiectasia.
4. Tenderness.
5. Motility.
6. The consistency of the swelling, especially whether it is smooth or irregular or lobulated and its degree of softness or hardness.
7. Its margin, whether well or ill defined.
8. Fluctuation, which must be sought for in two planes.
9. Occasionally transillumination, for example in differentiating a hydrocele from a solid testicular tumour.
10. Whether a bruit is audible over the swelling.

These findings help to differentiate the type of pathology of the swelling: for example, whether it is more likely to be inflammatory or neoplastic and, if the latter, whether benign or malignant. But such differentiation cannot always be made with certainty, because chronic inflammatory swellings may be as hard and as nodular and as fixed as any malignant growth.

The third stage diagnosis is the special pathology. This can only rarely be made clinically with certainty, histology being usually necessary. Many swellings are like attractive girls, you do not know their true nature until you take them out, and even then you may not be certain.

Lack of method in discussing a diagnosis is often due to misconceptions as to the meaning of this word. An attempt will be made in each of the sections of this book to point out and emphasize that diagnosis is always a matter of stages; that in the majority of cases it is only a stage 1 diagnosis, the anatomical, which can be made with any certainty on clinical examination; that any discussion of the diagnosis attempting to carry it beyond this stage must be prefaced by phrases such as 'may be'; and that probabilities must always be considered before possibilities.

ENLARGED LYMPH NODES

Enlargement of cervical lymph nodes should always be sought with the examiner standing just in front of and later behind the sitting patient. It is better to use a slow and gentle sliding or rotatory motion of the palmar aspect of the finger tips rather than heavy pressure. When feeling for enlarged cervical lymph nodes the free hand is used to control the patient's head. The sternomastoids divide the neck into anterior and posterior triangles. It is essential to be methodical and have a definite fixed order for palpation of each of the individual groups of nodes – the occipital, the post- and pre-auricular, the submandibular, the submental, the anterior triangles and posterior triangles (both superficial and deep), and the supraclavicular. When one is feeling for enlarged glands from behind, the patient's head should be flexed forward and both sides of the neck felt simultaneously. In feeling for the submandibular glands the head should be flexed laterally, but not rotated, to the side being palpated. The lateral aspect is often best felt by tilting the patient's head towards the same side. Feeling for supraclavicular nodes in the scalene triangle just above the clavicle should include hooking a finger around the tendonous part of the sternomastoid.

If enlarged nodes are found, their size, consistency, if fluctuant, or if tender, their motility, whether they are discrete or matted together, and whether or not they are attached to the skin and/or other structures, should all be determined. If any enlarged nodes are found in the neck, then the area of their lymphatic drainage must be carefully explored, and search made for other enlarged nodes in the axillae, epitrochlar and inguinal regions.

BRANCHIAL CYST

A branchial cyst is a congenital anomaly due to a persistent branchial cleft. It causes a circumscribed cystic swelling (which feels like palpating a half-filled hot water bottle) along the anterior border of the sternomastoid anywhere between the angle of the jaw and the suprasternal notch, but nearly always situated in the upper third of the neck. Most of the swelling is deep to the sternomastoid but projects beyond its anterior border. In the region of the margin of the sternomastoid a small dimple in the skin may be visible.

THYROGLOSSAL CYST

A thyroglossal cyst is a midline swelling due to persistence of the foetal thyroglossal duct and is situated between the hyoid and the suprasternal notch. Its other distinguishing feature is that it moves on protrusion of the tongue.

CAROTID BODY TUMOUR

A rare swelling of the neck seen in middle-aged or elderly people is a carotid body tumour which arises from chemo-receptor tissues and is situated in the region of the bifurcation of the carotid. It is potato-shaped, is movable horizontally but not vertically, and often exhibits well marked transmitted pulsation. Its importance to the physician is that it may cause spontaneous attacks of syncope, which may also be produced by pressure on the swelling.

THYROID ENLARGEMENT

There are only two endocrine glands which can be inspected and palpated readily, the testes and the thyroid. The latter is normally not visible except very rarely in very thin people, and in them such a swelling is localized to the region of the isthmus just below the cricoid cartilage. A thyroid swelling (goitre) is the commonest midline swelling in the neck. Most thyroid enlargements are readily visible, but hyperextension of the head may render such a swelling discernible even though it was not so previously. Any thyroid swelling can be more readily seen if the patient is asked to swallow. Many people can easily swallow their own saliva, but if they cannot they should be given a glass of water. If a swelling in the neck does not transiently glide upwards on deglutition, then either it is not a thyroid swelling or, if it is, it must be very large or due to a chronic thyroiditis or malignancy. Recognition of a thyroid swelling may be difficult in short-necked people and in children.

Thyroid palpation must always be gentle because digital pressure will otherwise cause coughing or a sensation of choking. The thyroid must be palpated with the patient sitting with his head slightly flexed and with the examiner standing at first in front and later behind the patient, as each procedure may give additional information. The thyroid must also be palpated while the patient is swallowing. If it is impossible to feel the lower border of the swelling, then evidence must be sought for retrosternal extension. It is very rare for any thyroid enlargement to be completely confined to the mediastinum with no swelling palpable in the neck.

Sometimes it is possible to determine the details of a thyroid swelling by palpation with the palm and fingers of one hand. But it is often possible to displace each sternomastoid in turn and at the same time to insert the finger tips deeply behind the muscle and so feel the lateral aspect of each thyroid lobe with the head slightly tilted to the side being examined. However, the consistency and the more exact limits of the swelling are often better determined by grasping the thyroid between a finger and the thumb of one hand while each upper lobe is displaced in turn from behind the sterno-mastoid by the fingers of the other hand, the manoeuvre being repeated on each side.

The pyramidal lobe is an upward finger-like projection from above the isthmus and may be enlarged either alone or together with other parts of the gland. The cricoid cartilage is sometimes very prominent in thin-necked people and must not be mistaken for an enlargement of the thyroid isthmus.

Palpation of any thyroid swelling should determine its borders; its size; which lobe or lobes are affected; tenderness; consistency, and whether or not this is uniform throughout the gland; whether the swelling is nodular (single or multiple), and whether it is irregular or smooth. The consistency and discreteness of each nodule must be carefully assessed. All these features will give clues to the likely pathology of the enlargement.

A solitary nodule of the thyroid may be a colloid nodule, a cyst, or a benign or malignant tumour. By palpation alone the differen-tiation between these is occasionally very difficult or even impossible. Any thyroid enlargement may, because it is huge or malignant or partially retrosternal, cause compression of the trachea, the superior vena cava or the recurrent laryngeal nerve, with appropriate symp-toms and signs which are described in another chapter. The trachea is not displaced laterally unless the enlargement of the lateral lobes is grossly asymmetrical. The trachea may be compressed, especially by a retrosternal goitre, from side to side, producing the 'scabbard trachea' with the principal axis of the ellipse antero-posterior and therefore better recognized on a postero-anterior than on a lateral chest X-ray.

Disfigurement, dyspnoea, dysphonia and dysphagia, in this order, are probable symptoms of any large simple parenchymatous (colloid) goitre. But this order is likely to be completely reversed if the lesion is malignant, and the dysphagia in these cases is due to enlarged lymph nodes in the neck or the superior mediastinum and not to pressure by the thyroid itself. Malignancy of the thyroid is nearly always confined to one lobe. Patients with malignant thyroids are usually euthyroid but may be thyrotoxic but never myxoedematous unless the result of therapy.

Chronic thyroiditis is nearly always of the Hashimoto* type and generally starts in the forties producing a large, very firm and fixed thyroid swelling which may have a bossy surface. Histologically it is characterized by a marked lymphoid infiltration with fibrosis as a

*H. Hashimoto (1881–   ), a Japanese surgeon.

secondary and lesser phenomenon. The sufferers are often myx-oedematous but may be euthyroid but never thyrotoxic. It is regarded as an auto-immune disease. Riedel's* chronic thyroiditis is a very rare condition seen usually in youngish females and produces identical clinical signs with the Hashimoto variety. Its distinction is histological, showing a very marked fibrosis and but little lymphoid infiltration.

Subacute thyroiditis is always an inflammatory lesion often complicating an acute infection such as mumps. A painful thyroid swelling with signs of mild thyrotoxicosis develop and both are transitory.

Percussion of the thyroid is useful only as a possible guide to retrosternal extension and should be performed with the neck fully flexed forwards. It is rarely a helpful sign. A systolic bruit over the gland is very good evidence of marked vascularity and so, indirectly, of thyrotoxicosis.

Other conditions

Any arthritis of the cervical spine causes limitation of some neck movements and often spasm of neck muscles. Limitation of all or any of the neck movement may be due not only to arthritis but also to meningitis or meningeal irritation or spasm of the neck muscles secondary to any neck lesion especially if inflammatory.

Spasmodic torticollis is a unilateral spasm of the sternomastoid causing an involuntary turning of the head away from, but a tilting towards, the affected side.

Distension and pulsation of the neck veins and arteries are dealt with in Chapter 14. Involuntary movements of the head, wasting of the neck muscles and meningismus are discussed in Chapter 16.

---

*Bernhard Riedel (1846—1916), a German surgeon, described the condition in 1896.

11 Dermatology

Every physician should have a sound knowledge of dermatology. Unfortunately far too many physicians, because of their inability to recognize common skin conditions, react to their own ignorance by an almost complete apathy and lack of interest in the subject causing them to lapse into the bad habit of either completely ignoring skin lesions or leaving their diagnosis entirely to specialists. An interest in dermatology can make a very significant contribution to the doctor's training in correct observations.

The reader may well ask, 'What is a skin disease?' The reply should be, 'Any skin lesion, including such conditions as purpura, herpes zoster, scleroderma and jaundice', because by such a conception the doctor will better appreciate the breadth and importance of dermatology. In fact probably only a minority of skin lesions are of purely dermatological interest and of no concern to the general physician. Many diseases have cutaneous manifestations. Conversely a wide knowledge of general medicine is essential for a good dermatologist and should be more important to him than an understanding of auto-immune factors and immuno-fluorescent investigations. 'Nature is neither husk nor kernel but all is one.'

There are two principle ways, not necessarily mutually exclusive, of describing skin conditions. The first, which is recommended for the general physician, is in purely descriptive terms as recognized on inspection and palpation. The second method is in terms of histopathology and although this is the more scientific approach it is outside the scope of this elementary account.

Always use orthodox and simple words and terms in your descriptions, avoiding the common error of the tyro who either attempts to be smart and diagnoses a condition with which he is completely unfamiliar or uses tautological or waffling terms such as 'skin rash' as though such phrases constituted a serious contribution to diagnosis. The word 'dermatitis' without a qualifying adjective is a controversial one variously used to mean any skin lesion, or an inflammatory skin lesion as opposed to a dermatosis (which etymologically is a very peculiar word), or eczema. So it is far better not to use the word except preceded by an adjective such as 'contact' or 'morbilliform' etcetera.

A history should include the duration of the rash, the site where it was first noticed, how it has developed, whether itchy, aggravating and relieving factors (including sunlight), the nature of any treatment for it which he has had and its effect, and the names of any other drugs which he has had (including any used locally) during the past six months, occupation, previous skin lesions, and any family history of skin disease.

The patient should be examined in a good light, preferably not artificial because this interferes with colour appreciation. Whenever feasible the whole body must be inspected even if the patient complains of only a localized lesion.

Descriptive pattern

Descriptive dermatology has for many decades followed a fixed pattern to which all non-specialists should adhere rigidly including the precise order of the headings: colour, morphology, sites and secondary phenomena. Only the briefest outlines are discussed here.

COLOUR

Colour can be described in ordinary English words such as red, bluish etcetera, or by Latin and Greek terms such as erythematous, or by romance descriptions such as ham-coloured. This possible three-pronged method of description also applies to the morphological features which are discussed later but the use of ordinary English words should always be preferred.

MORPHOLOGY

By morphology is meant whether the lesions are macular, papular or vesicular or any combination of these, and their shape and size.

Macules

Macules are lesions which are not raised above or depressed below the skin surface and are like stains on a white cloth. Apart from colour, size and shape it should be noted if the lesions are discrete (well defined) or ill defined (blotchy), often due to confluence of lesions.

Papules

Papules are solid raised lesions and their colour, size (which may vary from small and called miliary, to large and called nodules) and shape (which may be pointed, flat-topped, branching, or large and flat plaques) should be noted. Skin nodules are discussed later.

Vesicles

Vesicles (blisters) are raised lesions containing fluid. Their colour, size and shape must be described, and they are also subdivided according to the contents. Large vesicles are called bullae, and when huge 'hydroa', as for example in the skin lesion known as hydroa aestivale, which may be seen in congenital porphyria (aestivale meaning appertaining to summer). Pustules are vesicles containing pus and the term haemorrhagic vesicles is self-explanatory. The majority of vesicles start as such but occasionally are produced by breakdown because of infection of pre-existing papules.

The commonest cause of bullae is either burns or scalds but the conditions in which they occur of special interest to the general physician are:

1. Conditions in which light sensitivity occurs including albinism, pellagra, the various porphyrias, and drugs (especially barbiturates, phenothiazines and the sulpha group including the oral anti-diabetic agents). It is often stated that lupus erythematosus and pemphigus vulgaris are examples of light sensitivity, but although sunlight exacerbates these conditions it does not play a role in their aetiology.
2. Stevens–Johnson syndrome, which has been described previously, is a condition characterized by bullae of skin and mucous membranes, conjunctivitis which is often severe and associated with oedema of the eyelids and urethritis. Sometimes red macular lesions which are widespread may be the dominant skin lesion and the bullae few. All the cases described originally were in male children but it is now known that the condition can occur in either sex at any age. Sulpha and cytoxic drugs and irradiation may cause identical lesions. The syndrome is sometimes called erythema multiforme exudativum or bullosa.
3. Pemphigus vulgaris and its variant pemphigus foliaceus (which is associated with widespread desquamation) is characterized by bullae of skin and mucous membranes, the bullae exhibiting a specific histology. The mucosae are involved early and may be initially. It is seen mainly in the middle-aged, and a distinctive feature is that at any one time bullae which are fully distended and others which are flaccid and with little fluid in them are present.
4. Eczema, especially in its acute phases, causes vesicles which may be large especially when due to chemical contact (discussed later).
5. Herpes zoster and herpes simplex.
6. In impetigo the dominant lesion may be bullae.

SITES OF LESIONS

The sites of lesions is of great importance as similar lesions may be produced by different diseases, the main differentiating feature being the different sites of election. It is for this reason that the physician should be reluctant to make a final diagnosis until he has inspected the patient's whole body.

SECONDARY PHENOMENA

Secondary phenomena include desquamation, crusting, lichenification, hyperkeratosis, ulceration, scars, and teleangiectasia.

Desquamation

Desquamation is a shedding of the horny layer of the skin and the resultant scales may be fine and powdery or large and flakey and they may be sticky and adherent or easily removed. Desquamation is a very common feature of skin diseases especially the non-infective varieties. Ichthyosis (fish skin) may be a feature of several skin lesions but can be the sole disturbance involving the greater part of the body and is then usually genetically determined and the large scales are dry as is the whole of the skin.

Crusts

Crusts (scabs) occur when serous, purulent or haemorrhagic exudate derived from ruptured vesicles dries on the skin surface. They are a commonly seen feature in impetigo and in eczema.

Lichenification

Lichenification is characterized by thickening of the skin and marked increase in the normal skin markings so that it comes to resemble the bark of a tree or coarsely grained leather. It is a constant feature of chronic eczema but it may also occur with many chronic skin diseases.

Hyperkeratosis

Hyperkeratosis (cornification) is due to an increase in the horny layer (stratum corneum) producing papules which may be only very slightly raised and appear to be macular, but their papular nature can be felt, the skin feeling roughened like velvet as compared with silk. On the other hand the lesions may be large and markedly raised, looking limpet-like. Hyperkeratosis is often associated with lichenification of the same area but it must be emphasized that these are two separate features.

The commonest cause of hyperkeratosis of the soles in some parts of the world is the habit of walking barefoot. Blackish or dark brown hyperkeratosis of the palms and soles may be due to chronic inorganic arsenical poisoning. Keratoderma (or hyperkeratosis) blenorrhagica is a condition in which large areas of blackish or dark brown hyperkeratosis occur on the palms and soles. The lesions are often markedly raised and the commonest cause used to be gonorrhoea (blenorrhoea is the French word for gonorrhoea) but nowadays non-specific urethritis is the commonest aetiology. Psoriasis only occasionally affects the palms and soles and when it does so the resultant lesions are atypical resembling keratoderma blenorrhagica and then is usually called pustular psoriasis. When typical psoriform lesions occur on the palms and soles the diagnosis of secondary syphilis should always be considered. Hyperkeratosis of the palms and soles is occasionally a genetically determined condition and is then sometimes called tylosis. On but scant evidence it has been reported and often quoted that this condition is associated with a liability to cancer of the oesophagus, which information should never even be hinted at to the patient because no prophylactic action is possible.

With vitamin A deficiency in adults but not in children greyish or blackish papules develop around the hair follicles of the limbs and the papules have keratotic plugs which separate leaving pits. The affected areas are itchy, dry and scaly. The fully developed picture is called phrynoderma (toad skin).

A common cause of brownish hyperkeratotic papules which are often branched and multiple are viral warts. They most often occur on the back of the hands and fingers, soles of feet and around anus and genitalia. In the last two sites they resemble condylomata of secondary syphilis (described later).

Seborrhoeic warts, often called senile warts, are benign neoplasms, being basal cell papilloma, and are seen only in the elderly, especially on the face and trunk. They may form plaques. They are always surrounded by similar but much smaller lesions and this fact may be an important diagnostic clue. Another special feature is that their surface feels greasy. They are of no significance except cosmetically.

Ulceration

Ulceration of skin should always be described in full detail with reference to numbers, size, shape, margin, edge (wall), base (crater), and the condition of the surrounding skin. The shape is usually circular or elliptical but is occasionally serpiginous (snake-shaped) with healing in some parts and extension in others. The margin if everted and raised above the normal skin surface is strongly suspicious of malignancy. The edge may be sloping towards the base or be undermined or vertical (punched out) as shown in the diagrams.

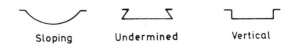

Sloping   Undermined   Vertical

Most skin ulcers have sloping edges. Undermined edges are typical of tuberculous ulcers but may occasionally be seen as a result of bed sores. Punched out ulcers are typical of tertiary syphilis. The base is often covered with a crust which when removed usually shows pinkish granulation tissue. In syphilitic ulceration the base is covered with a dirty yellowish slough. The surrounding skin may be pigmented, hyperkeratotic and lichenified in chronic lesions, and in acute lesions red macules with vesicles are likely. With infection with pseudomonas pyocyaneus the surrounding skin contains greenish pustules.

Scars

Scars are nearly always the result of healed previous ulceration or pustular lesions. Scars have little or no pigment, hair or elastic tissue, whatever their cause. Some scars have special features which may be an indication of their cause. The scars of a previous herpes zoster are segmental and unilateral. The scars of healed syphilitic gumma are thin and soft (cigarette or tissue paper). The scars seen especially over the patellae in pseudo-xanthoma elasticum may also be of this type. The scars of lupus vulgaris are often deep and cause gross tissue distortions such as ectropion. Irradiation scars are always surrounded by teleangectases. The scars associated with sinuses, especially tuberculous and actinomycotic, are deep and puckered, irrespective of healing. Anaesthetic scars should suggest the possibility of leprosy.

Teleangiectasia

A teleangiectasis is a cluster of dilated capillaries and venules. They may or may not be raised and if large enough it may be possible to demonstrate the sign of emptying. (If the centre of the lesion is compressed, preferably with a glass slide, it will be seen to blanch.) They are a common feature with liver disease and then occur on the face and chest, but never below the chest. Hereditary teleangiectasia of skin and mucous membranes is described in the chapter on alimentary diseases. Teleangiectases are however a common secondary phenomenon in many skin diseases and may then be marked and readily mistaken for the primary lesion. Some commonly seen examples of this are with lesions due to excessive sunlight or light sensitivity; irradiation; scleroderma (including the localized form); dermatomyositis (especially around the nail skin margin); lupus erythematosus (when it may not only surround the local lesions but also occurs on the palmer aspect of the digits); acne rosacea; lupus pernio; polycythaemia (especially on face and digits); and necrobiosis lipoidica (described in next chapter).

History and symptoms

SKIN NODULES

Nodules are large papules but the differentiation is arbitrary. Nodules are often present in addition to other skin lesions but an important consideration for a general physician is the occurrence of skin nodules without any other skin lesion. The conditions to discuss and consider are:

1. *Secondaries from the bronchus.* Secondaries in the skin and subcutaneous tissues are common immediately over a primary site such as the breast and also in the abdominal skin, especially in a scar following surgery or exploration of an intra-abdominal malignancy, but these are examples of local spread. The colour of skin metastases is variable but they are always, at least initially, very firm. Subsequent ulceration is common.

   A special consideration is melanomatosis because in this condition skin secondaries are common. The clue is their colour which is slate colour, dark brown or black. The primary sites causing the skin metastases are choroid of eye, subungual, gastro-intestinal (especially rectum) and skin. Primary melanoma malignum may arise in an adult in a melanocytic naevus (mole) which has been present since infancy or childhood and should be suspected by the development of itching, darkening colour, bleeding, rapid increase in size, new satellite lesions or enlargement of the local lymph nodes. However the primary melanoma malignum of the skin may start in previously normal skin.

2. *Reticuloses,* especially lymphadenoma and lymphatic leukaemia. Such nodules are always itchy and the pruritus may precede the skin involvement. They may occur anywhere on the body but have a predilection for the abdomen. They commonly ulcerate and there may also be purpuric lesions in the vicinity.

3. *Chronic inflammatory lesions* such as tuberculosis, syphilis (tertiary), leprosy, sarcoid, leishmaniasis and other tropical diseases. Chronic inflammatory nodules often ulcerate.

4. A special consideration is when the nodules are confined to the region of bony prominences and tendons and then they can be usefully subdivided into two groups (*a*) those associated with arthritis, namely rheumatoid, rheumatic fever (only in young people with heart involvement), osteoarthritis and gout, (*b*) those occurring independently of arthritis. The two most important conditions in the latter group are xanthomata (cholesterol deposits) and calcinois (calcium phosphate deposits). Xanthoma nodules when large are called xanthoma

tuberosum (like potatoes). Plaque lesions are common especially on the trunk. Xanthoma are nearly always very easy to recognize because of their colour, which may be of any shade of yellow from lemon, to reddish yellow or yellowish brown. The great majority of patients with xanthomas have a normal blood cholesterol. It is unusual for any of these nodules to ulcerate. Xanthoma of the eyelids are known as xantholasma.

Calcinotic nodules can be readily recognized because of their whitish colour and this will be obvious if the nodules ulcerate which is a commonly occurring feature. In many cases there are widespread nodules but the patients are not hypercalcaemic and there is no evidence of any disturbance of calcium metabolism. Calcinotic nodules, nearly always confined to the hands, may be seen with scleroderma and then an additional feature, Raynaud phenomenon, is often present. Theoretically any patient with persistent hypercalcaemia may have calcinosis but actually this is most unusual.

Adenoma sebaceum (epiloia)

Adenoma sebaceum is a genetically determined condition characterized by nodules which are confined to the cheeks, nose and chin. In fact the lesions do not arise from sebaceous glands but are vascular fibromata (sometimes described as example of hamartoma). The initial lesions are small red papules which slowly increase in size become confluent and produce huge nodules (tuberose). In a minority of cases darkish brown roughened plaques are present on the trunk, usually in the lumbar region. This is called the shagreen (shark) patch. The most interesting feature of this disease is that most of the patients also have widespread benign tumours which are all primaries. These may be subungual fibromata, rhabdomyomata, renal adenomas, phakomata (whitish plaque lesions arising from retinal neuroglia), and multiple small benign brain gliomata or localized areas of dense glial proliferation and these lesions may cause mental retardation and epilepsy. This association of skin and brain lesions was first described by Bournville in 1880 and the combination is sometimes called tuberose sclerosis but others use this term as a synonym with adenoma sebaceum. Cerebral calcification may be seen radiologically. Chest symptoms are unusual but some of these patients have bilateral ring shadows on a chest X-ray which presumably are due to bronchial dilatations, but the mechanism of this is disputed.

Neurofibromatosis (von Recklinghausen disease)

In neurofibromatosis nodules are never the sole skin lesion. Neurofibromatosis is a genetically determined condition characterized by pleomorphic skin lesions (macules, papules and nodules) and café au lait zones which are well defined light brown macular lesions which are present in 100 per cent of cases. The oft-quoted opinion that there must be at least six of these café au lait lesions and that they must be more than 1.5 cm to be of diagnostic value is absurd. Initially the macules and papules are red but gradually become flesh coloured. The nodules may become huge and may be sessile or pedunculated. Their number varies from very few to literally hundreds, and they may occur anywhere over the body. Ulceration and malignant change rarely occur. Many of the patients also have lentigo, which are lesions looking identical with freckles but are not affected by sunlight. When the nodules occur along the course of a superficially situated peripheral nerve their nature should be obvious and such lesions may cause sensory, lower motor neurone or mixed findings, their exact nature depending on the nerves affected. But often the nodules do not appear clinically to have any association with nerves but they are in fact also neurofibromata from sensory nerve endings and this variety of the condition is sometimes called molluscum fibrosum.

Neurofibromatosis is often associated with congenital anomalies of the thoracic cage (including spine) and limbs. Apart from involvement of any peripheral nerve, including components of any of the nerve plexuses, any cranial nerve, but especially the eighth, may be affected. An important association is that of neurofibromatosis and pheochomocytoma of the suprarenal.

PORTMANTEAU WORDS

A common and useful practice is to convert a noun which represents a dermatological clinical entity into an adjective which is merely an abbreviated way of describing the important features of that disease and such words also form the basis of the differential diagnosis of that particular clinical entity. Put in another way, the difference between the noun and the adjective and therefore between the disease and its mimics can be more dramatically expressed by the analogy which distinguishes between a mess of blood and a bloody mess. Such commonly used words are morbilliform psoriaform, impetiginous, pemphigoid and eczematous.

Morbilliform

The basic lesion of morbilli (measles) are brownish red large blotchy confluent ill-defined macules mainly on the face, neck and trunk. But if a patient had a similar rash confined to or mainly on his limbs, and excluding non-dermatological associated findings, the condition is unlikely to be measles but very likely to be due to drug toxicity, this being one of the commonest types of drug rashes.

Psoriaform

Psoriasis is a condition of unknown aetiology characterized by red flat papules with silvery scales involving the extensor aspects of limbs, the scalp and trunk. Psoriaform means identical lesions which are not due to psoriasis. For example, typical psoriaform lesions on the soles and palms are more likely to be due to secondary syphilis than to psoriasis. In psoriasis the lesions may be very small or form large confluent bizarre-shaped lesions especially on the trunk. In the scalp the unaffected areas, unlike in seborrhoeic dermatitis which commonly affects the scalp, are completely normal. Psoriaform involvement of joints and nails are discussed in a later chapter.

Impetiginous

Impetigo contagiosa is a condition affecting mainly the younger age groups and is characterized by pustular lesions and honey coloured sticky crusts and is due to a staphylococcal and occasionally a streptococcal infection. Impetiginous lesions are commonly seen in eczema, herpes simplex and herpes zoster.

Acneiform

Acneiform indicates any lesion in which small pointed papules dominate. Acne vulgaris is a condition characterized by small reddish pointed papules and pustules together with comedoes (blackheads) and a seborrhoeic condition of the surrounding skin. The lesions are mainly on the face, neck and trunk. Similar lesions, often of identical distribution, may be a feature of intoxication with bromides, iodides and steroids. In those conditions comedoes are unusual and seborrhoea is often absent. In Cushing syndrome the skin often exhibits an identical rash.

Acne rosacea is characterized by reddish discoloration and small red papules and pustules on the nose, cheeks and occasionally the chin and forehead, but never other parts of the body. Teleangiectases are always present and often they are a prominent feature. At least initially it represents an excessive and usually persistent vasomotor reaction (flushing) in response to emotion, gastric irritants (including alcohol) and changes of external temperature. The involvement of the nose may be very marked and it becomes thickened, bulbous and fleshy with visible prominence of the follicular orifices and is then called 'rhinophyma'. The importance of acne rosacea to the general physician is that although only a minority are due to excessive alcohol its presence should always make him consider this as a cause of either liver disease or peripheral neuritis.

Pemphigoid

Pemphigus vulgaris has been described previously. Pemphigoid is a term usually used to mean bullous eruptions of skin and mucous membranes from any cause. Some dermatologists confusingly use the term as a noun and in a very limited way to indicate a clinical entity in which identical lesions occur but of unknown aetiology and not fitting into a described pattern and lacking the specific histology of pemphigus vulgaris.

Specific conditions

ECZEMA

Acute eczema is characterized by bright red macular blotchy ill-defined large areas on which papules and vesicles develop. Later as the lesion become subacute and chronic the vesicles develop in one of two alternative ways. (a) They ooze their fluid and become crusted (impetiginous) and may become pustular; this is often described as 'wet eczema'. (b) The vesicles dry up with the production of the secondary phenomena of hyperkeratosis, lichenification, desquamation and often extensive areas of brownish pigmentation; this is 'dry eczema' and will obviously have an entirely different appearance from either acute or 'wet eczema'. This differentiation into wet and dry depends largely on the site of the area affected. If it occurs on areas normally associated with sweating such as groins and axillae then the lesions are likely to be 'wet'. Eczema is always itchy and the pruritus may precede the skin lesions and is then sometimes called 'neurodermatitis'.

Apart from classifying eczema into acute and chronic, or 'wet' and 'dry', other differentiations used are infantile and adult, allergic and non-allergic, or exogenous and endogenous.

Infantile eczema is common both in infancy and childhood and involves especially the face, neck and limb flexures. It is usually (probably always) allergic and hence is often referred to as eczema or allergic eczema. The evidence for this is very strong:

1. There is often a family history of an acknowledged allergic condition especially asthma or hay fever.
2. The child often later himself develops hay fever or asthma and then the usual sequence of events is that as the child grows older the eczema spontaneously improves but asthma or hay fever develops and gradually gets worse.
3. There is often a single known allergen which is usually a food.

In adults the evidence for any typical eczematous lesion being allergic is often poor. Two closely related problems with regard to eczematous lesions in adults are: Must the condition be definitely allergic before it is called eczema? What is the definition of allergy? The latter point is discussed in Chapter 3.

Some attempt to avoid the quibbling engendered by the word eczema and avoid it when dealing with rashes in adults. It is claimed that immunoglobin studies give the answer, true eczema being then defined as a genetic tendency to produce IgE globulins (reaginic antibodies). Some call this group of conditions 'atopic dermatitis', a term which was coined in 1923 and literally means 'strange or out of place'. Unfortunately its author used the terms allergy and hypersensitivity as synonyms.

A common cause of eczematous lesions in adults (? true eczema) is due to contact with various chemicals, including many used industrially, in the home, cosmetically and in dermatological therapy. In most of these cases the skin reaction represents a toxic or hypersensitivity phenomenon and not allergy. Some prefer to call these group examples of contact dermatitis, or name the offending chemical and add the word dermatitis.

Fungus infections cause eczematous lesions and whilst these are commonest in the groin and feet the true nature is often missed when they occur on other parts. In children but not in adults fungal infections of the scalp are common. Fungus infections very rarely involve the face primarily.

Over the lower half of the legs especially in those with either varicose veins or chronic pitting oedema eczematous lesions with ulceration and hyperpigmentation are common.

EXFOLIATIVE DERMATITIS

Exfoliative dermatitis is a condition characterized by a widespread redness of the skin together with desquamation and often also with oedema of the skin and vesicles. Its causes which are of interest to the general physician are:

1. Severe cases of light sensitivity which has been discussed previously (see bullae).
2. Chemicals: (*a*) by injection, such as arsenic and gold, and (rarely) antibiotics; (*b*) given orally; this is rare except with those drugs previously mentioned which may be associated with light sensitivity reaction; (*c*) used locally on the skin; this applies especially to keratolytic agents such as tar, dithranol, salicylates, etcetera.
3. Lymphadenoma: in this condition the skin lesion may precede the other manifestations of the disease.
4. Leukaemia; the same applies as to lymphadenoma.
5. Generalized skin diseases such as psoriasis, eczema etcetera, but in these cases the exfoliative dermatitis is often iatrogenic being caused by over-enthusiastic use of keratolytic agents to remove the scales, or ultraviolet light therapy.

SKIN LESIONS IN LYMPHADENOMA AND LEUKAEMIA

The following skin lesions may complicate or be the presenting feature of either lymphadenoma or leukaemia. Pallor, jaundice (nearly always obstructive and due to lymph nodes in portal fissure but may rarely be haemolytic), exfoliative dermatitis, purpura, nodules, urticuria and a mild non-genetically determined form of ichthyosis. Any of these lesions may be aggravated by alcohol and, apart from pallor or jaundice, are always itchy, and the itching may precede any other manifestations.

MYOCOSIS FUNGOIDES

Myocosis fungoides was first described by Alibert* in 1806 long before pathogenic fungi were recognized and the name was given from the derivation of 'fungoides' meaning 'mushroom'. It is seen mainly in the fifth and sixth decades and is characterized by reddish brown, purplish or plum coloured scaly well-defined plaque lesions often of bizarre shapes and occurring most often in the scapular regions or buttocks and very itchy. As they develop the lesions become more and more nodular and ulcerate.

The typical plaque lesions may be preceded by premycotic lesions which may be eczematous, psoriaform or seborrhoeic and the clue to their real nature may be an unusual site or itchiness of a psoriaform lesion. However, the premycotic label is often made by hindsight after the typical lesions of mycosis fungoides have developed. Although histologically because of infiltration with lymphocytes, plasma cells, eosinophils and abnormal histiocytes mycosis fungoides bears some resemblance to either lymphatic leukaemia or lymphadenoma but the consensus of opinion is that the disease is a separate entity.

PRURITUS

Pruritus is itching and this provokes a strong desire to scratch which in itself is a peculiar mixture of pain and pleasure. In some skin lesions any secondary phenomena may be the result of scratching. About 50 per cent of all skin diseases are itchy, notable exceptions being psoriasis and secondary syphilis. Apart from those dermatological disease entities pruritus may be caused by the following: urticuria, exfoliative dermatitis, lymphadenoma, leukaemia, obstructive jaundice from any cause (the itching may precede the jaundice), uraemia, polycythaemia vera, neurosis, 'senile' (seen in elderly people for no apparent cause and often considered to be entirely psychogenic), psychoses (melancholic psychotics spend much of their time scratching), and miliaris (prickly heat). Widespread pruritus occasionally occurs during pregnancy and clears up after labour but is liable to recur with each succeeding pregnancy. In diabetics pruritus is nearly always localized to the genitalia.

*J. L. M. Alibert (1768–1837), a French dermatologist.

LUPUS ERYTHEMATOSUS

Lupus erythematosus is due to a fibrinoid necrosis of collagen tissues and may remain a localized skin condition or have widespread manifestations. The condition was first described as a local skin disease as far back as 1838 but its generalized effects were not generally accepted until the 1920s. It affects mainly young women. The localized lesion is characterized by a well-defined red area which initially is macular but becomes raised (plaque) and remains discrete. The area develops a fine desquamation and roughly its centre becomes increasingly atrophic (devascularized, pale and losing normal skin markings) whilst the periphery becomes teleangiectatic. The lesions do not ulcerate except as a result of injudicous local therapy. There may be a single large lesion or multiple small ones and they occur mainly on the normally exposed areas of the body especially the face. The term 'discoid' is used in two different ways: (*a*) to describe the most usual lesion which is raised and round, the shape of a disc; (*b*) as a term for that variety of the condition which is confined to the skin. A butterfly distribution involving nose and cheeks is fairly common. A Raynaud phenomenon involving the digits often occurs.

When the condition is confined to the skin it is impossible to predict if it will remain so or not. It is important to appreciate that only a minority of the cases ever develops systemic manifestations and when this happens the interval between the first signs of the skin condition and the generalized disease varies from a few months to many years. A condition closely resembling systemic lupus erythematosus can occur as a consequence of therapy with hydrallazine, anti-convulsants, propranalol, isoniazid, and procainamide.

SCLERODERMA

Scleroderma is a condition characterized by a fibrinoid necrosis of the collagen of the skin producing whitish plaques or depressed areas which are usually ill-defined but which especially on the face may be linear and well-defined. The affected skin loses its normal markings and becomes tense, stretched and tight which can be demonstrated by the difficulty experienced when trying to pinch it or move it over underlying structures. The lesions especially on the face and limbs are surrounded by teleangiectases and especially on the face they may be more prominent than the primary lesion. Purplish pigmentation is common around the lesions. The hands (sclerodactyly) and face are the commonest sites. In the hands, which are often involved alone, gross flexion deformity with consequent loss of movement results and calcinosis and Raynaud phenomenon may be additional features producing a superficial resemblance to an arthritic hand, but the absence of joint swelling is the important clue. In the face a comparative immobility and lack of facility of emotional expression causes a resemblance to the Parkinsonian facies. In the face and limbs wasting of the underlying muscles may be present.

A minority of patients with scleroderma have non-cutaneous manifestations including defects of motility and contractility of the gastro-intestinal tract especially the oesophagus, myocardial involvement, and in the lungs a progressive bilateral fibrosis with multiple ring shadows especially in the lower zones shown radiologically. The patients who have non-cutaneous complications are needlessly and pompously sometimes designated 'systemic sclerosis'.

DERMATOMYOSITIS

Dermatomyositis is a condition characterized by fibrinoid necrosis of the collagen tissue of skin and voluntary muscles. Usually the skin lesions occur first and the commonest is fairly widespread violaceous or heliotrope blotchy macules especially on exposed areas and often affecting the eyelids and knuckle areas. Teleangiectases, fine scaling and skin oedema are common secondary phenomena. Teleangiectases involving the skin around the nail margins is an important feature. The macular lesions which are transitory resemble a light sensitivity reaction or lupus erythematosus. Pyrexia is common at the commencement of the disease and in those cases which become chronic lesions which resemble or are identical with scleroderma develop. In children but not in adults, calcinosis may develop and in adults a Raynaud phenomenon of the digits is common. Pain, tenderness and later wasting of the voluntary muscles, usually of proximal distribution, occurs early in the condition and may be very extensive and the dominant clinical feature. In scleroderma histological evidence of voluntary muscle involvement is often present but obvious clinical evidence is unusual. But there is a great similarity between the two conditions and it has often been disputed whether they are really two separate clinical entities. In adults dermatomyositis may be associated with malignancy, especially of breast, bronchus or pelvic organs, but this does not occur with scleroderma. The figures quoted for the frequency of this association vary from 6 to 60 per cent. In children there is no association with malignancy.

SKIN TUBERCULOSIS

Tuberculous skin lesions can be divided into two groups: (*a*) those types of lesion in which tubercle bacilli can usually be demonstrated; (*b*) those in which they cannot, these being the non-caseous and non-ulcerative lesions. The first group is represented by lupus vulgaris, scrofula, the occupational type and the generalized papular type.

Lupus vulgaris
Lupus vulgaris is characterized by small red papules occurring especially on the face, arms and buttocks and which vary in size from very small (miliary) to nodules. They become confluent and their centres caseate producing greenish 'apple jelly' nodules. At an early stage of their development the nodules ulcerate. The condition often spreads to the nasal and palatal mucosa later causing destruction of the nasal cartilage and hard palate. As a result of these features a severe case shows gross facial disfigurement.

Scrofula
Scrofula is tuberculous involvement of the skin secondary to sinuses caused by tuberculous disease of lymph nodes, bone or joint.

Occupational
In butchers, pathologists, milkmaids and veterinary surgeons tuberculous warty lesions especially on the back of the hands and which later ulcerate used to be much commoner than nowadays.

Generalized
Widespread reddish papular lesions which vary in size from very small (miliary) to nodular occur mainly on the face, forearms and buttocks and if they ulcerate tubercle bacilli can be found in the papules.

Tuberculides
Tuberculides are those skin lesions which are presumed to be tuberculous but from which the bacilli cannot be demonstrated and therefore proof is lacking. Within this group are generalized papules, as above, but without ulceration; erythema nodosum; lupus pernio and Bazin's disease.

Erythema nodosum
Erythema nodosum is a condition characterized by red nodules usually confined to the legs but occasionally on the arms and very rarely elsewhere. Other causes apart from tuberculosis are rheumatic fever, drug toxicity (especially sulpha group), sarcoid and ulcerative colitis.

Lupus pernio
Lupus pernio is characterized by violaceous ill-defined plaques on the nose, cheeks and ears and fingers with frequently teleangectases over the plaques. Its appearance and development is independent of climatic conditions.

Bazin's disease
The French dermatologist Bazin (1807—78) described a condition which he maintained was not tuberculous and almost entirely confined to young women with fattish legs and characterized by blueness, induration and ulceration of the legs, all three components being essential. The condition may resemble pernio (chilblains) but in the latter induration does not occur.

SKIN LESIONS IN SARCOIDOSIS
The various skin lesions which may occur in sarcoidosis are identical with the tuberculoides described above and this indicates that any of those conditions may be tuberculous, or due to sarcoid or be a clinical entity.

SYPHILITIC SKIN LESIONS

Primary
The primary lesion (chancre) consists of a red papule or papules which have a well-defined and cartilagenous feel and which eventually ulcerate. The usual site is penis or vulva. Rarely they are visible on the cervix uteri and extra-genital lesions may occur on lips, anus or nipple.

Secondary
The secondary syphilitic skin lesions are great imitators of other dermatological conditions. They occur four to six weeks after the chancre and, although they make take various forms, the commonest and most distinctive consists of coppery-red or dull red (ham coloured) well-defined round or elliptical macules anywhere on the body but especially the trunk. The condition is not itchy and typically no lesions apart from the macules are present. Such a rash is often referred to as 'the roseolar'. Occasionally the lesions later become papular and scaly and especially around the anus and genitalia may become warty and teeming with spirochaetes and are called 'condyloma'. The occasional occurrence of a psoriaform lesion of the palms and soles due to secondary syphilis has been mentioned previously.

Tertiary
Gummatous tertiary lesions of skin and mucous membranes which ulcerate and subsequently break down with the formation of typical syphilitic ulcers used to be very common. They may arise primarily from the skin or the skin may be involved secondary to disease of an underlying structure, usually bone.

THE SKIN IN LEPROSY

Leprosy affects the skin and peripheral nerves. The skin lesion are of three main types.

1. Indeterminate, starting as a single shiny depigmented macule on any part of the body. Later multiple lesions occur especially symmetrically over the trunk. The macules are much easier to recognize in coloured races. They are not anaesthetic and may clear spontaneously. Myco-leprae organisms cannot be isolated and the diagnosis of leprosy is unlikely to be correctly made except by an expert.
2. Tuberculoid leprosy is seen in those who have a high resistance to the infection. In addition to the macules, small and large papules develop and later these become anaesthetic. Healing and repigmentation occurs in the centre of the lesions and myco-leprae cannot be recovered from them.
3. Lepromatous leprosy is characterized by widespread and numerous ill-defined depigmented macules and papules which may be nodular. The lesions become anaesthetic and from them myco-leprae can be obtained. The skin, especially of the face, often becomes extremely thickened, corrugated and greasy (the leonine facies). The lesions often spread into the nose and mouth destroying the nasal cartilage and producing nodules and erosion of the hard palate.

GENERALIZED SKIN HYPERPIGMENTATION

Generalized skin hyperpigmentation may be due to bilirubin and occurs in all types of jaundice, the shade of yellow varying from a lemon as frequently occurs in haemolytic jaundice to a deep green which is most often seen with biliary cirrhosis. With jaundice the mucous membranes are always discoloured. The presence of large amounts of reduced haemoglobin causes purplish discoloration (cyanosis) of the skin and mucous membranes. With methaemaglobinaemia and suphaemaglobinaemia due to inorganic nitrites, organic nitrates, aniline dyes, some sulpha compounds and occasionally a congenital enzyme defect, the whole body becomes bluish purple but mucous membranes are not affected.

Addison's* disease is characterized by pigmentation of the skin and mucous membranes together with hypotension and gastrointestinal symptoms. The pigmentation which may be a very light or dark brown is especially marked in those areas usually not clothed, in areas normally well pigmented such as the nipples, and areas

*Thomas Addison (1793–1860) was born in Newcastle, graduated in Edinburgh and became a physician at Guy's (London). He wrote his paper entitled 'The constitutional and local effects of disease of the suprarenal capsules' in 1849.

irritated by belts, cuffs and collars. The mucous membranes are invariably affected and this is most easily recognizable in the mouth and there the pigmentation is always spotty and never diffuse. It is only very dark-skinned people who normally have pigmentation inside the mouth.

Chronic inorganic arsenical poisoning may cause dark brown spotty hyperpigmentation on the trunk, especially the back, which is sometimes described as raindrop pigmentation. Silver intoxication causes a bluish-grey or slatey-grey discoloration of skin and mucous membranes. Quinacrine causes a yellowish or yellowish-green pigmentation especially of exposed parts simulating jaundice but the mucous membranes are never affected. Eating large quantities of carrots, tomatoes, or other vegetables and fruits may cause lemon-yellow or orange-yellow pigmentation which is only occasionally generalized and is usually localized to the palms and soles and the face, principally the naso-labial grooves, but never involving mucous membranes. The condition is called carotinaemia.

Ochronosis causes deposition of blackish pigment in the cartilages and in the nose and ears which will be easily visible. Occasionally it affects the rest of the face but is very rarely more generalized. Acanthosis nigricans is a condition characterized by blackish papules which are usually small and pointed but may be larger and they occur especially over the abdomen, axillae and around the mouth. In adults it may be associated with intra-abdominal malignancy or intra-abdominal tuberculosis other than of the suprarenals. In young people the condition has no significance.

LEUCODERMA (VITILIGO)

Leucoderma is characterized by well-defined areas of depigmentation occurring especially on exposed areas but the genitalia are often affected. The extreme example of leucoderma is albinism which always involves the whole of the body and is associated also with lack of pigment in hair and eyes. Leucoderma is much easier to recognize in dark-skinned people, and in paler people the condition may become more obvious after exposure to prolonged sunshine. It may be genetically determined but is often of obscure aetiology. It may be a feature but is unusual in myxoedema, hyperthyroidism and Addison's disease and in the last named the associated hyper-pigmentation will produce a peculiar piebald appearance. In these endocrine conditions an auto-immune mechanism is held to be the cause. Leucoderma sometimes is present with pernicious anaemia. Skin scars other than keloids are always depigmented and leucoderma is also a feature of scleroderma and of leprosy. In secondary syphilis an area of leucoderma localized to the neck (corona veneris) may develop. Leucoderma which may be extensive can be caused by hydroquinone derivatives used in processing natural rubber.

URTICURIA

Urticuria (nettle rash or hives) is characterized by transient localized exudation of fluid into the dermis producing weals (white raised lesions surrounded by a red flare, which are not vesicular). It is always very itchy. Angio-neurotic oedema is generally considered to be a giant form of urticuria but surprisingly the lesions are not itchy and some do not use the term unless mucous membranes, especially the lip, are affected. The causes of urticuria are:

1. A definite allergen which may be (*a*) ingested (shell fish, strawberries, eggs etcetera and rarely drugs given orally), (*b*) injected (especially insect bites and sera and very rarely antibiotics, morphine and pethidine), (*c*) due to local contact especially with nettles and primulas.
2. Although urticuria is often described as a feature of collagen diseases actually it is very rare with any of them except polyarteritis nodosa.
3. It occurs occasionally with lymphadenoma.
4. It may rarely be a consequence of helminth infestation.
5. Physical causes have been described but they are rare and include pressure with a blunt instrument seen in anxiety states and thyrotoxicosis (dermatographia); exposure to cold and then it may be associated with either cryoglobinaemia or cold agglutins in the serum; and as a reaction to marked heat or sunlight.
6. Cholinergic urticuria is seen in young adults following marked exercise which produces marked sweating and is called cholinergic because a similar condition can sometimes be produced by cholinergic drugs.
7. Urticuria pigmentosa is a rare condition characterized by itchy reddish brown macules (looking like freckles) and papules often associated with considerable teleangiectatic reaction and always first appearing in childhood. The condition is associated with a marked increase of the normal mast (basophil) cells of the corium of the skin and there may be hepatosplenomegaly. The lesions after several years may regress spontaneously.
8. Chronic urticuria is an unusual condition for which a definite allergen is rarely discovered. Its cause is obscure.

PURPURA

When discussing the dermatological manifestations of many conditions purpura is often forgotten, but it is a skin lesion although its prime cause may be vascular or haematological. It is characterized by spontaneous haemorrhages into skin, mucous membranes and occasionally into viscera. That it is always spontaneous is very important and is the sole distinction from haemorrhages due to trauma including in haemophilia and related blood dyscrasias.

Purpuric lesions may be small and discrete (petechiae) or large and ill-defined (ecchymoses). Fresh lesions are bright red but they become increasingly darker and this is seen particularly with ecchymoses when they may become blackish and the physician may fail to recognize them as purpuric. The easiest lesions to recognize as purpura are petechial, but insect bites especially caused by fleas, may mimic them unless it is noticed that the centre of the lesions where the bite occurred is always darker than the periphery. Angiomata, especially when small, may mimic purpura but if any one of the three following features are present then the condition is never purpura, namely: raised, pallor on pressure (sign of emptying which is best done with a glass slide), or the presence of dilated capillaries and venules radiating from a central feed vessel (a 'spider').

The approach to purpura must always initially at least be purely clinical and not haematological and the following causes of purpura (secondary purpura) must always be first sought and considered.

1. Drug intoxication has become perhaps the commonest cause of purpura today. A very large number of drugs can, at least occasionally, cause purpura and among these are gold, organic arsenic, sulpha compounds, thiouracil, carbamizole, salycylates and other analgaesics, iodides and sometimes antibiotics. So, in any patient with purpura the first task must be to exclude a drug causation and not blather about obscure theories or platelet abnormalities.

2. Septicaemias, including meningococcal and brucellosis and infective endocarditis and also with the haemorrhagic severe forms of smallpox, scarlet fever and diphtheria. It may also be present in glandular fever. In all these conditions, except perhaps in the last named, the patients will invariably be very ill and have high fever, and septicaemia should immediately be suspected; haematological investigations other than blood culture can be a dangerous waste of time.

3. Bone marrow replacement by secondaries, myelomatosis, leukaemia, lipoidoses, and myelofibrosis. In these conditions almost invariably other signs are present and form important diagnostic clues to the cause of the purpura.

4. In scurvy purpura is the commonest manifestation and then the spontaneous haemorrhages are often confined to the lower limbs and the effect is commonly the production of large blackish echymotic areas. Bleeding gums are not as often seen in scurvy as some descriptions would have us believe.

5. Senile purpura does exist but is far less common than is often reported and diagnosed, the mistake being caused by a lack of appreciation of the fact that purpuric lesions are always spontaneous and that elderly people and also the obese often bruise even with trivial trauma to which the elderly are particularly prone. Genuine purpura does sometimes occur in the

elderly and then is always confined to the back of the hands and forearms and is always associated with thin atrophic inelastic skin with loss of turgor in the affected area and always loss of subcutaneous fat. Senile purpura is always of the echymotic type and is persistent causing dark pigmentation of the affected parts.

Having excluded these known (secondary) causes only then should resource be made to haematological investigations. Primary purpuras are subdivided into the primary thrombocytopenic purpuras and the primary non-thrombocytopenic purpuras which are sometimes called anaphylactoid purpuras or by various eponyms according to the main site of haemorrhages.

ASSOCIATION OF GASTRO-INTESTINAL AND SKIN LESIONS

In this brief account the associations are listed without detailed descriptions many of which are given elsewhere in this book.

Ulcerative colitis

Purpura (often due to drugs but may be due to scurvy); morbilliform eruption especially on limbs due to drugs; phrynoderma due to vitamin A deficiency; bilateral ulceration of legs; erythema nodosum (usually in women with severe active disease); perianal abscesses and fistulae; pyoderma gangrenosa characterized by red papules and vesicles which become pustular and surrounded by localized and later spreading skin gangrene, often first on digits but may occur anywhere on body and be widespread.

Malabsorption syndrome

In malabsorption syndrome there may be skin manifestations of any vitamin deficiency but especially of C; liability to widespread seborrhoeic dermatitis; and dermatitis herpetiformis. An interesting fact is that some patients with dermatitis herpetiformis who have no evidence of steatorrhoea, have histologically the same small bowel lesions seen in the malabsorption syndrome.

Peutz—Jegher*

The small bowel lesions associated with Peutz—Jegher syndrome may cause malaena or intussusception.

Crohn's disease†

Crohn's disease may be associated with perianal fissures and abscesses; and abscesses and sinuses of the abdominal wall; and the skin lesions described above as complications of ulcerative colitis very occasionally occur.

*J. L. Peutz from Holland wrote his paper in 1921 and H. Jegher of the USA wrote his paper in 1949.
†B. B. Crohn (1884–   ), a New York physician.

Cancer of gastro-intestinal tract
Very occasionally cancer of stomach or bowel may be associated with either acanthosis nigricans or dermatomyositis.

Hereditary teleangiectasia
Hereditary teleangiectasia is often associated with angioma of any part of the gastro-intestinal tract which may bleed.

Polyposis coli
Polyposis coli is an inherited condition in which the polyps often become malignant. It may be associated with multiple disfiguring sebaceous cysts which first appear in childhood.

Scleroderma
In scleroderma the musculature of the gastro-intestinal tract, especially the oesophagus, is often affected causing defects of motility and contractility.

Ehlers—Danlos* disease
Ehlers—Danlos disease is a genetically determined condition in which the skin, especially of the neck, axillae and groins, feels very smooth and can be pulled out from its underlying structures and stretched like a piece of elastic and when released it immediately returns to its normal position. Late in the disease the skin may become very lax and wrinkled and hang in folds. Bruising, haematomas and gaping lacerations occur with minor injuries, especially over bony prominences. The lacerations heal with tissue paper scars and the haematomas become organized producing soft nodules particularly over the knees.

Skeletal abnormalities and hyperextensability of joints are sometimes present resembling Marfan syndrome. The gastro-intestinal involvements are marked liability to herniae, eventration of the diaphragm, achalasia cardia and megacolon. The essential pathology is a defect of collagen tissues.

Pseudo-xanthoma elasticum
Pseudo-xanthoma elasticum is an inherited disease which clinically has a close resemblance to the above. It is characterized by yellowish papules which are usually small in the neck, axillae and groins, which do not consist of cholesterol and hence the term 'pseudo-xanthoma'. Over the same areas at an early stage of the condition the skin becomes lax and markedly wrinkled or develops into large inelastic redundant folds. Gastro-intestinal symptoms including bleeding are common. A large percentage of the patients have angioid streaks in the retina (described in the neurological chapter).

*Edvard Ehlers (1863—1937), a German and H. A. Danlos (1844—1912), a Frenchman, described the condition independently in 1901 and 1908 respectively.

12 The Limbs

Size and shape of hands

Congenital anomalies of the hands such as polydactyly, syndactyly (fusion of some fingers) and arachnodactyly (long thin spider-like fingers and toes) may occur by themselves but are often present with other congenital abnormalities. Marfan's* syndrome in its complete form is characterized by arachnodactyly, congenital dislocation of the lens, a high arched palate, skeletal deformities of the bony thorax, abnormal laxity of ligaments, allowing marked hyperextension of joints, and congenital heart lesions (usually coarctation or patent atrial septum). Those with Marfan syndrome are nearly always thin with dolichocephalic skulls and long thin faces with prominent supraorbital ridges. Polydactyly may be accompanied by retinitis pigmentosa and dystrophia adiposa genitalis. A flexion deformity of the interphalangeal joints of the little fingers, which is always bilateral, is a fairly common congenital lesion.

In achondroplasia the hands are small and podgy with all the fingers of almost equal length. At rest the hands are held with the middle and index fingers firmly adducted; the ring and little fingers are also adducted, but the ring and middle fingers are very widely separated, hence the term 'trident hand'.

In mongolism, although all the fingers are small the little finger, due to a rudimentary or absent second phalanx, is especially so, and it is curved with an ulnar convexity. Although the fingers are short the palm is broad and flat. The palm often shows a well marked transverse crease, contrasting with the sole, which shows a marked crease between the hallux and the adjacent toe. The study of normal and abnormal patterns of the fine ridges of the palms, soles and fingers (dermatoglyphics) is a new development; it has been demonstrated that in mongols the lines across the distal part of the palms are unusually horizontal but the details and the changes seen in other diseases cannot be appreciated unless the normal variations and the technical jargon which has been invented are known, and these facts are of very little interest except to specialists in this field. In cretinism the fingers are short, broad and spatulate and the thumb is often deformed. In acromegaly the hands are large and

B.-J. A. Marfan (Parusuan physician) wrote his paper in 1896.

spade-like and the fingers lack the normal tapering, their ends being bulbous; on X-ray the terminal phalanges show enlargement of their peripheral and distal ends and, more important, the distal margin shows multiple fine hair-like lines instead of the normal well-defined border (tufting). In hyperparathyroidism the ends of the fingers are often bulbously enlarged. This condition can be readily distinguished from arthritis of the terminal interphalangeal joints because the swelling is not confined to the joint line. In pseudohypoparathyroidism the fingers, especially the fourth and fifth, are very short. The condition is usually seen in blondes of poor intelligence and, because of the associated hypocalcaemia, these patients may exhibit carpo-pedal spasm. Carpo-pedal spasm, which is characterized by painful involuntary flexion of the metacarpal joints and adduction of the thumbs across the palms, is an important manifestation of tetany. Squeezing the arm, for example with a sphygmomanometer cuff pumped up to about 200 mm and kept at that level for about five minutes, may precipitate the spasms (Trousseau's* sign). Facial spasms may be precipitated by percussing the facial nerve at roughly its point of emergence from the parotid (Chvostek's† sign).

Moist warm hands, which may be tremulous, are an important feature of thyrotoxicosis, but many normal people have moist hands in a warm environment. In myxoedema the skin of the hands, especially over their dorsal aspects, is cold, dry and rough. Conversely, if the hands are smooth and moist the patient is extremely unlikely to have myxoedema, while if they are cold and dry, thyrotoxicosis is very unlikely.

Deformity of hands

Flexion deformities of the fingers associated with limitation of movement are common features of certain neurological lesions, sclerodactyly, Dupuytren's‡ contracture and arthritis. The classical neurological deformity of the hands is the claw hand (*main en griffe*). This is characterized by wasting of the small muscles of the hands supplied by the ulnar nerve, together with hyperextension at the metacarpo-phalangeal joints, especially of the ring and little fingers, and flexion at the interphalangeal joints. The commonest cause of a unilateral claw hand is an ulnar nerve lesion, often due to injury. The most frequent cause of a bilateral claw hand is syringomyelia, but rarer causes are peripheral neuritis and peroneal muscular

*A. Trousseau (1801–67), a French physician.
†F. Chvostek (1835–84), an Austrian surgeon.
‡ Baron G. Dupuytren (1777–1835), a French surgeon.

E

atrophy. The resemblance to rheumatoid arthritis will be accentuated if the arthritis is associated with subluxations producing hyperextension at joints.

Sclerodactyly (*see* Chapter 11), especially when it is associated with calcinosis and a Raynaud phenomenon, may mimic both arthritis and a neurological lesion.

With sclerodactyly, which usually forms part of a much more widespread disease, the skin is hardened and inelastic, appears unduly stretched, and cannot be readily pinched between finger and thumb. This often causes flexion deformity of the fingers with limitation of their movements. The condition may be associated with Raynaud's syndrome and with calcinotic nodules in the subcutaneous tissues which may ulcerate and resemble tophi.

In Dupuytren's contracture there is fibrosis and thickening of the palmar fascia and secondarily of the flexor tendons, causing a flexion deformity of the metacarpo-phalangeal joints, especially of the ring and middle fingers. The thickened fascia can always be felt and usually seen. This condition can also be readily differentiated from arthritis by the absence of joint swelling. The lesion is nearly always bilateral, although often asymmetrical, and is much commoner in men than in women. It may be occupational, for example in gardeners, but does occur in cirrhosis of the liver (especially alcoholic), in diabetes and in gout with a greater frequency than can be accounted for by coincidence. The aetiology in many cases is obscure, although a genetic basis is reputed to be the cause in some people.

All types of arthritis of the hands cause deformity and limitation of movement of the fingers, but the feature distinguishing this group of conditions from all the others producing these two signs is the presence of swelling of the joints in arthritis. In the vast majority of cases this swelling can be readily appreciated on inspection alone. In any arthritis of the hands, but especially the rheumatoid type, there may be wasting of the muscles and Raynaud's syndrome, and these signs create a further resemblance to neurological lesions. Ulnar deviation may occur with any form of arthritis of the hands, although it is most common in rheumatoid.

The three commonest types of arthritis affecting the hands are rheumatoid arthritis, osteo-arthritis and gout, and a very important feature differentiating them is the distribution of the arthritis. Rheumatoid arthritis involves the metacarpo-phalangeal joints and the proximal but not the distal interphalangeal joints. The joints are often not involved symmetrically. Osteo-arthritis affects the distal interphalangeal joints and is often associated with bony nodules along this joint line (Heberden's* nodes). Osteo-arthritis may also

---

*William Heberden (1710–1801), a London physician. His account of the nodes was published posthumously in 1802.

involve other joints of the hands, but is then always secondary to repeated trauma which is often occupational. The metacarpo-phalangeal joint of the thumb is often affected in this way. In osteo-arthritis, angulation deformity of the distal interphalangeal joints is sometimes more obvious than the swelling. Gout may affect any joints of the hands, and the presence of tophi is the only proof that the condition is definitely gout.

Arthritis affecting the proximal and distal interphalangeal and metacarpo-phalangeal joints is common, especially in elderly people; and is most often due to combined osteo- and rheumatoid arthritis, but may be caused by gout or psoriasis. Any arthritis of the hands may affect the carpal joints. Although this lesion may be severe as shown radiologically, it cannot be recognized clinically. However, arthritis of the tarsus, when due to either gout or Charcot's disease (secondary to peripheral neuritis or tabes dorsalis), may produce marked swelling of the dorsum of the foot and may be associated with ulceration of the toes or heel or dorsum of the foot due either to tophi or peripheral vascular disease. Any arthritis anywhere which does not also involve the hands is extremely unlikely to be rhuematoid arthritis.

Nodules over bony prominences including the knuckles have been discussed in Chapter 11. In osteo-arthritis such nodules are confined to the joint line of the distal interphalangeal joints. The size of the nodules does not help in the differentiation between rheumatoid and gouty arthritis but ulceration of nodules occurs only with gout but not with rheumatoid arthritis or osteoarthritis.

A chronic dactylitis which has never been acute is characterized by swelling of the greater part or the whole of one or more fingers. The swelling is not confined to the region of the joints. It may be smooth and cigar-shaped or nodular. Tuberculosis and syphilis used to be two common causes, but today probably the commonest cause is gout. The correct aetiology may be easily overlooked because the swelling often occurs while the arthritis is very mild and may be missed, and the finger may even be amputated under the mistaken diagnosis of a tuberculous dactylitis. Bursae over the olecronon and occasionally prepatellar are often present in rheuma-toid arthritis and in gout.

Involvement of the phalanges, metacarpals and metatarsals in sarcoidosis is common, but it should be easy to demonstrate that the swelling produced in the bone does not involve the joint. X-ray will show a single well-defined area of rarefaction of the affected bones. The condition is often associated with lupus pernio of the fingers, which exhibit a purplish discoloration which, unlike that seen both in pernio and in Raynaud's syndrome, is unaffected by cold.

The nails

CLUBBING

Clubbing of the fingers is an important sign in aiding diagnosis and should always be looked for. In recent years this has, too often, quite unjustifiably been dismissed as of little or no importance. Clubbing of the fingers was known to Hippocrates, and over 2,000 years of clinical experience cannot so lightly be cast aside.

The essence of clubbing is increased curvature of the nails in both planes, horizontal (from side to side) and longitudinal (axially). The difficulty is to say what constitutes 'increased curvature', because nails are normally curved. In a marked case there can be no doubt, but in a slight case such an opinion is nothing more than a clinical impression. It is for this reason that comparatively recently it has been emphasized that the increased curvature of the nails is often preceded by a filling in of the normally obtuse angle between the proximal end of the nail and the adjoining soft tissues, which is best observed by looking at the finger in profile at the level of the observer's eye. It is this 'profile sign' which is open to objection as an important sign and not clubbing, because it is often even more difficult to assess than increased curvature.

With clubbing, in addition to the increased curvature, the nails are smooth. A reputed early sign of clubbing is increased fluctuation between the nail bed and the nail plate best demonstrable by the physician pressing the nail of one index finger on the lunula of the finger under suspicion and the nail of his other index finger pressing the distal part of the patient's same nail and by varying the pressure imparting a rocking movement. This is a very difficult sign to appreciate. The nails may be brittle but with normal colour and lustre. Clubbing is not painful except occasionally when due to carcinoma of the lung, especially of a peripheral type. The increased curvature of the nails is later followed by an increase in all the soft tissues of the end of the finger, giving rise to an appearance which has been variously described as 'drumstick', 'serpent's head' and 'parrot's beak'. This is never seen except when the clubbing is marked.

At a further stage the condition may be complicated by the development of pain and swelling of the joints of the hands and feet, which may later involve the wrist and ankles and, rarely, spread to the elbows and knees. This condition of joint involvement has been given many names, but the term 'hypertrophic pulmonary osteo-arthropathy' (coined by Marie* in 1890, minus the word 'pulmonary') is probably the best. An important point to realize is that clinically it will closely resemble rheumatoid arthritis, but the presence of clubbing of the fingers will give a clue

*Pierre Marie (1853–1940), a French neurologist.

to the real nature of the joint lesion unless, of course, it be true that the patient has two diseases, rheumatoid arthritis and another unassociated condition – for example, bronchiectasis – causing the clubbing.

Radiological examination of the joints will differentiate between rheumatoid arthritis and hypertrophic osteo-arthropathy with certainty because, although both show diminution of joint spaces (extremely difficult to assess unless marked), the latter will exhibit in addition a bilateral symmetrical periostitis at the ends of the bone. The emphasis is therefore that, in the great majority of cases, the clubbing goes through the following phases, in chronological order: (1) filling in of the angle between the nail and the nail-bed; (2) increased curvature of the nail in two planes, which in itself constitutes the actual clubbing; (3) increase of the soft tissues at the ends of the fingers; (4) hypertrophic osteo-arthropathy. However some clinicians do not agree that hypertrophic osteoarthropathy represents a severe form of clubbing, pointing out: (1) some patients have very marked clubbing without hypertrophic osteo-arthropathy; (2) occasionally hypertrophic osteo-arthropathy is associated with only a minor degree of clubbing; (3) clubbing is often asymmetrical but hypertrophic osteo-arthropathy never is. In spite of these facts I do not consider that it is justifiable to regard the two as entirely different conditions.

Causes

Clubbing is an important physical sign because of the great help it may offer in diagnosis. Its common causes are as follows:

1. It is caused by chronic lung infection, such as tuberculosis or bronchiectasis. Nowadays it is frequently taught that clubbing does not occur in pulmonary tuberculosis, but this is wrong. The truth is that clubbing in pulmonary tuberculosis is seen only with chronic disease and should never be regarded as an early manifestation of the condition. Neither chronicity nor infection is necessary to produce clubbing and, for example, it may occur in acute infections, such as lung abscess or empyema, and may then develop within two or three weeks of the onset of the disease. Nor is infection necessary, because clubbing may be seen in peripheral carcinoma of the lung unassociated with any superadded infection. In spite of what is often written to the contrary, the author does not believe that clubbing ever occurs with uncomplicated bronchitis or emphysema.

2. It may be seen in cyanosed congenital heart disease, for example Fallot's tetralogy. In neither non-cyanosed congenital heart disease nor acquired heart disease does clubbing develop unless there be a superadded infective endocarditis. Clubbing

may also occur with aneurysms of the thoracic aorta and in these cases it frequently is unilateral, affecting the fingers of the right hand only.

3. It occurs with chronic diarrhoeas, either of an infective type (for example, chronic dysentery and ulcerative colitis) or of a non-infective type (for example, the idiopathic steatorrhoeas). With diarrhoea, chronicity but not infection is essential to the production of clubbing.

4. It occasionally occurs in cirrhosis of the liver. It is fairly commonly seen in biliary cirrhosis, but is unusual with the much commoner portal cirrhosis.

5. It may be a familial condition, and then it is frequently grossly asymmetrical and, surprisingly, increases with age.

6. It is sometimes seen in myxoedema, particularly iatrogenic, and is found especially in association with exophthalmic ophthalmoplegia.

7. A rare form of idiopathic non-familial severe clubbing, seen especially in young healthy adolescent boys, has also been described. There is no point in giving this a special name.

Acromegaly and hyperparathyroidism, both of which produce changes in the terminal phalanges, may cause enlargement of the ends of the fingers and this may superficially resemble clubbing, but there should be no difficulty in differentiation.

KOILONYCHIA

Koilonychia is characterized by the nail surface losing its normal convexity and becoming flat or even concave. The nails are thin, ridged and very brittle and lose their normal lustre. There is only one important cause of this, namely iron deficiency anaemia.

LEUCONYCHIA

Normally the half-moon (lunula) at the proximal end of the nail is its only white part. In many normal people a lunula is not visible. Leuconychia is the presence of whiteness of the whole of the nail or of white flecks or bands. Some clinicians limit the term to those cases in which the entire nail becomes white. To lay people such white lines or spots are an indication of ill health, but there is only a small element of truth in this. The commonest cause of white flecks or bands is minor local injury.

White transverse bands, which may form ridges or depressions, initially starting near the lunula, progressing with nail growth (normally 0.5 to 1.2 cm per week) towards the free margin are called Beau's* lines. These may occur in any febrile illness, but their most important diagnostic significance is that when found in a

*Joseph H. S. Beau (1806–65), a French physician.

patient with a prolonged fever of obscure aetiology where no temperature chart is available, they indicate that the fever is of an undulant type (*see* Chapter 6).

Leuconychia may occur in chronic inorganic arsenic poisoning and in hypo-albuminaemia, especially when this is caused by cirrhosis of the liver but occasionally when it is due to the nephrotic syndrome and in these conditions leuconychia may be seen in the form of white bands or whiteness of the whole nail. Some do not regard the nail abnormality in these cases as a true example of leuconychia claiming that the whiteness is not in the nail itself but in the nail bed. A large number of other conditions are reputed very rarely to cause leuconychia.

HAEMORRHAGES

The commonest cause of haemorrhage into the nail is injury. Spontaneous haemorrhages are a rare occurrence in any condition associated with an abnormal liability to bleed. Splinter haemorrhages are linear and longitudinal and grow out towards the free margin with growth of the nail. They come in crops and are usually regarded as pathognomonic of infective endocarditis, but they have been described in septicaemias from other causes and in various severe anaemias. Transverse linear haemorrhages are probably pathognomonic of trichiniasis. They differ from splinter haemorrhages not only in being transverse but also in that they do not occur in crops. In dermatomyositis, dilated blood vessels in the nail bed give the nail a heliotrope colour; in addition, the skin at the nail margins shows punctuate atrophy, dilated capillaries and minute haemorrhages.

RIDGES

Longitudinal ridges (reeding) are nearly always the result of local injury, but they are common in koilonychia and also with any peripheral vascular disease of any type and then the longitudinal ridging is often associated with splits along the nail margin. The nails become brittle and the thinning of the nail plate allows the colour of the nail bed to show through better than normally, so that the nail appears to be unduly reddish-blue, contrasting with the later appearance of white patches due to onycholysis, which is a loosening or separation of the nail from its bed which may be due to trauma, psoriasis, fungal infection, or paranychia. Eunuchs often have very prominent nail ridges causing the nails to be shaped and patterned like a shell (onychauxis).

Pigmented longitudinal lines or bands are common in coloured races and have no significance. In hepato-lenticular degeneration the lunulae may exhibit an azure bluish tint. A similar discoloration may be seen as a result of phenolphthalein habituation. The nails may become bluish-black with chloroquine overdosage.

BRITTLENESS AND OTHER SIGNS

Causes of undue nail brittleness are iron deficiency, hypocalcaemia, fungus infection of the nails, psoriasis, repeated injury (including injudicious manicuring and nail-biting), repeated application of nail varnishes, and prolonged hand immersion in water, especially if the water contains added chemicals. In the majority of people, however, the real cause is never found.

Psoriasis often affects the nails, which become pitted, discoloured (with yellowish or brownish blobs) and very brittle. Onycholysis is a common late manifestation and this may produce a yellow line between the separated and the attached portion of the nail and later the whole nail may become a yellowish brown colour. Psoriasis is very rarely confined to the nails but when it is the distinction from fungus infection is impossible except by microscopy. The earliest sign of fungus infection of the nails, which is often but not necessarily associated with fungus infection of hands or feet, is usually the appearance of brownish blobs of discoloration starting at the free edge and later spreading to the whole nail, which becomes pitted and very brittle and often exhibits onycholysis. With fungus infections and psoriasis the nail involvement is often grossly asymmetrical and some fingers may be completely spared.

Partial or complete absence of some or all of the nails is a rare congenital anomaly which may be associated with other congenital lesions, especially with absent or rudimentary patellae.

Evidence of nail-biting is often a very good indication of the patient's psychological make-up. Dirty nails reflect poor standards of hygiene.

Teleangiectases of the nail folds with ragged cuticles is a common feature of dermatomyositis and an occasional finding in sclerodactyly and lupus erythematosus.

The rare yellow nail syndrome is a surprising combination of yellow or yellowish-green discoloration, together with a mild lymphatic oedema of the lower limbs and a sterile plural effusion. Its cause is unknown.

EPITROCHLEA LYMPH NODES

The epitrochlea lymph nodes are proximal and slightly anterior to the medial epicondyle and are best felt with the patient's elbow partly flexed and supported by the physician's palm. Enlarged, firm and well-defined (shotty) lymph nodes at this site are a common finding in secondary syphilis. They may be enlarged secondary to infection of the hand or arm or as part of a generalized lymphadenopathy.

Involvement of large joints

ARTHRITIS

The three fundamental signs of any arthritis are swelling, deformity and alteration of movement (nearly always limitation) and of these three signs, except in the case of the shoulders and hips, swelling is the most important because, as indicated previously, many conditions other than arthritis, including upper motor neurone lesions of the limbs, may cause both deformity and limitation of movement. Moreover it must always be borne in mind that in many patients who complain of difficulty in walking the cause is not neurological but skeletal. It is true that arthritis in its early stages may cause pain without any visible swelling but except in the shoulders, hips, spine and sacro-iliac joints, the diagnosis of arthritis clinically is problematical and never certain without the presence of swelling.

Arthritis can be classified into two main groups, periarticular and degenerative.

Periarticular arthritis

In this form the changes are primarily in the sinovial membrane and capsule and as a consequence radiological signs in the early stages consist only of a mild degree of diminution of the joint space and rarifaction of the bone ends, both features being difficult for the non-specialist to appreciate. Sometimes in this type of arthritis instead of the rarified bone ends retaining their normal shape and margins they may exhibit radiologically a scooped out area of erosion, with consequent loss of the bone margins extending over the whole width of the articular surface. This contrasts with gout in which typically the erosions are limited to the lateral aspects of the joint margin. Included in the group of periarticular arthritis are rheumatoid arthritis, rheumatic fever, and non-purulent arthritis due to infections such as gonococcal, non-specific urethritis, brucellosis, dysentery and meningococcal septicaemia. Effusion into the joints is a common feature of periarticular arthritis. Arthritis is a common complication of haemophilia and is due to injury which is often trivial, and it might therefore be expected that the radiological appearance of a haemophiliac joint would be identical with an osteoarthritic joint but surprisingly it resembles the rheumatoid joint and its final stage causes a fibrous ankylosis without any osteophytes.

Degenerative arthritis

In the degenerative forms, of which by far the commonest is osteoarthritis, the lesion affects primarily the bone cartilage on the surface of the joints, causing new bone formation (osteophytes) and, radiologically, osteophytes with diminution of the joint space and sclerosis, with only a minor degree of rarifaction, of the bone ends. Effusion does not occur with this type of arthritis. A joint injury may cause an effusion into the joint and that joint much later may become osteoarthritic.

Swelling of a joint can nearly always be readily recognized by inspection and palpation rarely helps in this decision. A supposed differentiation between 'snowball' crunching and creaking felt on palpation of joints when they are moved is unreliable diagnostically.

In any patient with arthritis of a large joint the hands must be carefully inspected as the correct cause of the arthritis is often given by them. A Charcot* (neuropathic) joint is characterized by swelling with excessive range of painless movement. This is a far better description than the commonly used phrase 'disorganized joint' because the term is difficult to define and to demonstrate. Except in the case of the spine and shoulder swelling is an essential feature of a Charcot joint because with the two commonest causes of this, namely tabes dorsalis and severe sensory peripheral neuritis, an excessive range of joint movement may be due to the hypotonicity even in the absence of any arthritis. It is not necessary for all movements to be excessive because either huge osteophytes or dislocation may interfere with some movements; for example, in the knee flexion and extension may be limited with a great deal of painless lateral movement possible. A common complication of a Charcot joint is dislocation. The X-ray is identical with a severe osteoarthritis but dislocation favours a Charcot joint. In syringomyeia Charcot joints may develop in the shoulder or elbow but are very rare elsewhere. In the shoulder the diagnosis can be very difficult because of the absence of swelling and any disability can be accounted for by the neurological involvement of the muscles around the joint. Charcot joints of the tarsus have been described previously.

BOWING OF LEGS

Bowing of the legs can be easily missed when the patient is lying down and becomes more obvious when the patient is walking. There are three main medical causes of bowing namely, Paget's disease, rickets and syphilis (congenital or acquired). The clinical approach to this problem of differentiation should be as follows. If the patient is less than middle-aged then the bowing is not due to Paget's disease. If however the patient is middle-aged or older, then any of the three conditions may be the cause because many with rickets do survive even to old age. If the bowing is unilateral it is not due to rickets but rickets is always bilateral, syphilis often bilateral but may be unilateral, and Paget's disease often unilateral but may be bilateral. In a middle-aged or elderly patient increased warmth of the tibia assessed by palpation is a diagnostic sign of great importance

*Jean Martin Charcot (1825–93), a French neurologist.

because if accomplished by bowing it is pathognomonic of Paget's disease. It can be more readily appreciated if the bowing is unilateral. Bilateral bowing associated with stunting of growth indicates that the condition started in infancy or childhood, indicating either rickets or congenital syphilis. In rickets the bowing is typically lateral, involving the lower half of the tibia; in syphilis it is anterior, affecting the upper half of the tibia (sabre tibia); while Paget's disease typically causes forward and lateral bowing of the whole of the tibial shaft. But these differences in the character of the bowing are usually very unreliable diagnostically. These three conditions may also cause bowing of the forearms and then the differential diagnosis should be considered in an identical manner.

OEDEMA OF LOWER LIMBS
The main causes of oedema of the lower limbs are cardiac, renal or liver failure and venous or lymphatic (lymphoedema) obstruction. The most important single sign differentiating venous from lymphatic oedema is that the latter pits only very slightly or not at all on digital pressure. An additional pathognomonic feature with lymphatic oedema, which however is not always present, is a peau d'orange change in the skin. With venous obstruction there may be discoloration and collateral veins but either or both are often absent. With thrombosis of the deep calf veins an important sign is the production of severe pain in the calf on forcible dorsiflexion of the foot.

The great importance of distinguishing between venous and lymphatic oedema is the relatively good prognosis of the former and the bad prognosis, as regards its likely disappearance, of the latter. A patient may have both venous and lymphatic oedema in the same limb, as occurs with pre- and post-operative cancer of the breast and with pelvic neoplasms (benign or malignant), and the determination which is dominant is important prognostically. The condition of 'white leg of pregnancy' (phlegmasia alba dolens) used to be very common. It follows parturition and abortion especially if instrumental and is caused by a parametritis with pelvic lymphangitis and phlebitis. Initially the patient is febrile and develops marked swelling of one or both lower limbs which pits on pressure and may be very extensive but the venous element usually spontaneously regresses leaving a permanent brawny lymphatic oedema.

Milroy* in 1891 described a series of patients all of whom were relatives (twenty-two of ninety-six members of six generations) who had lymphatic oedema of one or both lower limbs which was first noticed at birth or early infancy, and who were otherwise

*W. F. Milroy (1855–1942), a New York physician.

healthy. In its entirety as described by Milroy this has probably never been seen since. But lymphatic oedema of one or both lower limbs starting about puberty in girls and not genetically determined is fairly common and is named lymphoedema praecox. A mild degree of lymphatic oedema of the legs of obscure cause is sometimes seen in Turner syndrome, and also with the yellow nail syndrome.

ULCERATION OF LEGS
Ulceration of the legs is a common finding and the main causes are as follows:
1. Varicose ulcers are always on the lower half of the leg and are shallow with sloping walls, and they are associated with an acute or chronic eczematous involvement of the surrounding skin. Varicose veins in the limb may be few or many and a history of phlebitis is not always present.
2. So-called 'gravitational' ulcers occur in patients with chronic leg oedema, especially when due to chronic cardiac failure. In these patients venous thrombosis may be a factor. These ulcers are in every way identical with varicose ulcers and their differentiation is often impossible.
3. Syphilitic ulcers (gummatous) may occur anywhere on the leg but are often over the upper half. Their appearance has been described in Chapter 11.
4. Bilateral shallow ulcers of the legs are a complication of (a) rheumatoid arthritis (b) ulcerative colitis (c) the haemoglobinopathies.
5. Necrobiosis lipoidica diabeticorum is a chronic condition seen only in adults and is characterized by yellowish shiny plaques or small nodules usually with teleangiectases over the lesions which later become ulcerated. The condition which is confined to the legs is badly named because the yellowness is not due to lipid and the lesion often occurs in non-diabetics.
6. Tuberculous ulceration of the legs which can be proved to be so is either a patch of lupus vulgaris (an unusual site) or may form part of the more generalized papular-necrotic lesions. Bazin's* disease which may be a tuberculide has been described in Chapter 11.
7. Diphtheritic ulceration with the typical membrane on its base is unusual, but an epidemic of this was present in some Mediterranean countries during the Second World War and many of the patients developed peripheral neuritis which was often confined to the affected leg.
8. Decubitus ulcers may occur over pressure points in bedridden patients.

*A. P. E. Bazin (1807–78), a French dermatologist.

9. The so-called 'tropical' ulcer of the leg is usually due to Vincent's spirochaete; this causes pustular lesions on the front of the legs which become confluent and later ulcerate. The edges of the ulcer may be everted and a foul-smelling blood stained discharge is frequent on the ulcer base and around its margin which is also dark red and swollen. These ulcers often become chronic and then lack any distinguishing features. There are many parasites and protozoal infections which may cause gummatous lesions of the legs complicated by ulceration in tropical and subtropical countries.

Peripheral arterial diseases of functional or obstructive type and including diabetic cause skin ulceration but this does not involve the leg, which anatomically extends from the knee to the ankle joint, but affects the toes and heel and occasionally the dorsum of the foot. The exception is that occasionally peripheral vascular disease may produce ulceration localized to the region of the internal malleolus. Perforating ulcers due to sensory peripheral neuritis or tabes dorsalis occur not on the leg but on the plantar aspect of the foot. Peripheral vascular diseases and neurological involvement of the lower limbs are more fully described in later chapters.

13 The Respiratory System

Anatomy of the chest

An ability to name the ribs numerically is of great importance when attempting to localize a chest lesion either clinically or radiologically. Anteriorly the junction of the manubrium and the sternum proper is the level of the second rib articulation, and this is the landmark used rather than the first rib because its costo-chondral junction, being covered by the inner end of the clavicle, is difficult to feel. Each interspace is numbered by the rib above. Posteriorly each rib articulates with the identically numbered thoracic vertebral body. The 'vertebra prominens' is the seventh cervical, and the others can be counted from this; the upper articulation of each body corresponds numerically to the rib attached to it, the first rib articulating with the first dorsal vertebra, and so on. Obliquity of the ribs varies enormously from the almost horizontal with the barrel chest to the marked sloping with long thin chests.

Congenital anomalies of the ribs are very common, usually being recognizable only on X-ray. If the anterior portion of one of the upper ribs is forked, it may radiologically simulate a cavity. Cervical ribs, unilateral or bilateral, are common and vary in size from a small bony excrescence to a fully developed rib.

There are important anatomical landmarks in the chest which must be known. The great fissure passes obliquely from the fourth dorsal spine to the sixth costo-chondral junction anteriorly. The surface marking frequently given as commencing at the second dorsal spine is that found in the deflated lungs of the cadaver. The horizontal fissure, which is only on the right side, passes horizontally from the fourth costo-chondral junction to meet the great fissure in the mid-axillary line. Whenever one is examining a chest or a chest radiograph, the position of these fissures should always be borne in mind and the relationship of any signs to them carefully noted. By this means it should be possible, clinically and radiologically, to locate the site of any pulmonary lesion and also to differentiate between lesions of the lung itself and those in the pleura or the mediastinum; any single large opacity which has not the shape or position of any segment or lobe is probably not in the lung. The interlobar fissures are also important potential spaces for pathological processes, especially effusions of all types.

The oblique fissures are not normally visible on a postero-anterior X-ray, but may be seen on a lateral view without being indicative of any pathology. However, the horizontal fissure is fairly often seen at the level of the fourth rib on a postero-anterior film because its plane is tangential to that of the X-rays. If not displaced, it is of no pathological significance.

The lower surface markings of the lungs on deep inspiration commence at the sixth costo-chondral junction anteriorly, passing obliquely to the tenth rib in the anterior axillary line and then horizontally to the upper border of the twelfth dorsal vertebra.

The trachea bifurcates at the level of the junction of the manubrium and the body of the sternum, where the second rib articulates with the sternum anteriorly, which is equivalent to the upper level of the fourth dorsal vertebra posteriorly. The right main bronchus is slightly larger than the left and comes off at a less acute angle than the left (hence septic material and other foreign substances are more likely to be inhaled into the right lung than into the left). On the right the main bronchus divides into the upper, middle and lower lobe stem bronchi. The right upper lobe bronchus subdivides into three main divisions – apical, anterior and posterior. The middle lobe bronchus comes off anteriorly from the main right bronchus and divides into lateral and medial main divisions. The lower lobe bronchus subdivides into the apical, medial basal (cardiac), anterior basal, lateral basal and posterior basal divisions (*see Figure 1*).

The left main bronchus divides into upper and lower lobe bronchi. The upper lobe bronchus has upper and lower divisions, the former dividing into an apico-posterior and an anterior division. The apico-posterior branch is continued as the apical division, and from it arises the posterior division. The lower division, which corresponds to the middle lobe bronchus of the right lung and is often known as the lingula bronchus, subdivides into superior and inferior branches. The left lower lobe bronchus divides in the same fashion as the right except that it has not got a medial basal branch.

In a small number of normal people the azygos vein enters the superior vena cava at an abnormal angle, producing a cleft in the upper lobe and forming the so-called azygos lobe. This has not got an independent blood or bronchial supply. It is seen on a postero-anterior X-ray as a thin, delicately curved line extending downwards and medially and ending in a small blob.

Cyanosis

Cyanosis is far easier to recognize with good natural lighting rather than with artificial especially fluorescent light. With severe anaemia from any cause a marked degree of unsaturation of the arterial blood is essential before cyanosis can be recognized clinically. The

PULMONARY SEGMENTS

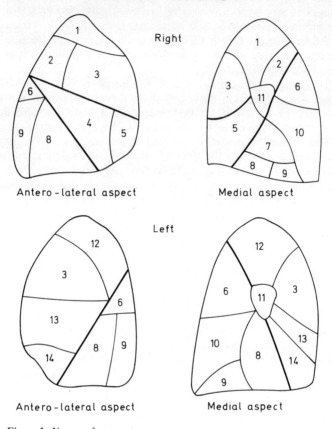

Figure 1. *Names of segments*

1. *Apical upper lobe.*
2. *Posterior upper lobe.*
3. *Anterior upper lobe.*
4. *Lateral middle lobe.*
5. *Medial middle lobe.*
6. *Apical lower lobe.*
7. *Medial basal lower lobe.*
8. *Anterior basal lower lobe.*
9. *Lateral basal lower lobe.*
10. *Posterior basal lower lobe.*
11. *Hilum.*
12. *Apico-posterior left upper lobe.*
13. *Superior of lingula.*
14. *Inferior of lingula.*

The great and lesser fissures are marked with a thicker line.

clinical recognition of cyanosis in any patient depending as it does on visual impression requires a good deal of experience. Cyanosis is a bluish discoloration of the skin and mucosae due to an increase in the amount of reduced haemoglobin in the capillary blood. This definition excludes a bluish discoloration caused by abnormal pigments such as sulphaemoglobin or methaemoglobin, which may result from a congenital enzyme defect or from the toxic action of inorganic nitrites, organic nitrates, aniline dyes, some sulpha compounds or phenacetin (with the last named the discoloration is greyish rather than blue). With these abnormal pigments the striking feature is the presence of an apparent cyanosis in a patient who is not dyspnoeic on exertion, and the diagnosis can be confirmed by blood spectroscopy.

Central cyanosis is caused by an excess of reduced haemoglobin entering the aorta and may be due to: (1) extensive disease of the lungs or thoracic cage; (2) a right-to-left shunt bypassing the lungs; (3) polycythaemia vera, in which there is an excess of reduced haemoglobin because of the red cell increase. Central cyanosis causes blueness of the lingual and buccal mucosae and the tarsal conjunctiva. Cyanosis of the exposed labial mucosa is far less conclusive. The hands are usually warm and not cyanosed. Cyanosis of the fingers when the person is in a warm atmosphere is never central. Clubbing and a secondary polycythaemia are often present. Central cyanosis is always accentuated by exercise and is usually associated with a high cardiac output, which may be suggested by a large-volume pulse. It is absurd, however, to diagnose a high cardiac output on these clinical findings alone, as this is a measurement which can be determined only by special techniques.

Peripheral cyanosis is caused by either heart disease (with low cardiac output) or peripheral arterial disease, either obstructive or spasmodic. In shock the sudden fall of blood pressure and cardiac output is associated with cyanosed, cold and clammy extremities. In both these conditions, a diminished blood flow through the capillaries allows an excessive time for extraction of oxygen from the blood and thus an excessive production of reduced haemoglobin. Peripheral cyanosis affects mainly the peripheral parts of the limbs, which are cold and not the naturally warmed lingual and buccal mucosae. However, the distinction between central and peripheral cyanosis is not always clear-cut on clinical grounds alone, there often being an element of both, so beware of basing your diagnosis on such a finding. It is important when attempting to make this differentiation that the patient is not cold, because normal people and those with purely central cyanosis will exhibit blueness of the fingers and toes under such conditions.

Central cyanosis indicates a low arterial oxygen saturation which falls below 85 per cent (normal 95 per cent). With peripheral cyanosis the oxygen saturation does not fall below 85 per cent. By hypoxia is meant an oxygen deficiency of such a degree as to be insufficient for proper tissue metabolism. Hypoxaemia is a reduced partial pressure of the oxygen in the blood which if marked will cause cyanosis. Cyanosis may be mild or absent in patients with obstructive airway disease until a late stage of the disease although the dyspnoea on exertion is severe. Such patients are facetiously referred to as 'pink puffers' and the explanation is that a vigorous respiratory drive causes hyperventilation which is sufficient to maintain a relatively normal blood milieu. This is in contrast with those patients who have diminished respiratory drive and hypoventilation causing cyanosis which will be intense if heart failure supervenes. These are 'the blue bloaters'.

Examination of the chest

Examination of the chest should always follow the standard pattern of inspection, palpation, percussion and auscultation. If possible the patient should be examined while sitting, preferably on a stool or a hard chair.

INSPECTION

On inspection any abnormality of the skin is noted. Apart from papular and nodular lesions due to secondaries, especially from the bronchus, or reticuloses such a lymphadenoma, skin lesions over the chest are unlikely to have any association with lung lesions. However, pulmonary actinomycosis may present as a swelling of the chest wall and later as a sinus (empyema necessitans). Enlarged veins over the chest should never be ignored as although by themselves they often have no significance, they are always suggestive of superior vena caval obstruction, and confirmatory signs of this should be sought.

Swelling and tenderness of the ribs and sternum are often found in myelomatosis, in leukaemias and also with secondaries. Unfortunately these important findings are often missed. Paget's disease may be suspected and even confidently diagnosed if there is deformity and enlargement of the clavicles. Marked tenderness and swelling of the costo-chondral joints of the upper ribs, and sometimes also of the sterno-clavicular joints, may be due to a self-limited condition of unknown aetiology, Tietze's* disease. Swelling of the sterno-clavicular joints is commonly seen in rheumatoid arthritis and gonococcal arthritis and rarely in non-specific urethritis.

Chest deformities

Flattening

Flattening of any part of the chest may be present and this may be secondary to pulmonary disease, to disease of the ribs or to scoliosis (postural or structural). However, unilateral gross pulmonary disease

---

*Tietze (1864–1927), a Breslau surgeon.

can itself cause scoliosis. If the scoliosis is the primary deformity, then the chest is usually flattened anteriorly on the same side as the convexity of the scoliosis, while if the scoliosis is secondary to lung disease, the chest flattening is on the same side as the concavity of the spinal deformity, but this distinction is not important. Flattening of the chest anteriorly or posteriorly over the upper or lower zone or both, when secondary to pulmonary disease, indicates a chronic lesion, either a fibrosis or collapse of the underlying lobe, but the presence of such flattening should always favour fibrosis rather than collapse.

'Barrel'

A 'barrel deformity' of the chest is characterized by an increase in the antero-posterior diameter with a dorsal kyphosis; the ribs and clavicle are more horizontal than normal, the supraclavicular fossae are filled in, and the subcostal angle is greater than the normal 90 degrees. The last can be readily estimated by placing each hand along the lower costal margin with the palms pressing against the under-surface of the lower ribs and the finger-tips of both hands touching. The normal ratio between antero-posterior and lateral chest diameters is roughly 5 to 7, but with a barrel deformity the ratio approximates to unity. Such chest deformity is found in, but is not synonymous with, emphysema.

'Pigeon'

A 'pigeon chest', pectus carinatum, is characterized by marked prominence of the upper part of the sternum and adjacent costal cartilages; the lower sternum is usually also prominent but occasionally is depressed (*see below*). The ribs are usually unduly sloped and gross kyphoscoliosis is common. There may in addition be a Harrison's sulcus, which is a groove directed outwards and slightly downwards over the lower chest anteriorly and which is reputed to be along the line of diaphragmatic attachment. Such a chest deformity indicates rickets or chronic chest infection in childhood or, of course, both. Rarely it may be a congenital anomaly. The presence of a Harrison's sulcus favours rickets.

A prominent sternum may be secondary to a gross kyphosis, for example due to tuberculosis of the upper dorsal spine.

'Funnel'

A depression of the lower end of the sternum occurring without other chest deformity is often called a funnel chest, pectus excavatum or trichterbrust. It is then nearly always congenital and is reputed to be associated with and perhaps due to a short central diaphragmatic tendon. This deformity is occasionally occupational, for example in cobblers. If it is found in association with any other chest deformity, the likely aetiology is rickets.

'Rickety rosary'
Permanent knobbly projections of the costo-chondral junctions are commonly seen as a result of rickets and are usually associated with other deformities of the ribs or sternum.

Any deformity of the ribs or sternum is likely to be associated with a spinal deformity, and may also cause the following in order of frequency: (1) cardiac displacement rendering clinical assessment of cardiac size very difficult; (2) a systolic bruit over the praecordium, which in itself is of no significance; (3) right-sided cardiac failure. However, the frequency of cardiac complications has been greatly exaggerated.

Degree of chest movement
The degree of chest movement on deep breathing, and whether or not it is symmetrical, should always be noted, and this is best assessed whenever possible with the patient lying flat and the physician standing at the foot of the bed. Another method, if the patient is lying flat, is for the physician to examine the chest from either side of the patient and with his eyes level with the manubrium. If the patient is sitting his chest movement can be assessed by looking over the patient's shoulders at the upper parts of the chest anteriorly so that they are observed tangentially. Asymmetry of chest movement indicates that the disease is unilateral and on the side showing diminished movement or, if bilateral is greater on that side. Any disease of the underlying lung or pleura will interfere with chest movement in the affected area, and gross symmetrical diminution of chest expansion as a whole may be a very important clue: even the only evidence of emphysema or bilateral fibrosis or ankylosing spondylitis. Normal chest expansion in an adult, when measured round the maximum circumference of the chest and recording the difference between deep inspiration and deep expiration, should be at least two inches.

Women make more use of their intercostal muscles than their diaphragm, and therefore their respiratory movements are predominantly thoracic, while in men they are mainly abdominal.

In any patient with peritoneal irritation or gross abdominal distension from any cause, respiration becomes entirely thoracic. Ankylosing spondylitis, paralysis of intercostal muscles, or severe pleural pain may make respiration entirely abdominal.

PALPATION
Palpation is used to measure chest expansion by placing the observer's hands symmetrically on each side of the chest and asking the patient to breathe deeply. The thumbs are placed almost vertically immediately to either side of the midline, and the fingers are held as horizontal as possible and pointing outwards. With practice this

technique will be found to be more helpful than placing the thumbs together horizontally and the fingers vertically. Some find it more helpful to keep the fingers flexed but the young physician is advised to try various methods and discover which he finds the easiest and most helpful. Possibly it may depend on his finger span. The performance is repeated both anteriorly and posteriorly over the upper, mid and lower zones of the chest. When assessing movement posteriorly the patient should be leading forward slightly with his hands clasped on top of his head.

Determining the position of the apex beat on palpation must always be an important part of the examination of the chest, as the apex beat may be shifted to the left by collapse or fibrosis of the left lower lobe or by a right pleural effusion or pneumothorax, and displaced to the right by a left pneumothorax or pleural effusion or by collapse or fibrosis of the right lower lobe.

For reasons explained previously, each individual rib and the sternum must always be felt for swelling and tenderness. Tenderness of the sternum is very common in acute primary blood diseases, especially leukaemia.

Position of the trachea

The position of the trachea should never be ignored as it constitutes one of the most important clinical signs in chest disease. It may be the only clue, for example, to fibrosis of an upper lobe. Students today, too often like their teachers, depend on radiographs to determine the position of the trachea. With practice, however, a correct location of this can be made in the great majority of cases, and the realization that the technique is difficult to master should make the student practise all the more.

The patient's neck should be slightly flexed and not rotated, so that the chin remains in the midline of the body. The commonly advised method is to insert the index and middle fingers in the suprasternal notch and then attempt to feel for tracheal displacement. The author has found hooking the index fingers, one on each side, around the tendon of insertion of the sterno-mastoid immediately above the clavicle, with the palmar aspect of the fingers against the tendon and the nail pressing against the lateral wall of the trachea, to be a better method. It is frequently easier to appreciate the tracheal position with the patient sitting up. Sometimes there is a visible undue prominence of the clavicular head of the sterno-mastoid muscle on the side to which the trachea is deviated, but this sign is not likely to help when the position of the trachea is equivocal clinically. If there is doubt as to whether or not the trachea is deviated, it is advisable to regard it as being central.

Large swellings in the lower part of the anterior triangle of the neck or in the superior mediastinum may compress the trachea or, if unilateral or grossly asymmetrical, may push it over to the opposite side. A thyroid swelling is the only neck swelling which commonly causes lateral tracheal displacement. The trachea may be deviated to the side of the lesion in fibrosis or collapse of an upper lobe. It is rare for the trachea to be displaced by a pleural effusion or a pneumothorax, however large it may be.

To talk about deviation of the trachea and of the heart is far better than to use the much vaguer term 'mediastinal shift' which is frequently employed. The emphasis must be that it is only lesions of the upper lobes which will cause deviation of the trachea and lesions of the lower lobes or pleura which will cause deviation of the heart. If the fibrosis or collapse be only of a segment of the lobe or bilateral, then deviation of the trachea or heart is very unlikely.

Axillary lymph nodes

The details concerning enlarged lymph nodes in the neck (*see* Chapter 10) also apply to the axillae.

The examiner should be facing the seated patient and should support the patient's arm. When feeling the right axilla the support should be with the examiner's right hand, using his left hand for the actual palpation. The opposite hands are used for palpation of the left axilla. The palpating fingers must be flexed and slightly cupped and the palpation should start as high in the axilla as possible, the fingers being slowly brought lower while exerting a constant gentle pressure against the chest wall. Excessive abduction of the arm must be avoided because this will interfere with deep palpation. The posterior, lateral and pectoral groups of nodes should be felt for in turn, and the whole procedure should then be repeated while the examiner is behind the patient. Enlargement of the pectoral group is sought for by inserting the fingers beneath the pectoral muscle. The subscapular group in the region of the posterior axillary fold is better approached from behind, with the patient's arm raised to a right angle and supported by the physician holding the wrist or elbow with his free hand.

Palpation for enlarged lymph nodes in the neck, supraclavicular fossae and axillae is an essential part of every chest examination.

The breasts

Examination of the chest in men as well as in women must always include careful palpation of the breasts to exclude a carcinoma. Any chest lesion may be secondary to this. The breasts, including the nipples, should be inspected for symmetry and skin changes.

The breasts should be palpated with the palmar aspect of the fingers and the palm itself, using one hand only, this being moved in a rotatory manner while exerting at first gentle and later increasingly firm pressure against the chest wall. Examination of each quadrant must be carried out in turn. Especially if the breasts are pendulous, it is better for the patient to be sitting and leaning slightly forward.

It often helps if in addition the breasts are also examined with the patient's hands clasped behind her neck or on top of her head and with her arms horizontal and each elbow supported in turn by the examiner's non-palpating hand. Stand on the patient's right side to examine her right breast and on her left for her left breast. Any swelling of the breast that can be felt with the flat of the hand is probably neoplastic. Fibro-adenosis (known for many years as chronic interstitial mastitis), can be readily palpated only when the breast is felt between fingers and thumb. A single well-defined swelling is very likely to be neoplastic (simple or malignant) and multiple ill defined lumps to be non-neoplastic. Peau d'orange involvement of the skin is an early sign of malignancy. Retraction of the nipple occurs with malignancy and following a breast abscess, but is significant only if it is of recent origin, because it may occur in an otherwise normal breast. The nipple and the underlying tissues should be gently palpated for lumps and for thickening of the duct.

Gynaecomastia is the presence in males of breast tissue. Obese men commonly accumulate fat in the breast region, but this must not be mistaken for true gynaecomastia. The latter occurs in Cushing's syndrome from whatever cause, and very rarely with tumours of the testis (especially teratoma and chorionepithelioma), in thyrotoxicosis and in Addison's disease. It may be seen in intrathoracic malignancy even in the absence of endocrine therapy or endocrine metastases. Gynaecomastia is a usual but not a necessary accompaniment of Klinefelter's syndrome. It is occasionally found in liver disease and sometimes in renal failure, especially when treated by dialysis. Therapeutic agents which may cause it are oestrogens, spironolactone, and rarely digitalis. Patients with leprosy complicated by testicular atrophy often have gynaecomastia.

Vocal fremitus
Vocal fremitus, the transmission of voice sounds felt by the examiner's hand when the patient loudly repeats some such phrase as 'ninety-nine' or '1,1,1' without stopping and in as deep a voice as possible. The corresponding parts of the right and left side of the chest are compared in rapid succession. This should never be a laborious procedure, because repetition of it and hesitation on the examiner's part is not likely to help but rather to cause further doubt. In any case, vocal resonance is easier to assess and always exhibits the same alterations as vocal fremitus. Because of the possible unequal sensitivity of the physician's hands, the same hand is used for both sides and not both hands on opposite sides simultaneously.

PERCUSSION
Percussion of the chest is often done very badly. The technique must be so uniform and automatic that the physician can concentrate on

the note elicited and not on the method of percussion. The various notes obtained on percussion are essentially comparative, and therefore every aspect of percussion must be identical each time it is performed.

It is important not to keep on tapping one area many times, because each tap will produce a different note and more uncertainty. Try to develop the technique whereby an opinion on the percussion note can be given after, at most, two taps. Moreover, always compare the corresponding part of the chest on the opposite side. It is always better to percuss with the patient sitting up rather than lying down, because the latter position may produce false signs. However, if the patient is too ill to sit up even when supported then percussion posteriorly should be done with the patient rolled on to each side in turn, but then only gross differences between the two sides should be considered significant. The percussion note elicited varies in different parts of the chest and the note, for example, at the base of the lung should never be compared with that over the clavicle. It is immaterial whether percussion is carried out over the ribs or the interspaces, but it is imperative to do the same on both sides and so compare like with like.

When percussing it is important that the pleximeter finger be applied accurately and with sufficient firmness but not pressed too hard and, moreover, that it be applied in precisely the same manner on the opposite side of the chest. The pleximeter finger should never lie across a rib but should be entirely in an interspace or entirely along the rib percussed. The percussion stroke must be made with the pad and not the tip of the finger; it must be made from the wrist, must strike at right angles to the pleximeter surface and must be short, sharp and decisive, the percussing finger being raised immediately the pleximeter finger has been struck. In comparing two areas the force of percussion must be the same at each site. It is advantageous to percuss directly with the flexed middle finger the centre of each clavicle in turn, and to percuss both lung bases with all fingers of one hand without using the other fingers as pleximeters and then later to percuss these areas in the more conventional fashion.

The percussion note normally varies over different parts of the chest, being least resonant at the lung bases. What constitutes the normal note at any area can be learnt only by a great deal of practice. One should always proceed from resonant to dull and not the reverse because it is easier to appreciate this order of change. Percussion over the manubrium should always yield a resonant note, dullness indicating a superior mediastinal swelling.

In addition to taking cognizance of the character of the note elicited, the degree of resistance appreciated by the pleximeter finger should be carefully observed. In percussing posteriorly the patient's head should be flexed, his shoulders drooping and his arms folded loosely with his hands on the opposite shoulder tips. Do not forget to percuss the axillae: it is amazing how many people, when examining chests, forget to percuss and to auscultate the axillae and so perhaps miss the only important positive signs.

The percussion over any given area may show increased or diminished resonance compared with what it normally should be in that area. Hence, a unilateral lesion is much easier to diagnose than a bilateral one because in the latter case there is no longer any means of comparison. A hyper-resonant note is lower in pitch and definitely more vibrant than normal resonance. A tympanitic note is higher pitched than normal and has a ringing quality. An amphoric note is similar but with a metallic quality. Dullness indicates definite pathology, but resonance does not imply the absence of pathology. Light percussion is necessary to determine the lung margins anteriorly and laterally but heavy percussion is necessary posteriorly. During quiet respiration the lower lung border is in the line of the sixth rib in the midclavicular line, the eighth in the midaxillary and the tenth in the scapular line. The upper borders of the lungs should be percussed over the trapezius muscles. By tidal percussion is meant a method for detecting the increase in the limits of the area of resonance over the lower borders of the lungs in deep inspiration compared with deep expiration and when such a difference can be detected it indicates satisfactory ventilation. It is a very difficult sign to demonstrate.

In some medical schools it is taught that the word 'dullness' implies the presence of effusion and terms like 'absolute dullness', 'stony dullness' and 'flatness' are frowned upon, although they all have a long usage and are usually regarded as synonyms. Such quibbling is an abuse of the English language, because the word dullness in any connotation implies a comparison. However, this objection can be overcome by using the phrase 'impairment of percussion' and always preceding the term by one of the qualifying adjectives slight, moderate or marked, recognizing the great difference between the slightly impaired percussion note, for example, of a fibrotic lung and the marked impairment over a pleural effusion.

The advice of a distinguished clinical teacher should be followed:

'We must not explore the chest by percussing our ideas into it; we must rather give our attention to listening to what comes out. The principal task in the course of percussion is to encourage the beginner in an honest method of investigation, and to guard him against the intrusion of previously formed judgments' (F. Müller*).

*Friedrich von Müller (1858–1941), a German physician.

AUSCULTATION

On auscultation of the chest, the physician should demonstrate to the patient exactly how he wishes him to breathe — deeply but not noisily, with his mouth open to minimize any sounds produced in his nose, but not holding his breath at the height of inspiration and not attempting to force expiration. Coughing after deep breathing is often helpful as it may bring out crepitations not previously heard. A diaphragm should not be used for chest auscultation because it is likely to cause misleading findings.

Classification of breath sounds
The classification of breath sounds is the same the world over and follows a nomenclature originally stated by Laennec in 1819. There are two groups of breath sounds, vesicular and bronchial.

Vesicular breath sound
A vesicular breath sound may be diagrammatically represented ∧ , which illustrates that the inspiratory sound is followed immediately without an interval by a shorter expiratory sound. It is reputed to resemble the noise made by wind rustling in the trees, which is perhaps more poetic fancy that fact. What vesicular breath sounds actually sound like, and the same applies to all breath sounds, can in fact be learnt only by hearing them frequently.

Vesicular breathing has several subdivisions as follows:
1. Normal vesicular breathing, as described above.
2. Puerile, in which the breath sound is merely louder than normal. This is found in children and in adults with thin chest walls, and in either case is of no significance.
3. A prolongation of the expiratory phase. This type of breath sound is frequently referred to as 'harsh'. Perhaps a better term is 'prolonged expiration', but if the word 'harsh' be used at all it must be used only in compliance with the above definition and not otherwise. Such a breath sound may be diagrammatically illustrated ∧ and is found in patients with partial bronchial obstruction from whatever cause. The commonest cause is bronchitis, but asthma or any other obstructive lesion will also produce this type of breath sound.
4. Cog-wheel, a jerky interrupted breath sound diagrammatically represented ‚⁓ˏ which is frequently heard in patients who are not breathing satisfactorily during auscultation, for example due to nervousness. This type of breath sound is heard in normal people and is of no significance.

Bronchial breath sound
The important difference between a bronchial and a vesicular breath sound is one of quality, a bronchial breath sound always having a blowing quality; in addition, the expiration is prolonged

and there is a short gap between inspiration and expiration. It is important to note that it is the blowing element which is the most important of all the three differential attributes described. A good way to imitate bronchial breathing is to place the tongue against the roof of the mouth and quietly to blow in and out through the open mouth. It can also be imitated by whispering the word 'who'.

Listening over the trachea, which is often advised, produces a loud, intense, very low-pitched type of bronchial breathing such as is not often heard clinically and therefore may give the beginner an erroneous conception as to what to expect. In actual fact, as stated above, the best way and the only truly satisfactory way for beginners to learn what this or any other breath sound is like is to listen to patients exhibiting these various phenomena, because it is virtually impossible to imitate or describe them adequately. A bronchial breath sound may be diagrammatically illustrated ∥\ .

Bronchial breathing is found over consolidation but may also be found over collapse, over an effusion or pneumothorax, or over a cavity. The breath sounds are classified according to pitch, high-pitched sounds being designated tubular. Tubular breath sounds are reputed to be pathognomonic of consolidation and not to occur in any of the other conditions named above. Whether this is really so or not is impossible to say, because what may be high-pitched to one person may not sound high-pitched to another, and if the examiner is virtually tone deaf, as many doctors are, then it would be better not to indulge in any finesse of subdivision according to pitch.

Low-pitched bronchial breathing is called cavernous, and if it has a superadded element as though blowing over the neck of a jar it is called amphoric (*amphora* is Latin for jar). The only way to imitate this is to blow intensely over the neck of a jar and note the sound produced; if anything like that is heard when listening to a chest, that breath sound should be designated amphoric. If one blows softly, the resultant sound very closely resembles cavernous rather than amphoric breath sounds, but the essential though subtle difference between these is the metallic quality of the amphoric sound. Both cavernous and amphoric breathing are suggestive of cavitation, but are not pathognomonic because either may also occur with consolidation and, occasionally, with a pneumothorax.

'Broncho-vesicular breath sound'. This term is sometimes used for a type of breath sound representing, so to speak, a half-way house between true bronchial breathing and harsh vesicular breath sounds. It is described as one in which, although inspiration is blowing and expiration is prolonged, there is no gap between the expiratory and inspiratory phases as in true bronchial breathing. Sometimes this type of breath sound is called 'indeterminate', but it is important to note that it is usually the listener who is indeterminate (not being able to make up his mind) rather than the sound itself. Broncho-

vesicular breath sounds can normally be heard near the midline over the upper part of the chest, but elsewhere they are pathological and their significance is the same as that of bronchial breath sounds. Sensible physicians do not auscultate in the region of the midline of the chest either anteriorly or posteriorly.

'Diminished air entry'. This phrase is frequently used, but the simpler descriptive term 'diminished intensity of breath sound' is preferable. It is very important to realize that in any pathology of the lung (including pneumonia) or pleura the breath sounds may be slightly, moderately or markedly diminished in intensity.

Adventitious sounds

The great difficulty concerning adventitious sounds is that there is no single classification which has had general recognition, with the result that there is great confusion. It is possible to know one's way around a big city such as London without knowing the names of the streets, but the difficulty will arise when conversing with other people about London's topography. If three different people call the same road by three different names, then intelligent discussion concerning, for example, how to get from one place to another becomes impossible. The same applies to adventitious sounds in the chest. Each individual pundit may well be able to recognize and correctly interpret the adventitious sounds which he hears; but if three different authorities call the same adventitious sounds 'rales', 'moist sounds' and 'crepitations' respectively, then what is the listener — particularly if he is a student — to make of it all? This subject will remain difficult and students will remain confused until some authoritative body lays down what should be taught. The author has found that a simple classification into pleural rub, rhonchi and crepitations is quite sufficient.

Pleural rub

A pleural rub is a squeaking sound like that produced by a new pair of shoes. It is usually localized to a fairly small area, is increased by pressure of the stethoscope and does not disappear on coughing. It can usually be felt with the palm of the hand. In contrast, rhonchi are occasionally palpable, but when they are it is over a large area. Crepitations are never palpable. A pleural rub can be imitated by pressing the palm of one hand against the ear and slowly rubbing the back of that hand with the fingers of the other. A pleural rub indicates a pleurisy — that is, a lesion of the pleura, not necessarily inflammatory — and disappears with the development of an effusion.

Rhonchi and wheezing

Rhonchi are continuous sounds which diminish on coughing and are audible during the greater part of inspiration and expiration. It is impossible to describe them accurately in words, but the condition of bronchitis is so common and the opportunity of hearing rhonchi is, therefore, so frequent that familiarity with them can be easily acquired. Rhonchi are produced in the bronchi and indicate partial bronchial obstruction, of which the commonest cause is bronchitis. They may be subdivided according to pitch, high-pitched rhonchi being called sibilant and low-pitched ones sonorous. The latter will be heard when the large bronchial tubes are involved, and the former when the smaller calibre tubes are affected. The classification of rhonchi into types has therefore got some value, although this is limited. Rhonchi, when marked, may be audible without the use of a stethoscope, and they are also occasionally palpable.

Wheezing is a high-pitched abnormal sound which can be heard without stethoscopic aid in patients with broncho-spasm especially during an acute attack or any other obstruction to a main bronchus. It can often be heard distinctly by the patient and often by those standing nearby. Wheezing and asthma are not synonymous and all that wheezes is not asthamatic. Sometimes it is well heard when the stethoscope bell is put in the patient's open mouth. No accurate word image can be given of this or of many other auditory phenomena. Some regard the description of a wheeze as a low-pitched rhonchus as incorrect and classify it separately from the other adventitious sounds.

Crepitations
Crepitations are interrupted sounds heard mainly at the height of inspiration and the beginning of expiration, and are accentuated and even brought out by coughing. Again the best way to know what crepitations are is to listen to a chest which contains these sounds, but a way of imitating them is to rub together the hairs near your ear. This gives a very accurate reproduction but, unfortunately, not all crepitations have exactly this crackling quality.

Crepitations are produced by fluid, whether transudate or exudate, in the alveoli and therefore indicate a lung lesion, which may be of any nature. In bronchiectasis crepitations are heard, but this is because bronchiectasis is associated with collapse and/or consolidation of the alveoli distal to the lesion, and therefore there is a pulmonary lesion as well as the bronchial one. If objections be raised to this interpretation, then a more acceptable statement might be that crepitations indicate a lesion of the lung or bronchiectasis. Crepitations, unlike rhonchi, are never palpable and are never heard without a stethoscope.

Attempts have often been made to subdivide crepitations into many descriptive types, and the resultant nomenclature is usually confused and often extremely personal to the author. Statements are frequently made such as that in pulmonary oedema and bronchiectasis the crepitations are always of a coarse type, whereas in pneumonia, especially during the phase of red hepatization, they are fine; that over a cavity the crepitations are frequently 'tinkling' or metallic, and that with extensive fibrosis they are 'creaky and dry'. Now these descriptive terms are all very well, but if they are used it is important to be very careful not to make the terminology fit a preconceived notion of the pathology. For example, having decided that the patient has got bronchiectasis many clinicians would call any of the crepitations they heard 'coarse', because that is what they have been taught the sounds should be and they are not prepared to describe what they actually hear. By 'coarse' is usually meant sounds of mainly low frequency or pitch, and by 'fine' those of high frequency. But the subdivision of types of crepitations is a dangerous practice and more likely to lead one astray than to be of help.

Rales
The term 'rale' has purposely been avoided in this book because this is a word which, more than any other in chest diseases, is differently used by different clinicians. If this word is employed, it is imperative to define it exactly and state its significance. Laennec himself used the word rale as referring to the noisy breathing of many dying patients ('the death rattle'), the word being the French one for 'rattle', but when talking to students in front of patients he used the exact euphemistic Latin word 'rhoncus' and he thus considered the two words to be synonymous. Unfortunately the first translation of Laennec's memorable monograph stupidly ignored his views and confusion has reigned ever since.

To describe any adventitious sounds as 'moist' is usually making the description fit in with a preconceived notion of the pathology. For example, the clinician, having correctly diagnosed congestive cardiac failure, conjures up a vision of air bubbling through oedematous lungs, and so he is determined to describe any adventitious sounds he hears at the bases as moist. After all, how can a 'moist sound' be described in ordinary English?

Vocal resonance
Vocal resonance is the same as vocal fremitus but is elicited on auscultation instead of palpation. It also must be performed by rapid comparison of the equivalent part of the chest on each side. Increased vocal resonance is sometimes referred to as bronchophony; when it is markedly increased, the voice sounds can be very well heard when the patient merely whispers, and this phenomenon is called 'whispered pectoriloquy'. Aegophony is a bleating nasal quality in the vocal resonance which is frequently heard over the upper limits of a pleural effusion and, rarely, over consolidation.

Consolidation is usually but not invariably associated with increase of vocal resonance, and the same applies to cavitation. In the latter, whispering pectoriloquy may be heard, but this is not pathognomonic because it may sometimes be found over con-solidation. In all other pathologies of the lung and pleura the usual finding is a diminution of vocal resonance, such diminution being slight or marked, and all such impairment usually being directly proportional to the degree of impairment of the percussion note.

Diagnosis of chest conditions

The first stage diagnosis in respiratory disease is a combined patho-logical and anatomical one: bronchitis, emphysema, thickened pleura, pleural effusion, pneumothorax, consolidation, fibrosis, collapse or cavitation, and determining exactly where the lesion is. The physical signs elicited indicate the general pathology and its site but no more, and this constitutes the first stage of diagnosis.

The second stage is special pathology — that is, the cause of the pleural effusion, collapse or other condition. This is rarely possible with certainty on clinical examination alone, and frequently is not possible even on radiology. It is therefore necessary to attempt to diagnose the general pathology for certain and to postulate from the history, the site of the lesion and the associated features the likely cause of that pathology (special pathology), always discussing probabilities first and possibilities last of all.

In cases of bronchitis and also of emphysema, another pathology is frequently present and capable of being diagnosed — for example, bronchitis plus consolidation, or bronchitis plus emphysema plus bronchiectasis. In other conditions it is, in the great majority of cases, impossible to diagnose more than one pathology with certainty. Whereas two pathologies, such as consolidation and collapse, may occur in the same lobe, or pleural effusion and collapse at the same base, clinically it is possible to diagnose only one of these and no attempt should be made to be clever and diagnose both, because the result is more likely to be wrong than right. In special circumstances two different pathologies can be diagnosed in two different parts of the same lung with more certainty — for example, collapse of an upper lobe because of gross deviation of the trachea on that side and an effusion at the same base.

THICKENED PLEURA

The physical signs of a thickened pleura are that respiratory move-ments, percussion note, vocal fremitus and resonance, and breath sounds are all slightly impaired over the affected area without displacement of the heart or trachea. Radiographic examination usually shows a hazy and ill-defined opacity which, in the lateral view, will be a very small shadow compared with that shown in the

postero-anterior view because of the comparative lack of thickness
of the lesion when seen in profile. The normal pleura is not visible
on X-ray. Screening will demonstrate with greater certainty that the
opacity is in the pleura. The exception to the above radiographic
appearance is that when the thickened pleura has become calcified,
it is then shown in the postero-anterior view as a very dense shadow
with well-defined margins and often a bizarre shape, and it is this
latter point which frequently gives the clue to the real nature of the
opacity. The lateral view will again show that the opacity is not
lobar or segmental.

The diagnosis of thickened pleura must always be considered
clinically whenever one or more of the physical signs is slightly
impaired; but thickened pleura is only rarely a complete or satisfactory diagnosis by itself either clinically or radiologically because
it is, in the great majority of cases, associated with fibrosis or collapse
of the underlying lung, and it is this other lesion which is more
important than the thickened pleura.

Calcification of the pleura may result from any type of exudative
effusion, especially empyema or haemothorax. It may also be
associated with extensive and marked pulmonary fibrosis, especially
when due to tuberculosis.

PLEURAL EFFUSION

The physical signs of pleural effusion are that:
1. there is a shift of the heart towards the opposite side unless
   the effusion is small or encysted (the trachea is very unlikely
   to be displaced unless the effusion is extremely large;
2. movement over the area is diminished and the percussion
   note markedly impaired;
3. the breath sounds are usually grossly diminished;
4. there may be bronchial breathing, which is rarely intense and
   usually distant;
5. vocal fremitus and resonance are markedly diminished over
   the area except over the upper limits of the effusion (not
   above it as often stated), where the vocal resonance has a
   bleating nasal quality called aegophony. Aegophony can be
   imitated by counting aloud and then suddenly pinching both
   nostrils with the fingers while continuing the count.

Percussion

Some further percussion signs are of importance. The impaired
percussion note over an effusion, compared with that found in
collapse or consolidation, has the quality of the note elicited and
the resistance felt on percussing a solid brick wall in contrast to those
encountered with a wooden table. Such marked impairment of
percussion is a *sine qua non* of effusion, and if it is not found,

fluid is unlikely to be present. If this rule were remembered, fewer mistakes would be made. It is no use trying to be ambitious or smart and disgnosing a small pleural effusion because it is impossible to do so, since at the very least half a pint of fluid must be present. On the percussion note alone, in most cases, a correct diagnosis of pleural effusion can be made.

On the other hand, it is necessary to know other signs because of the occasional more difficult cases where other conditions, for example collapse, may closely simulate fluid. It is for this reason, and this reason alone, that other percussion signs are described and must be understood. Unless the effusion is encysted or there is a hydropneumothorax — that is, air as well as fluid — the upper limit of the impaired percussion note will exhibit a characteristic shape, highest in the axilla, with a remote resemblance to the letter S (Ellis's* S-shaped line). This can be elicited only with the patient sitting up, and signifies that the marked impairment of the percussion note is not of lobar distribution. The absence of an S-shaped line indicates either that one is not dealing with an effusion at all or that, if an effusion be present, it is either encysted or associated with air.

Triangular areas of slightly or moderately impaired percussion note, over which breath sounds, vocal fremitus and resonance may be diminished, are found posteriorly above an effusion and also over the opposite base. These areas of impaired percussion note are not, it must be observed, in themselves in any way diagnostic of pleural effusion, but it is important to realize that they do occur and are of no significance. If one did not know this, one would be tempted to diagnose incorrectly an additional pathology above an effusion or at the opposite base.

In a moderate-sized pleural effusion above the areas of impairment of percussion and below the clavicle there may be hyper-resonance, even amounting to tympany, which has been called Skodaic resonance, boxy note or relaxed lung note. In a patient with a pleural effusion, the absence of such hyper-resonance below the clavicle would suggest that the effusion was either very large or only small. More important, however, is the fact that tympany above the level of an effusion is not by itself strong evidence of a hydropneumothorax.

In a large left pleural effusion there will be diminution of the normal area of gastric tympany, which is situated over the lower ribs anteriorly and is bounded by the spleen to the left, the liver margin to the right, the lung margin above and the costal margin below. The correct way of eliciting this sign is with the patient sitting up. It is a sign which is rarely of value but on occasion may help, for example in differentiating between a pleural effusion and a

*Calvin Ellis (1826–83), an American physician.

F

collapse of the whole left lower lobe, especially in a case where it is difficult or impossible, owing to obesity or emphysema, to determine the position of the apex beat. Moreover, the physical signs of such a collapse may be accentuated by an associated paralysed diaphragm and thus even more closely simulate those of effusion.

The interpretation of the significance of the bronchial breathing sometimes heard over a pleural effusion is controversial. It is commonly taught that these breath sounds indicate a consolidation of the underlying lung, but the author does not think that any such inference should be drawn. He has frequently heard bronchial breathing over a primary tuberculous pleural effusion where there has been no question whatsoever of consolidation of the underlying lung. Such an explanation of bronchial breathing must have been wrong in those cases, and the author suspects that it is equally incorrect in most other cases. The true reason why such breath sounds are heard is unknown and cannot be explained in terms of physics.

It is extremely unusual to hear any adventitious sounds over a pleural effusion, although sometimes crepitations may be heard above and also on the opposite side of the effusion. Therefore, if adventitious sounds are heard over an area of marked impairment of percussion, the diagnosis of an effusion is likely to prove incorrect.

Radiography

A radiograph of a pleural effusion shows a homogeneous dense opacity with an ill-defined upper limit which is higher laterally, with shift of the heart to the opposite side and filling in of the costo-phrenic angle. The shape and extent of the opacity may be largely an optical illusion. The lateral view always shows filling in of the costo-phrenic angle posteriorly unless the effusion is encysted.

When all these signs are present on a radiograph there can be no doubt of the diagnosis, but if the effusion is small or encysted, some of the X-ray signs are often not present and a differential diagnosis from collapse and consolidation must be considered. The lateral view is usually decisive, showing that the opacity is not of lobar or segmental distribution.

The most frequent sites of encysted effusions are between the lobes, along the costal surface of the lung, and between the lung and the diaphragm. It may be difficult to differentiate between a middle lobe lesion and an encysted effusion in that area. The commonest cause of an encusted interlobar effusion is cardiac failure.

If there is air as well as fluid, then the upper limit of the opacity will be horizontal (fluid level).

Types of pleural effusion

It is important to realise that the physical signs, clinically and radiologically, of an effusion are the same whatever the nature of the fluid, and therefore the question as to its cause can be answered only when the features of the fluid have been determined by paracentesis. The fluid may be obviously purulent (empyema), or it may be milky (chylous), haemorrhagic or straw-coloured (serous). The differentiation of chylous effusions into pseudochylous, chyliform and true chylous is an extremely artificial one and should not be perpetuated.

Chylous effusions are seen where there has been injury or obstruction of the thoracic duct. The latter condition is usually produced by enlarged glands, which may be (1) neoplastic, for example from carcinoma, of the bronchus or stomach or in reticuloses such as lymphadenoma; or (2) inflammatory, as in tuberculosis. Injuries to the thoracic duct may occur at or soon after birth, sometimes due to over-enthusiastic resuscitation. Such chylous effusions are often incorrectly regarded as idiopathic. Filariasis is a rare cause of chylous effusions.

The commonest cause of a haemothorax is injury. However, the most frequent cause of spontaneous haemothorax is malignancy, although it occasionally occurs in tuberculosis, in primary blood disease (for example, leukaemia and primary purpura) and in pulmonary infarction. With any spontaneous haemothorax the amount of haemoglobin in the fluid is always very small, the effusion being bloodstained rather than blood.

The features which should arouse suspicion that a pleural effusion is malignant are (1) that it is a spontaneous haemothorax, and (2) that it recurs very rapidly within a few days after each successive tapping. Sometimes malignant cells can be demonstrated in the pleural fluid by special techniques and this would, of course, prove the diagnosis.

A serous pleural fluid may be either a transudate or an exudate. The latter has a high specific gravity, above 1.015, due to its high protein content which is usually above 2 grammes per cent. In fact, the history and also the signs outside the respiratory system nearly always enable an exudate to be distinguished from a transudate without much difficulty. Right-sided pleural exudates may occur with subphrenic or amoebic liver abscess. Transudates may occur in cardiac failure, severe anaemia, renal disease, hepatic cirrhosis and severe malnutrition, and Meigs'* syndrome (the association of a benign ovarian tumour with ascites and/or a hydrothorax). If the fluid is an exudate and is lymphocytic, with no organisms demonstrable on the film or by culture, one must be strongly suspicious that the effusion is tuberculous because of the known after histories of such patients, the majority developing overt pulmonary tuberculosis within five years.

The difficulty is sometimes encountered that a patient has had a lot of antibiotic therapy prior to paracentesis and that this may

*J. V. Meigs (1892–   ), an American obstetrician, described the syndrome in 1954.

have rendered what otherwise would have been an empyema into a sterile effusion, but in that case polymorphs rather than lymphocytes are found in the centrifuged deposit. Systemic lupus erythematosus and also pulmonary infarction may cause a sterile serous effusion of an exudative type. Rheumatoid arthritis may occasionally cause a sterile serous lymphocytic effusion resembling a tuberculous effusion but its distinctive feature is the very low sugar content of less than 30 mgm per cent.

Biopsy of the parietal pleura has proved useful in the diagnosis of neoplastic and tuberculous pleural lesions when performed by an expert using a special needle.

Eosinophils in a pleural effusion, particularly if associated with blood eosiniphilia, should arouse a suspicion of helminth infestation, especially hydatid. Eosinophils in any effusion make the diagnosis of malignancy unlikely.

PNEUMOTHORAX

A pneumothorax is the presence of air in the pleural cavity. This may be spontaneous or induced (diagnostically or therapeutically). Injury to the chest rarely causes a pneumothorax because both the visceral and the parietal layers are almost invariably torn by a fractured rib, resulting in air escaping from the lungs through the pleura into the subcutaneous tissues and producing surgical emphysema.

With a penetrating injury resulting in an open chest wound, a pneumothorax or a haemopneumothorax will occur. Here air entering freely through the chest opening produces mediastinal flutter, the mediastinal contents deviating to the healthy side on inspiration and to the opposite side on expiration. This is sometimes called a sucking pneumothorax and is very serious.

The severity of the symptoms in any pneumothorax depends on the rate as well as the degree of alteration of the interpleural pressure and also the existence of previous extensive lung disease. These days when physicians are always on the look out for evidence of coronary thrombosis or pulmonary infarction as the cause of chest pain associated with dyspnoea and shock the possibility of a spontaneous pneumothorax is often overlooked. A spontaneous pneumothorax may occur with an apparently healthy lung and is then usually due to the rupture of a subpleural bleb or bulla resulting from a congenital defect or previous bronchiole obstruction by inflammatory material.

The physical signs of a pneumothorax can be briefly described as hyper-resonance with silence. Movement of the area is diminished. The heart is shifted to the opposite side only if the pneumothorax is large and of high pressure. The hyper-resonance, which may amount to tympany (comparable with the note elicited normally over the centre of the abdomen), extends over an area which is not of lobar or segmental distribution. Breath sounds, vocal fremitus and vocal resonance are all impaired. Occasionally, however, bronchial breathing, usually of an amphoric type, is heard over the pneumothorax. The author believes that this is of no significance and that the commonly stated interpretation − namely that such breath sounds indicate that the pneumothorax is an open one, that is, that there is a pleuro-bronchial fistula − is incorrect. His evidence for this view is that he has frequently heard bronchial breathing in patients with an artificial pneumothorax in whom there could have been no question of the presence of a pleuro-bronchial fistula. Sometimes over a pneumothorax the breath sounds, any adventitious sounds and the vocal resonance all have a ringing quality which may be very suggestive to the experienced listener.

The additional sign which may be helpful in difficult cases is the coin sound. If one coin be placed on the front or back of the chest and the surface struck with the edge of another coin, and at the same time the clinician auscultates over the front of the chest if the percussion is performed posteriorly and at the back if it is done anteriorly, he will hear a metallic, bell-like sound described like that made by a blacksmith striking his anvil, a note which very few of us have ever heard. The only other pathology which will give these signs is a huge cavity. Occasionally, with a left-sided pneumothorax, a clicking sound or an extremely loud knocking or crunching noise synchronous with the heart may be heard. It is quite unlike a pleural rub or cardiac bruit. It indicates a pneumothorax and/or mediastinal emphysema, and is most often heard in patients who also have surgical emphysema of the neck.

A pneumothorax may be an extremely difficult condition to diagnose clinically even though the radiograph shows very gross changes. Mistakes are less likely to be made if careful examination of the trachea is carried out, because deviation of the trachea is extremely rare even with a large pneumothorax. Though hyperresonance is to be expected, the degree of this is often so slight as to be missed by even the most competent clinicians. Do not, therefore, always expect a drum-like tympanitic note. Often the only physical signs are diminution of movement, breath sounds, and vocal fremitus and resonance, closely simulating fibrosis; but the positions of the apex beat and trachea, if you can be certain of these, will be a very important guide.

A large congenital cyst (pneumatocele) of the lung, a large emphysematous bulla or rarely, at the left base, a diaphragmatic hernia may also give rise to 'hyper-resonance with silence' and thus simulate a localized or shallow pneumothorax. These conditions can also closely resemble one another radiologically.

If a patient with a pneumothorax has an impaired percussion

note at the base, the explanation of this will in large measure depend upon the degree of the impairment. If it is marked, but only if it is marked, it is likely to be due to a pleural effusion complicating the pneumothorax. Absence of an S-shaped upper limit will suport this diagnosis, and if the effusion be moderate or marked in amount, a splashing sound (Hippocratic succussion) may be elicited on shaking the patient and listening with the ear near the chest wall. If a pneumothorax patient has only slight or moderate impairment of percussion note over the base or any other area, one must consider the possibility of either a thickened pleura or a paralysed diaphragm (which may have been performed as a therapeutic measure).

In any patient with a hydropneumothorax, the possible order of events must be carefully considered and not presumed. The case may be one of pneumothorax (artificial or, less likely, spontaneous) complicated by an effusion; it may be an effusion complicated by a pneumothorax, usually induced accidentally or purposely during aspiration; or the fluid and the air may have occurred simultaneously because of gas-forming organisms or a pleuro-bronchial fistula. The same principle, of course, must apply when considering a radiograph of a hydropneumothorax, and guesswork should not be indulged in.

A spontaneous pneumothorax may be open, closed or valvular ('tension pneumothorax'). Normally the intrapleural pressure is negative, that is, less than atmospheric, being about −2 to −7 cm of water on inspiration and expiration respectively.

In the open pneumothorax there is still free communication between the ruptured lung (usually of an emphysematous bulla) and the pleural cavity. In a closed pneumothorax such a communication, having been present, has become sealed off by deposition of fibrin over the rupture. In the case of a valvular pneumothorax the hole has such a pattern that air gets into the pleural cavity with each inspiration, but the hole closes during expiration, preventing air returning from the pleural cavity into the lung and thus causing a rapid increase of pressure in the pleural cavity. The way to distinguish clinically between these three types is not on physical signs but on the history. If the patient's condition has remained more or less the same since the onset of symptoms, it is likely that the pneumothorax is open, but if his symptoms have lessened, then the strong probability is that the pneumothorax has closed. However, increasing severity of symptoms should always make one strongly suspicious of a valvular pneumothorax. The notion that the presence of amphoric breathing helps in this distinction is fallacious.

It is never justifiable to insert a needle into a pneumothorax merely to measure the pressure or to determine the type of pneumothorax. The only indication for the insertion of a needle is when the symptoms strongly indicate a valvular pneumothorax, and then the procedure is done not primarily to measure the pressure but for the relief of urgent symptoms.

BRONCHITIS

Bronchitis is a bilateral lesion of the bronchi associated with expectoration. Hypersecretion of the bronchial mucous glands is often regarded as the essential primary feature. Moreover, in Britain it is usually considered that the hypersecretion is caused by atmospheric pollution, including occupational dusts and fumes and cigarette smoking, and that infection plays only a minor and secondary role in its aetiology. But even if we accept these unproven hypotheses, many problems still remain. Why is it usually a disease of men in the lower social groups? Why do winter exacerbations occur? Can it cause impaired respiratory function of significant degree in the absence of emphysema, bronchospasm or other pulmonary involvement? There is no practical value in differentiating those bronchitics who have expiratory airway obstruction and calling their condition 'chronic obstructive bronchitis' because this is either a transitory or permanent progression of any chronic bronchitic.

In bronchitis the sputum is often mucoid rather than mucopurulent, but this does not exclude a primary inflammatory aetiology. Bronchitis itself never causes frank haemoptysis or even streaking of the sputum.

The physical signs of bronchitis are prolonged expiration plus rhonchi, and this is true whether the bronchitis is acute or chronic. If any other physicial signs be present, the patient must have some other condition in addition to the bronchitis. For instance, if he has clubbing of the fingers, bronchiectasis should also be suspected. If in addition he has marked bilateral symmetrical diminution of chest expansion, emphysema should be suspected. If there are crepitations as well as rhonchi, then he must have a lesion of the alveoli as well as bronchitis – for example, bronchiectasis, pneumonia or pulmonary oedema. The physical signs of bronchitis are bilateral and usually symmetrical. If the signs are unilateral or grossly asymmetrical, one should always suspect a partial bronchial obstruction producing a valvular mechanism and thereby causing an obstructive emphysema. Bronchitis itself produces no positive radiographic findings, such changes as have been described being in fact due to an associated emphysema, bronchiectasis, present or past, pneumonia or pleural thickening, and not to the bronchitis *per se*. The common practice of basing a radiological diagnosis of bronchitis on a supposed prominence of bronchial and vascular markings is completely unreliable and deplorable.

ASTHMA

The word asthma is derived from the Greek, meaning 'panting' or 'laboured breathing', and was previously used to include any type of dyspnoea and from any cause. It is a condition characterized by a paroxysmal wheezing dyspnoea, mainly expiratory, which is due to bronchial obstruction produced principally by widespread bronchial spasm but also by the plugging of the bronchi with mucus. Asthma causes an intermittent and reversible airway obstruction. It may be difficult to differentiate asthma from an acute exacerbation of bronchitis which also causes wheezing and which in bronchitis may in some measure at least be due to bronchospasm. Immediate relief with steroids or bronchodilators is sometimes regarded as diagnostic of asthma but this may be inconclusive if the response is either slow or incomplete and in many asthmatics of long standing the attacks do not always respond quickly or completely. Paroxysmal dyspnoea may also occur in either cardiac or renal failure; the terms cardiac asthma and renal asthma are sometimes used, but these phrases are both better avoided.

Asthma may be due to one or several of the following aetiological factors:

1. Allergic — that is, an abnormal response to a foreign protein which has been inhaled, ingested or injected. This group is sometimes called extrinsic asthma.
2. Infective, when the term 'infective asthma' is sometimes used: the infection is of sinuses, tonsils or the bronchi themselves, but may indicate an allergic reaction to protein produced by the infecting organisms. This group is sometimes called intrinsic asthma or non-allergic asthma.
3. Genetic.
4. Environmental.
5. Psychogenic: this is probably never by itself the sole aetiological factor, and there is no specific personality make-up.

In Europe outside Britain, often no attempt is made to draw a sharp distinction between asthma and bronchitis; these are regarded as essentially the same disease with either cough and sputum or paroxysmal dyspnoea predominating, and all bronchitics are considered to be either actual or potential asthmatics.

EMPHYSEMA

Emphysema of the lung is a condition characterized by permanent distension of the alveoli, the walls of which are often ruptured. The types of emphysema are as follows:

1. Generalized hypertrophic emphysema, discussed below.
2. Compensatory emphysema, in which a segment or lobe distends to make up for the diminution of lung volume caused by contraction of another segment or lobe as a result of fibrosis or collapse.
3. Obstructive emphysema. This is produced by a partial bronchial obstruction which has a valvular effect, allowing air to get into the lung with each inspiration but not allowing air to escape during expiration, and thus causing over-distension of

the alveoli of that segment or lobe. The usual cause of this is a foreign body (*see* page 168) or neoplasm.

4. Atrophic emphysema (senile or small lung emphysema). In this type, although the lungs are not macroscopically voluminous as in the other varieties of emphysema, microscopically the alveoli appear to be enlarged. This is produced by the breaking down of some of the alveolar walls, causing confluence of adjacent alveoli. The condition is found at postmortem examination in elderly people and has no clinical significance.

5. Focal emphysema, a complication of pneumoconiosis (*see* section on pneumoconiosis).

Generalized hypertrophic emphysema
Generalized hypertrophic emphysema is usually referred to simply as emphysema. Some physicians regard widespread lesions of the lungs (especially fibrosis) as an essential concomitant of the alveolar distension. This is an unorthodox and unhelpful limitation of the term.

In the majority of cases the cause is chronic bronchitis and/or asthma, but undoubtedly, emphysema can occur without previous bronchitis or asthma. Some clinicians complicate the discussion by maintaining that emphysema can itself cause bronchitis, which is yet another futile 'hen and egg' argument. It is undoubtedly true that emphysema and bronchitis are closely allied. Other possible aetiologies – for example, the blowing of wind instruments, and congenital abnormalities of the thorax – which were previously discussed *in extenso,* are today considered of very doubtful importance. This view of the aetiology means that any patient who has had bronchitis and/or asthma for several years should always arouse suspicion that he has emphysema as well, even though physical signs are completely absent. On the other hand the converse is equally true, namely that if the patient has not had chronic bronchitis and/or asthma, it is unlikely that he has got emphysema.

The essential pathology of emphysema is loss of the elastic tissue of the lung. The most important effects of emphysema are:

1. Irreversible airway obstruction. The breakdown of elastic tissue with a resultant narrowing of the airway which causes increase resistance to airflow and the trapping of air within the alveolar. A reduced intrapleural negative pressure reflects the diminution of elastic recoil of the lungs. The airway obstruction may be secondary to the dilated alveoli or its cause (a futile hen-or-egg argument).

2. Because of the trapping of air, the residual lung volume (dead space) is increased at the expense of the vital capacity, which is invariably reduced except in the very earliest stages of the disease.

3. Diminution of the capillary bed, producing a decrease in the area available for gaseous exchange and an increased resistance to blood flow.
4. Pulmonary hypertension.
5. Depression of the respiratory centre, leading to hypoventilation and later to the development of cor pulmonale.
6. It may cause a rise in arterial carbon dioxide tension and a fall in oxygen tension.

Emphysema is the commonest cause of cor pulmonale, a condition characterized by right-sided cardiac involvement secondary to disease of the lung or pulmonary vessels (*see* Chapter 14). Cor pulmonale is more likely to occur if in addition to emphysema there is dilatation and infection of the bronchioles. An unexplained feature is that there is no correlation between the apparent degree of emphysema and the severity of the heart changes. It is extremely important, however, to realize that emphysema and cor pulmonale are not synonymous. Cor pulmonale is a complication of emphysema and is not necessarily present in every emphysematous patient. Thus it is possible to have even severe emphysema without cor pulmonale, and there are other causes of cor pulmonale apart from emphysema. Moreover, emphysema is frequently found in middle-aged and older people who have in addition a coincidental hypertension, and in these patients any cardiac involvement present is just as likely to be due to this as to the emphysema and is, in fact, in most cases due to both.

On inspection the most important sign of emphysema is the diminution of chest expansion, and this is frequently the only physical sign. In moderate or severe cases there may be a mild degree of cyanosis, but marked cyanosis should always make one suspect coexistent pulmonary pathology (for example, pneumonia), cardiac involvement, or both.

Especially in those patients in whom bronchitic symptoms have been marked, cyanosis and symptoms of respiratory failure are likely to be the dominant features. In other patients, effort dyspnoea rather than cyanosis is present. But their facetious description as two distinct types, 'blue bloaters' and 'pink puffers', displays a childish delight in alliteration without due regard to accuracy.

Though emphysema itself will cause dyspnoea on even slight exertion, orthopnoea is very unusual unless there is in addition broncho-spasm, pneumonia or cardiac involvement. The accessory muscles of respiration may be in use, and abdominal respiratory excursion is often grossly diminished. Emphysema itself does not cause clubbing, and its presence should always arouse strong suspicion of the presence of some additional lesion such as bronchiectasis. An involuntary pursing of the lips is often seen during expiration, and this, by increasing the intra-bronchial pressure, may lessen the airway obstruction.

The patient may have a 'barrel chest'. However, it is very important to realize that a barrel-shaped chest and emphysema are not synonymous, as it is possible to have emphysema with a long thin chest and occasionally patients are seen with a marked barrel chest who have not got emphysema. Other deformities such as pigeon chest are sometimes seen coincidentally in emphysematous patients, but such deformities should not in themselves be considered as manifestations of emphysema.

In emphysema the apex beat is seen and felt with difficulty. Palpation also confirms the poor chest expansion.

The most important sign on percussion is a diminution of the normal areas of cardiac and liver dullness. The note over the whole chest is hyper-resonant, but this is extremely difficult to assess because the degree of increased note is usually only slight and the bilaterality of the disease gives no basis of comparison.

Tidal percussion, which has been described previously, is a difficult procedure which is rarely helpful in diagnosing emphysema.

Breath sounds are diminished in intensity and expiration is prolonged. Rhonchi, if present, are due to the associated bronchitis. A patient with emphysema experiences difficulty in breathing out rapidly and an excellent and easily performed way of demonstrating this, which is often as accurate and informative as many of the laborious and complicated pulmonary function tests, is to ask the patient to try and blow out a lighted match held about three inches from his lips whilst his mouth is held wide open.

Radiography
The radiographic appearance of emphysema can be extremely difficult to interpret with certainty even by an expert. It is characterized by an increased translucency of the lung fields with diminution of lung markings, especially of the arteries, which are reduced in size and number. Stated simply like this it all sounds very easy, but the degree of translucency and whether lung markings are well seen or not depend just as much on the X-ray exposure and the thickness of the patient's chest wall as on the actual condition of the lungs themselves. It takes a great deal of experience to be able to assess the adequacy of the radiological technique.

With regard to lung markings, it must be realized that radiologically the lungs normally have a delicate network or web-like reticular pattern produced by veins, arteries, lymphatics, bronchi, peribronchial stroma, and the division of alveolar septa. These striations are normally denser in the inner and lower lung fields and increase with age. Whether this pattern, especially the arterial markings, is normal, diminished as in emphysema, or accentuated as in pneumoconiosis may be obvious in marked cases but, when the changes are slight, it is extremely difficult for even an expert to be certain. On the other hand this does not justify the reluctance of some physicians, perhaps through fear of subsequently being proved wrong, to diagnose emphysema clinically or radiologically.

Emphysematous changes are more likely to be noticed on a radiograph if comparison is carefully made between the upper, mid and lower zones as well as between both sides, remembering that in muscular men the midzones may be less translucent than the others because of well-developed pectoral muscles. The X-ray changes may be most marked in either the upper or the lower zones.

Sometimes the radiograph shows ring shadows ('soap bubbles'); these are localized avascular translucent areas, usually 3–10 millimetres in diameter with well-defined hairline margins, and are due to blebs and bullae. These air spaces may be better visualized on a lateral view, when they are usually seen either between the heart shadow and the sternum or between the heart and the spine. Some regard differentiation between blebs and bullae as merely that of size, but others maintain that the visceral pleura is intact over bullae but not over blebs. Bullae are seen only in a small percentage of cases and when seen may be confined to one part of one lung and therefore not providing good evidence of a generalized disease which emphysema is. Bullae have to be differentiated from other causes of ring shadows, namely thin-walled cavities, pneumatoceles, and a localized pneumothorax.

The radiographs may also show evidence of a barrel-shaped chest, the ribs being more horizontal than usual and more widely spaced, the lower part of the chest splayed out and the diaphragm flattened and lower in position than normally because of the lung distension. In many emphysematous patients, especially in those with asthma, the heart shadow is narrower and more vertical than usual. If emphysema is complicated by cor pulmonale, but only if such complication be present, then enlargement of the pulmonary arc, the right atrium and the pulmonary arteries at the hila will be evident.

A further radiographic point is that whereas a bronchogram of a normal lung is like a tree in full leaf, that of an emphysematous lung is like a tree which has had its terminal branches lopped. The reason is that because of some unknown factor it is impossible to get the oil into emphysematous bullae. This fact may be useful in a radiological distinction between a large emphysematous bulla and a congenital cyst, which it is frequently easy to fill partially with the contrast medium.

Screening to demonstrate the poorness of lung deflation and the relative immobility of the diaphragm is the most accurate method for the experienced radiologist.

CONSOLIDATION

By consolidation is meant an area of pneumonia. The physical signs are diminished movement without shift of trachea or heart, a moderate impairment of percussion note with bronchial breathing which may be tubular in character, and vocal resonance and fremitus increased to a variable degree; often there are crepitations, and there may be a pleural rub over the area. Especially at an early stage of the disease, breath sounds may be diminished. An important point to realize is that frequently these physical signs are not all present; in fact, the diagnosis may have to be suggested on one physical sign alone, such as bronchial breathing or crepitations. Of course, in such a case other possibilities would have to be considered as none of these signs is individually pathognomonic. It is especially in virus pneumonias and in most bronchopneumonias that the physical signs are often minimal and bronchial breathing is frequently absent.

A radiograph shows either a patchy opacity (mottling) of segmental or lobar distribution or a homogeneous opacity, and in the latter case the differential diagnosis from collapse and encysted effusion should always be considered. Deviation of the heart or trachea excludes uncomplicated consolidation. A well-defined straight border to a homogeneous opacity favours collapse as opposed to consolidation, but on occasion, consolidations will also give this radiological sign. An encysted effusion will be excluded in a lateral view, which will show that the opacity is not of segmental or lobar distribution. It is often incorrectly stated by radiologists that a mottled opacity indicates a bronchopneumonia and a homogeneous opacity a lobar pneumonia. That this is not true can be demonstrated by the fact that a pneumonic opacity on one occasion may be homogeneous and two or three days later may be mottled or vice versa, and the notion that the pneumonia has changed from a lobar to a bronchopneumonic type is, of course, absurd. A pneumonia should not usually be regarded, clinically or radiologically, as a bronchopneumonia unless it is bilateral. Nowadays the differentiation between lobar and bronchopneumonia is no longer considered to be useful, pneumonias being better classified according to the organism responsible. In the pre-antibiotic era the distinction was important because lobar pneumonia when it resolved nearly always did so without any residual lung damage, whereas with bronchopneumonia permanent lung damage often resulted (*see* section on bronchiectasis).

An important point to realize is that neither the stethoscope nor a radiograph can indicate the organism responsible for an area of consolidation. Furthermore, consolidation may be secondary to bronchial obstruction – that is, consolidation and collapse may occur in the same lobe, but clinically and radiologically the signs are of one or the other and not of both. The diagnosis, therefore, of both consolidation and collapse of the same lobe, either clinically or radiologically, should never ordinarily be made unless there is a very strong evidence; for example, a patient with the clinical or radiological signs of a collapsed lobe who also has mucopurulent sputum must have infection as well as collapse.

A chronic or so-called unresolved pneumonia may be due to the following causes:

1. The organism, such as the tubercle bacillus, or a virus unresponsive to the therapy given. Most virus pneumonias are not amenable to antibiotic therapy and they may continue for six weeks or even longer. Lack of realization of this fact frequently causes quite unnecessary investigations to be undertaken.
2. The pneumonia is secondary to a partial obstruction of the bronchus.
3. There is a complication of the pneumonia, for example abscess or empyema.

MOTTLING

The radiological term 'mottling' is mentioned above. Following the Ministry of Health Circular,* it can be defined as multiple discrete or semi-confluent shadows, generally less than 5 millimetres in diameter. 'Miliary mottling' is where such shadows are bilateral, numerous, discrete, well defined and not exceeding about 2 millimetres in diameter. The term 'infiltration' is an ambiguous one and should not be used.

The causes of miliary mottling are as follows:

1. Miliary tuberculosis. Hilar gland enlargement is then very unusual.
2. Pneumoconiosis.
3. Sarcoidosis. Usually there is also bilateral hilar gland enlargement, and often bilateral fibrosis, and in addition to the miliary shadows there are others which are larger and less well defined and occasionally nodules.
4. Extensive bilateral pneumonia. The opacities are usually larger than 2 millimetres and not discrete, but any organism causing pneumonia may occasionally produce typical miliary shadowing. The pulmonary mycoses sometimes cause a miliary picture.
5. Miliary carcinomatosis is a rare form of pulmonary metastasis, usually secondary to a primary in the bronchus or stomach. Secondaries in the lungs usually cause a few large well-defined rounded homogeneous shadows. In miliary carcinomatosis a clue may be areas of rarefaction, or, less likely, sclerosis, of

*Ministry of Health, *The Standardization of Radiological Terminology in Pulmonary Diseases.* London: H.M. Stationery Office, 1952.

ribs and clavicles. Hilar gland enlargement is common but may not be present.

6. Pulmonary haemosiderosis secondary to mitral stenosis or as a rare idiopathic primary condition.

7. Polyarteritis. This should always be suspected if serial X-rays also show an increasing size of the left ventricle, the result of rising blood pressure.

Obviously the differentiation between miliary shadowing and mottling is not clear-cut, and miliary shadows may become confluent and thus indistinguishable from pneumonic mottling. Moreover, any mottled areas may conglomerate to form larger opacities which, if well defined, could be termed nodules. This commonly occurs in some of the pneumoconioses. The term nodulation should be used only when the areas are fairly well defined. In pneumonia there are often large areas of mottling, but most of these are ill defined and merge into each other. The only common causes of nodulation are pneumoconiosis secondaries and sarcoidosis.

In discussing the differential diagnosis of miliary shadowing, age, sex, occupation, and the presence of other radiological features such as enlarged hilar glands or bone changes (especially multiple areas of rarefaction) are important factors which must be taken into account.

COLLAPSE OF THE LUNG

Strictly speaking, the word atelectasis implies a lung which has never expanded — that is, a congenital lesion; but by common usage, and that is what determines language, the term has come to be synonymous with collapse. However, there is no special need to use the word at all.

Collapse of the lung may be due to its compression by a pleural effusion, a pneumothorax or, rarely, a large neoplasm, or may be of the absorption type due to bronchial obstruction. Such obstruction may be intra-, endo- or extrabronchial or any combination of these. When the word 'collapse' is used in relation to lung disease, absorption collapse is implied. The above statement also indicates the folly of diagnosing with any certainty effusion and collapse at the same base, because a pleural effusion of any size is always associated with a compression collapse of the underlying lung which will be indistinguishable, clinically and on radiographic examination, from an absorption collapse.

Physical signs

The physical signs of collapse can be briefly described as moderate impairment of percussion note with silence. The trachea is deviated to the affected side if the upper lobe is involved, and the heart is deviated if the lower lobe is involved unless the collapse is only partial or segmental. Percussion note, vocal fremitus and resonance, and breath sounds are all moderately impaired over the affected area. Sometimes there is bronchial breathing, occasionally with crepitations, over the area. Such findings are particularly common in post-operative collapse, hence such collapse was previously usually diagnosed as a post-operative pneumonia.

The radiograph shows a homogeneous, moderately dense opacity (except in the earliest stages when the opacity may be hazy and ill defined), with shift of the trachea if the upper lobe be affected and of the heart if the lower lobe be affected. The opacity usually has a well-defined straight border. When all these radiological signs are present, the picture is a pathognomonic one, but deviation of the heart or trachea will be seen only if the collapse is fairly extensive, and an involvement of only a segment or a partial collapse of the lobe will resemble the appearance of either consolidation or encysted effusion. The edge of a collapsed basal segment of a lower lobe must never be mistaken for the cardiac contour. This error will be avoided if it be remembered that the cardiac border is never a straight line. When the collapse is confined to one of the basal segments, the opacity may be visible only through the cardiac shadow by noticing a dense opacity with a straight oblique border within or immediately lateral to the cardiac shadow. A lateral view may help considerably as, in the case of collapse, the opacity will be shown to be of lobar or segmental distribution with contraction of that lobe or segment, often shown by displacement of a fissure.

Tomography is a technique whereby the lung can be visualized in serial sections, thereby minimizing the obscuring opacifications produced by overlying structures. Tomography or a bronchogram may prove the presence of a bronchial obstruction, but the former is often a preferable procedure, because the latter may further increase the collapse and therefore aggravate the patient's condition as well as interfering with the interpretation of subsequent films.

Middle lobe collapse
Because the right middle lobe bronchus originates at a very acute angle and is very nearly completely surrounded by lymph nodes, it is frequently obstructed due to enlargement of the hilar glands, often due to malignancy. Primary tuberculosis may affect the middle lobe bronchus because of either pressure by glands or endobronchial involvement. The resultant collapsed lobe often becomes bronchiectatic.

A patient with a collapsed middle lobe usually has a productive cough, sometimes wheezing, perhaps haemotyses, occasionally pleural pain and often recurrent bouts of fever due to recurrent lung infection. However, the clinical signs are nearly always minimal.

Middle lobe collapse radiologically produces a homogeneous dense opacity which has to be differentiated from consolidation and also from an encysted effusion. A lateral view is essential to prove that the opacity is of the middle lobe and is not a segment of either the upper or the lower lobe. But collapse of even the whole middle lobe may show no opacity in the postero-anterior view due to complete retraction of the lobe towards the hilum and compensatory emphysema of the other lobes. Even the right lateral view may be difficult to interpret because the shadow of a collapsed middle lobe may be superimposed on the heart and hilar shadows.

Often with collapse of the middle lobe a lateral view may not show any displacement or distortion of the fissure, and the lobe then will not appear to be contracted and the condition will be indistinguishable from middle lobe consolidation. If only the lateral division of the middle lobe bronchus is obstructed, a postero-anterior X-ray will show a diffuse, often not very dense opacity extending into the lower zone, with a relatively clear area separating it from the right cardiac border. The lateral view will show a triangular opacity posteriorly in the lower zone.

Obstruction of the medial division produces a diffuse opacity immediately adjacent to the right heart border, which in a lateral view is seen immediately behind the sternum and below the position of the horizontal fissure.

The lingula of the left upper lobe is the counterpart of the right middle lobe, and lesions of the former are common. A diseased lingula may show on a postero-anterior film as a shadow partially or completely overlapped by the heart shadow. The lateral view may show anterior displacement and accentuation of the fissure.

BRONCHIAL OBSTRUCTION

Collapse having been diagnosed, the next stage is to attempt to determine its cause, and it is important to remember that there are other causes of collapse apart from carcinoma of the bronchus. The collapse may, for example, be produced by a lesion within the lumen such as a foreign body, or by aspiration of septic material from the upper respiratory tract; by a lesion of the wall such as carcinoma of the bronchus; or by lesions outside the bronchus such as aneurysm or a mass of enlarged nodes (from neoplasm, reticulosis or inflammation). Bronchoscopy is usually an essential investigation to establish the cause. However, if one of the smaller bronchi is obstructed, it may not be possible to pass the bronchoscope far enough to demonstrate the lesion.

The effects of any bronchial obstruction on the lung depend on (1) the size and number of the bronchi involved; (2) the degree of obstruction, especially whether it is complete or valvular; (3) the nature of the obstructing material; (4) the speed with which the obstruction develops; and (5) the presence of infection distal to the obstruction.

INHALATION OF A FOREIGN BODY

The effects of inhalation of a foreign body into the air passages are described fully because the subject illustrates so many basic principles regarding bronchial obstruction.

Inhalation most commonly occurs (1) during anaesthesia (especially during dental and nose and throat operations); (2) in semi-comatose patients; (3) in those who indulge in the stupid trick of throwing things, for example peanuts, up in the air and catching them in their mouths; (4) in patients with bulbar palsy of any type; (5) in debilitated infants and children; (6) in careless people, usually children, who have the habit of putting small things such as coins or pins in their mouths; (7) in those who bolt their food, or drink large amounts of fluid while food is still in their mouth, especially if they have dentures.

Any foreign body, unless minute, will be held up in the larynx. Here it causes the sudden onset of choking, gagging and coughing and, later, stridor. No foreign body is likely to remain in the larynx for longer than a few minutes: it will either be coughed up with immediate relief, be inhaled into the trachea, or cause suffocation preceded by increasing stridor and cyanosis.

Any foreign body which has passed through the larynx is likely to drop unheeded through the trachea. But if the object be of such a shape — for example, a small button — that it can alter the position of its maximum diameter by rotating during its fall, it may become lodged in the trachea. Here again stridor will result. It may be possible also to hear a vibratory noise or thud on auscultation over the trachea. This is produced by the foreign body bobbing up and down with each respiration. The tracheal foreign body is likely to cause suffocation within hours unless it is either coughed up, when it may become lodged in the larynx, or inhaled into a main bronchus.

A foreign body is more likely to enter the right than the left main bronchus because the former is wider and comes off at a less acute angle. What happens later depends on the nature of the foreign body and its relative size compared with the obstructed bronchus. Vegetable (arachitic) foreign bodies, because they absorb water and swell within hours or at most days, cause rapid complete blockage of a large bronchus, with collapse of a segment or a whole lobe, resulting in retention of secretions and consequent infection. Thus, within a few days severe pneumonic symptoms and signs develop.

With other foreign bodies, their relative size compared with that of the bronchial lumen in which they lodge is most important. The question of the amount of infection introduced by the substance itself is often stressed but is of minor importance, as it is likely to be neither sterile nor teeming with highly pathogenic organisms.

Such a foreign body in a bronchus may allow air to enter and leave without hindrance (by-pass) and thus will not cause any pulmonary lesion. Or it may produce a check-valve effect, allowing air in but not out and so causing an obstructive emphysema of the distal lung. The striking physical signs then may be an asthmatoid wheeze, often best heard when listening at the patient's open mouth, and the presence of unilateral bronchitic signs. Hyper-resonance compared with the opposite side may be demonstrable.

On the other hand, the foreign body may produce a ball-valve mechanism, allowing air to escape from the lung but not to enter, or a stop-valve (corkage) effect, not permitting the passage of air either way. The result of either will be a complete absorption collapse. It must be understood that any one of the above mechanical effects can change into another, especially if the foreign body is inhaled further down into a smaller bronchus, so that although formerly it did not produce obstruction it will do so later; moreover, a check-valve mechanism may thus be converted into a ball-valve or stop-valve mechanism, with the consequences explained above.

When the foreign body lodges in the bronchus there is usually a long period, often of months and sometimes even of years, during which the patient is symptom-free (the 'long delusive interval'). After the lung collapses, it will sooner or later become infected, with resultant symptoms and signs of pneumonia or lung abscess. If the foreign body is not removed, permanent damage to the lung will develop, producing fibrosis and bronchiectasis or lung abscess with their own complications, both local and remote.

The details of all the possible physical signs which an inhaled foreign body may cause need not be enumerated because they are those related to the effect it has on the lung segment or lobe distal to it. It is important to realize that all which has been said about foreign bodies will apply equally to bronchial neoplasms, simple or malignant, which may have any of the same mechanical effects.

LUNG ABSCESS

The commonest cause of a lung abscess is bronchial obstruction due to a lesion of its lumen or wall or pressure from outside. Lung abscess is nowadays a rare complication of pneumonia. Any pyaemia, for example due to a pelvic infection, may be associated with multiple bilateral abscesses. The symptoms and signs of any lung abscess are identical with those of pneumonia or collapse and the X-ray appearance initially will also be the same as either of these. But later when the abscess ruptures into a bronchus the patient dramatically coughs up a large amount of foul purulent and often bloodstained sputum which may be followed by a temporary feeling of marked improvement. On X-ray the centre of the opacity becomes progressively less dense and later a fluid level develops. A tuberculous cavity is also really a lung abscess but the convention is to discuss lung abscess and tuberculous cavitation as two different conditions.

Surprisingly a fluid level does not develop in tuberculous cavities unless the disease has caused stenosis of a major bronchus.

FIBROSIS

The physical signs of fibrosis are essentially the same as those of collapse except that they are less in degree. In addition, the presence of flattening favours the diagnosis of fibrosis. The slightness of the physical signs is an important point always to be borne in mind. Often a fibrosis of an upper lobe is characterized merely by shift of the trachea and slight flattening, hence the great importance of being able to assess the position of the trachea correctly. The clinical diagnosis of fibrosis is very difficult.

The radiographic appearance of fibrosis is a non-homogeneous, usually streaky, opacity of lobar or segmental distribution, with shift of the heart if the lower lobe is involved and of the trachea if the upper lobe is involved, or there may be evidence of distortion of an interlobar septum. The radiological diagnosis of unilateral fibrosis should never be made unless there is evidence of traction on heart, trachea or septum. The main difference between the appearance of fibrosis and that of collapse is the more homogeneous opacity of the latter. Crowding together of the ribs on the side of the opacity compared with the other side would also favour fibrosis, and so would dilated bronchi or multiple small ring shadows indicative of bronchiectasis. The development of a single abscess cavity within an area of fibrosed lung is fairly common, but multiple cavities are unusual.

Causes of fibrosis

Having diagnosed fibrosis, the next state is to discuss the probable special pathology, and here the prime consideration must always be the localization of the condition. Fibrosis which is localized to or mainly involves an upper lobe should always make one think first of a tuberculous aetiology, whereas fibrosis localized to or mainly confined to a lower lobe should make one think first of bronchiectasis. However, it must be remembered that bronchiectasis may occur in upper and tuberculosis in lower lobes.

Pneumoconioses and sarcoidosis are important causes of fibrosis, but these are invariably bilateral and more or less symmetrical. It is often stated that pneumonia can cause fibrosis and this is true, especially of bronchopneumonia, but in these circumstances the fibrosis will invariably be associated with bronchiectasis, which should be diagnosed rather than talking about post-pneumonic fibrosis.

Two forms of diffuse bilateral interstitial pulmonary fibrosis of unknown cause are recognized, although they may be one and the same condition. The Hamman—Rich* syndrome occurs in children and has an acute or subacute onset. A similar condition, at least as regards the end result, but with a much more gradual onset, affects middle-aged males and females in roughly equal proportions and has been given many names including intrinsic fibrosing alveolitis, fibrosing alveolitis and idiopathic pulmonary fibrosis. The term 'intrinsic' is sometimes included to differentiate from the 'extrinsic' variety due to farmers' lung. Progressive dyspnoea and cyanosis develop, but there is little or no cough or sputum till late in the disease. Progressive cyanosis and clubbing develop. The chest shows gross diminution of expansion and possibly bilateral basal crepitations. Death is usually due to cor pulmonale. Initially, X-rays show a bilateral extensive ill-defined opacification of minor degree especially in the hilar area. Later there is linear streaking and bilateral mottling; the affected areas are usually small, but they may be large or even nodular. Later still, multiple ring shadows, often wrongly described as cysts, develop at both bases and mid zones. The condition may be mistaken for bilateral dry bronchiectasis, but bronchography demonstrates crowding and narrowing of the smaller bronchi and not dilatation. Lung function tests show that there is no airway obstruction. Histology shows marked thickening of the alveolar walls with intra-alveolar exudate containing macrophages, lymphocytes, and plasma cells. Later the alveolar architecture is destroyed and replaced by large areas of dense fibrosis which are separated by clear areas due to bronchial and alveolar distensions. Neither the histology nor the X-rays are pathognomonic and this condition has to be differentiated from other causes of bilateral fibrosis which may cause similar changes, namely, pneumoconiosis, sarcoidosis, rheumatoid arthritis, scleroderma, and systemic lupus erythematosus.

BRONCHIECTASIS

Bronchiectasis is a dilatation of the bronchi, which is nearly always permanent but occasionally is reversible. It should only rarely be regarded as a clinical entity, being rather an anatomical lesion with many possible causes.

For example, to the older clinicians tuberculosis was one disease and bronchiectasis an entirely different condition. But the real position is that bronchiectasis itself may initially be due to a tuberculous lesion. Enlargement of mediastinal lymph nodes due to a primary tuberculous process may cause bronchial obstruction, with resultant collapse and later bronchiectasis, even though the nodes themselves have healed; or a lobe which is fibrotic as a result of

---

*L. V. Hamman (1877—1946) and his contemporary, Rich, two American physicians, wrote their paper in 1944.

healed tuberculosis may show extensive bronchiectasis, and this explains why an apparently healed tuberculous lesion can still cause large amounts of tubercle-negative mucopurulent sputum or recurrent haemoptyses.

In fact, any condition which produces bronchial obstruction or pulmonary fibrosis may be associated with bronchiectasis. The phrase 'associated with' has been used purposely in order to avoid profitless quibbling as to which came first − the fibrosis, the collapse, or the bronchiectasis itself.

Bronchiectasis seen as post-mortem examination is characterized by:
1. dilatation of the bronchi with damage to the bronchial wall;
2. areas, small or large, of collapsed lung;
3. fibrosis of the affected segment or lobe;
4. frequently infection of the pulmonary segments supplied by the affected bronchi;
5. thickening of the overlying pleura.

The difficulty, a frequent one in medicine, is to attempt to place these changes in correct chronological sequence. In the great majority of cases the initial damage occurred in childhood as a result of bronchopneumonia, often complicating morbilli or pertussis. Exacerbations of symptoms in bronchiectasis are usually due to a complicating pulmonary infection and dry pleurisy rather than to extension of the bronchiectasis.

Except in the fairly rare bronchiectasis sicca, in which the only symptom is recurrent haemoptysis without mucopurulent sputum, the vast majority of cases give a history, usually from childhood, of recurrent bronchitis, frequently of recurrent dry pleurisy (dry because pleural adhesions prevent effusion), and often of attacks of pneumonia. Of recent years the view has been held by many that any damage to the bronchial wall is not of itself sufficient explanation for the dilatation, some additional factor being necessary. The factors most often invoked are:
1. Increase in intrabronchial pressure, often induced by stagnant exudate, for example that associated with bronchopneumonia complicating measles or pertussis.
2. Extrabronchial traction due to fibrosis.
3. Absorption collapse from any cause of bronchial obstruction, including mucopurulent sputum, with resultant increased intrathoracic negative pressure. This is due to the increased size of the pleural space, as a result of which mucus and exudate are likely to be sucked into collapsed alveoli and adjacent bronchioles, thus increasing and perpetuating the areas of pulmonary collapse. A collapsed lung is always very likely to become infected.

None of these factors excludes the others, although some physicians appear to consider them mutually exclusive.

That the symptoms of bronchiectasis often start in infancy is no longer regarded as evidence of a congenital aetiology. True congenital bronchiectasis, sometimes called 'cystic', does however occur, usually in association with fibrocystic disease (mucoviscidosis) or congenital dextrocardia.

Bronchiectasis is frequently associated with chronic sinusitis, and perhaps the inhalation via the nasopharynx of septic material from such a sinus constitutes an important factor in the production of the bronchiectasis, or at least in the maintenance of the infection.

There are no pathognomonic physical signs of bronchiectasis. The lower lobes are affected much more often than the upper. Clubbing is usually but not always present. Some signs of fibrosis or collapse may be demonstrable if the condition is predominantly unilateral. Often basal crepitations are the only sign. Rarely signs suggestive of cavity are present. Patients with bronchiectasis are very liable to recurrent pleurisy, and therefore it is not surprising that a persistent pleural rub over the area may be heard. Frequently the only physical signs are those of bronchitis, usually with emphysema.

A straight film may show:

1. No abnormality.
2. An area of fibrosis or collapse. If a basal segment is affected, the resultant area of collapse may produce a dense triangular shadow which is usually adjacent to the right cardiac border, with which it must not be confused. Sometimes the fibrosed or collapsed basal segment is retracted behind the cardiac silhouette and cannot be seen easily on the postero-anterior view unless it is well penetrated.
3. Increased hilar density, with radiating linear striations extending to the base.
4. Multiple small fluid levels.
5. Patchy opacities, often superimposed on any previous X-ray appearance and due to complicating pneumonia.
6. Rings with clear centres, usually within an area of fibrosis often described as 'honeycombing of the lung'. This term is undesirable and should be discontinued, as it is used by different authors in the following ways:
   (a) As a romantic description of the post-mortem appearances produced by multiple small saccular dilatations of the smaller bronchi and bronchioles.
   (b) As a romantic radiological description of ring shadows.
   (c) As a synonym for the extremely rare condition of true congenital bronchiectasis.
   (d) As a synonym for the lung changes sometimes found in adenoma sebaceum and pulmonary histiocytoses, which are conditions characterized by histiocytic proliferation of the reticulo-endothelial system and, in addition, by the formation of granulomatous lesions. Hand—Schüller—

Christian syndrome, Letterer–Siwe disease and eosinophilic granuloma are included in this group.

(*e*) As a synonym for an appearance often seen radiologically in patients with extensive marked pulmonary fibrosis from any cause. This is sometimes misleadingly designated 'cystic' in spite of the fact that the lesions are not cysts, which are encapsulated lesions containing fluid.

CAVITIES

The physical signs of a cavity are diminished movement; a cracked pot note on percussion; cavernous or amphoric breathing; crepitations, often of a metallic quality; whispering pectoriloquy, and post-tussive suction.

A cracked pot note is elicited by forcible percussion with several fingers during the height of inspiration, the note being accentuated by the patient having his mouth wide open. A good imitation of this note may be obtained by moistening the palms of the hands, clasping the two hands together and knocking the dorsal aspect of one hand against the knee. Post-tussive suction is elicited by asking the patient to cough, when a hissing sound is heard. This can be imitated by placing the tongue on the roof of the mouth and sucking air in rapidly through the open mouth. A cracked pot note or post-tussive suction will, it is true, never be heard unless the cavity is a large one, at least partially empty and communicating with a bronchus. However, this does not invalidate the important fact that both these signs in an adult are pathognomonic of a cavity and are the only pathognomonic signs.

The physical signs of a cavity are modified by the condition of the surrounding lung and pleura, the proximity of the cavity to the surface, its size, whether it is full of fluid or empty, and whether or not it communicates with a bronchus. Because of these factors, the physical signs of even a fairly large cavity may be nil, and with a small cavity are likely to be so. The presence of, for example, cavernous or amphoric breathing or whispering pectoriloquy, though not pathognomonic, should make one suspicious as to the possibility of a cavity, especially if the patient has a large amount of mucopurulent sputum.

To summarize, therefore, it can be stated that the finding of a cracked pot note or post-tussive suction allows a certain diagnosis of cavitation. In the great majority of cases, however, the presence of the condition can merely be suspected – for example, in a patient who has an area of pulmonary collapse or consolidation and who is expectorating a large amount of purulent or mucopurulent sputum. In patients with gross deviation of the trachea, cavernous or amphoric breathing and whispering pectoriloquy are very frequently heard, and though their presence should arouse one's suspicions of a cavity, the more likely cause of these signs is deviation of the trachea.

PNEUMOCONIOSIS

It is preferable to confine the term pneumoconiosis to permanent alteration in lung structure (mainly fibrosis) due to the inhalation of mineral dust, and not to include either bronchitis due to mineral dust but without pulmonary lesions or pulmonary diseases due to the inhalation of vegetable dusts such as shoddy cotton (byssinosis), cellulose from sugar cane (bagassosis), or from mouldy hay or grains (farmers' lung).

It is generally accepted that any dust can cause bronchitis without subsequent fibrosis, but the English legal definition for purposes of compensation does not include bronchitis without fibrosis. The compensation awarded is usually proportional to the degree of radiological change and not to the severity of symptoms. Coughing induced by chronic bronchitis caused by dust inhalation may minimize dust accumulation in the lungs and therefore the resultant fibrosis, but nevertheless may lead to the equally disabling condition of emphysema.

The effect of any dust on the lungs depends on:

1. The molecular size of the dust, which must be less than 5 microns to cause pulmonary lesions.
2. Its chemical composition.
3. Its amount. This chiefly depends on the time factor, but intermittent exposure to high concentrations for short periods may be even more dangerous than to low concentrations over much longer periods. The nature of the occupation is important: the more strenuous the labour, the more deeply the worker is likely to breathe and the more dust he will therefore inhale.
4. The presence or absence of superadded infection, especially tuberculosis.

The importance of the degree of solubility of the dust is controversial, and undoubtedly different people respond differently to the same dust. The classification of pneumoconiosis may be (1) according to the chemical nature of the dust – for example, silica, asbestos, iron (siderosis), carbon (anthracosis from coal), or graphite (a crystalline form of carbon); or (2) according to the occupation – for example coal workers, masons, metal grinders, potters, boiler scalers or foundry workers. In Great Britain, coal mining accounts for four-fifths of all cases, and potters and foundry workers together for nearly half the remainder. Pneumoconiosis may also be subdivided into simple, complicated, and silicosis proper.

Simple pneumoconiosis

This is seen especially in bituminous coal workers, but may also occur in haematite (iron) miners, graphite workers and boiler scalers, in all of whom the exposure to actual silica is slight or absent. Pathologically it is characterized by dust foci in the lungs up to 5 millimetres in diameter, with fine linear reticulin fibres spreading radially from each focus so that the resultant small nodules have a stellate appearance. The condition is called simple because it represents simply the effect of dust, uncomplicated by other factors. After many years' exposure the lungs also show focal emphysema, which consists of rings of dilated alveoli around the dust foci.

Radiographs show increased reticulation producing soft ill-defined shadows. With very good radiological technique, discrete, minute (0.5–1.5 millimetre), round bilateral opacities may be seen, especially in the mid zones. These are not as dense, as well defined or as large as in the other varieties of pneumoconiosis. Focal emphysema, unlike bullous emphysema, cannot be recognized on radiographs. Enlarged hilar lymph nodes are unusual. Increased reticulation – that is, increase of the normal lung markings – is very difficult to assess when of minor degree, even for an expert. The orthodox view is that all pneumoconioses cause increased reticulation, which is regarded as an essential finding. However, some experts deny the whole concept of increased lung markings as a valid radiological finding in the majority of cases.

Complicated pneumoconiosis (progressive massive fibrosis)

This often develops with dusts other than silica, such as carbon, and is commonly seen in coal miners. Its main distinctive feature is a massive progressive fibrosis, especially of the upper lobes and the apical segment of the lower lobes and multiple rounded or irregular opacities principally in the periphery of the upper lobes. *Post mortem* the lungs contain nodules about 1 centimetre in diameter, which may be few or many and are bilateral but often not symmetrical. These later coalesce into large hard rubber masses of dense black tissue. There is always in addition compensatory bullous emphysema of the remainder of the lungs. Such masses may cavitate because of superadded infection or ischaemic necrosis. Secondary infection is usually tuberculous, but the bacilli are often not demonstrable in the sputum, possibly because the cavities do not communicate with a bronchus. Lower lobe bronchiectasis and cor pulmonale often occur.

The radiograph of complicated pneumoconiosis shows an increased reticular pattern with ill-defined opacities of variable extent, size and density, seen especially in the upper and mid zones and often more profuse on the right side. Such opacities are sometimes difficult to distinguish from those of tuberculosis. Later they coalesce to form large nodules in which cavitation may occur. Gross emphysema of the lower lobes is usual. Caplan, a British physician, in 1953 described the co-existence in coal miners of rheumatoid arthritis and well-defined rounded pulmonary opacities of from 0.5 to 5.0 cm, especially in the lung periphery. Some of the nodules may cavitate or calcify. The precise relationship between these findings is controversial.

Silicosis

This is seen with a substantial exposure to free silica (silicon dioxide), for example in masons and quarrymen (especially those working with sandstone, granite or quartz), sand blasters in various types of mines, pottery workers, steel and other metal grinders, foundry workers, glass makers, and those making abrasive soaps and scouring powders. In Britain the condition is much less common than formerly. *Post mortem* the lungs contain hard shotty nodules which histologically consist of concentric layers of fibrosis around dust foci. Bullous emphysema and pleural thickening are also present. Tuberculosis is a common complication. Calcification of the nodules is common.

The radiograph shows increased reticulation and homogeneous well-defined opacities of an average diameter of 5 millimetres, especially in the upper zones. In the earliest stages of the disease these opacities are small, profuse and discrete, giving a miliary appearance, but later they coalesce forming nodules. Enlarged hilar lymph nodes are commonly seen. These may have rings or stippled areas of calcification, an appearance not seen with any other type of pneumoconiosis. Emphysematous bullae are also common.

The main symptoms of any pneumoconiosis are dyspnoea on exertion and mucoid sputum. The latter is often discoloured by the particular dust, but will be mucopurulent if there is superadded infection. Bronchospasm may be a prominent feature. Dyspnoea at rest will also occur if there is gross pulmonary infection or cor pulmonale.

On examination, obvious cyanosis is unusual unless the condition is extremely severe or is complicated by a cor pulmonale. Clubbing is often present but is far from constant. The physical signs in the chest itself are usually only those of bronchitis and emphysema, because bilateral fibrosis is very difficult to diagnose clinically. Any other signs are due to superadded infection.

Asbestosis

Asbestosis is a variety of a mixture of magnesium, aluminium, calcium or iron silicates which all occur naturally in fibres and the chrysotile (white) form (hydrated magnesium silicate) is the one most commonly used in cement, in thermal and electrical insulating and fire proofing materials. The asbestos fibre is much larger than 5 microns and so does not enter the alveoli but becomes lodged in the bronchioles, producing later extensive interstitial pulmonary fibrosis with gross pleural thickening and adhesions.

In the earliest phases of asbestosis, cough and dyspnoea are much more severe than would be expected from the X-ray changes. Following long exposure, extensive pulmonary fibrosis and nodules develop which, unlike in silicosis, cause ill defined radiological opacities. Pleural plaques develop which may become mesotheliomas and may also involve the peritoneum. Asbestos, especially the blue (crocidolite) variety undoubtedly predisposes to malignant disease of the pleura, lung and peritoneum. The precise pulmonary changes depend largely on the chemical composition of the asbestos fibres inhaled. People exposed to such dusts, whether they have radiological lung changes or not, often have asbestos bodies in their sputum (described later).

Asbestosis radiologically shows as widespread increase of reticular markings (fibrosis) especially in the lower zones with multiple smaller shadows and fine ill-defined opacities which produce a ground glass appearance. Often the cardiac border loses its usual well-defined differentiation from the lung shadowing and becomes shaggy. Pleural opacities are very common and except when they calcify are difficult to recognize on a postero-anterior film but may be more obvious on an oblique view. Any calcification is always maximum in the periphery of the plaques. The plaques occur mainly near the diaphragm.

COMPLETE DIAGNOSIS

It is important to realize that there are no physical signs of pulmonary tuberculosis, carcinoma of the bronchus or pneumoconiosis *per se,* but that each of these conditions causes signs dependent on the pathology or pathologies which that particular disease produced in the lung, pleura or mediastinum in that particular patient up to the time when he or she was examined. For example, both tuberculosis and carcinoma of the bronchus can cause any or all of the pathologies enumerated above, and therefore all possible combinations of physical signs may be encountered, depending on the dominant pathology. It is useless, therefore, to list the many possible clinical and radiological findings in either of these conditions. Moreover, in malignant lung disease it is often the signs produced by secondaries, especially glandular ones, which dominate the clinical findings.

The diaphragm

The diaphragm is a musculo-membranous septum separating the abdomen from the thorax. It consists of: (1) a sternal part which is attached to the posterior aspect of the lower end of the xiphoid; (2) a costal portion, attached to the inner aspect of the lower six costal cartilages, which also interdigitates with slips of the transversus abdominis; (3) a lumbar portion attached to the lateral arcuate ligament (which is continuous with the sheath of the quadratus lumborum) and to the medial arcuate ligament (which is continuous with the upper part of the sheath of the psoas). The lumbar portion divides into the right and left crura, the right being attached to the third and fourth and the left to the second and third lumbar vertebrae. From all these attachments the fibres of the diaphragm converge into a central tendon.

The diaphragm has three large openings:

1. The aortic, which is slightly to the left of the midline, lying between the crura and in front of the disc between the twelfth dorsal and first lumbar vertebrae. It is the lowest and most posterior of the three apertures and, in addition to the aorta, it transmits the thoracic duct and azygos vein.
2. The vena caval opening, which is situated in the central tendon. It is the highest of the three openings, and lies opposite the disc between the eighth and ninth dorsal vertebrae.
3. The oesophageal opening. This is in front of and a little to the left of the aortic opening, the right crus being between the two apertures. It lies opposite the tenth dorsal vertebra and transmits the oesophagus, the right and left vagi and the oesophageal branches of the left gastric artery.

As well as these large openings, the diaphragm has numerous small foramina and, from a clinical standpoint, it is important to know that there are in addition other potential openings. The latter are:

1. Two small deficiencies, one on either side of the xiphoid in the sternal portion. These are usually filled with fatty tissue, but either may be the site of a hernia, which is usually symptomless and first discovered as an opacity in the inferior mediastinum on routine chest X-ray. The opacity is nearly always homogeneous because the hernia contains omentum and not stomach or bowel.
2. A triangular area called the pleuro-peritoneal space, lying between the left crus and that part of the costal portion arising from the twelfth cartilage. This is deficient in muscle fibres and may be the site of another hernia, which often first presents in infancy with severe chest symptoms due to pressure effects.

THE PHRENIC NERVE

The diaphragm is innervated by the phrenic nerve, which arises from anterior primary divisions coming mainly from the fourth cervical segment, but usually also receiving a branch from the fifth cervical and occasionally from the third cervical segment.

The left nerve descends obliquely in the neck across the anterior surface of scalenus anticus and with the transverse cervical and suprascapular arteries immediately anterior to it. It then enters the thorax, passing between the subclavian vein and the first part of the subclavian artery, and crosses in front of the internal mammary artery, where it is lateral to the left common carotid. It next passes anterior to the arch of the aorta and the root of the lung, the vagus being posterior to the root. The nerve lies between the pericardium and the mediastinal pleura and reaches the diaphragm just lateral to the apex of the heart.

The course of the right nerve in the neck is the same as that of the left. It enters the thorax anterior to the second part of the right subclavian artery and passes anterior to the internal mammary artery. Descending in the thorax, it lies anterior to the root of the lung with the mediastinal pleura on its lateral side and the right innominate vein, superior vena cava from above downwards on its medial side. It reaches the diaphragm just lateral to the inferior vena cava.

The diaphragm is bilaterally innervated, and a unilateral lesion must be of a lower motor neurone type. Such involvement could be of the anterior horn cells — for example, poliomyelitis; of the nerve roots — for example, injury or compression by a mass of nodes; or of the trunk of the nerve in the neck or mediastinum — for example, compression by nodes or an aneurysm.

RADIOLOGY

Radiologically the right leaf of the diaphragm is normally about half an inch higher than the left, and this must always be taken into account when assessing paralysis or displacement of either cupola. Irregularities of the diaphragmatic outline, such as 'tentings' and apparent localized bulges, are in themselves of no significance and must not be interpreted as diaphragmatic or pleural pathology.

UNILATERAL DIAPHRAGMATIC PARALYSIS

Unilateral diaphragmatic paralysis is nearly always symptomless, but may cause (1) diminution of pulmonary function, but this is only of a minor degree and is unimportant unless there is severe lung or heart disease; (2) reduction of the explosive force of coughing.

The signs of such paralysis are elicited as follows:
1. The patient must be lying down with his head towards a window. The observer stands near the patient's legs, first on one side and then on the other. He will see with each respiration a small linear shadow or shallow furrow at an acute angle to the ribs, travelling down the lower part of the lateral chest wall almost to the costal margin and with expiration passing upwards to the sixth interspace, the total excursion being about 6 centimetres with ordinary and 9 centimetres with very deep breathing. This phenomenon, due to the 'peeling off' of the diaphragm from the chest wall, will be symmetrical on both sides unless there is (*a*) diaphragmatic paralysis or (*b*) gross diaphragmatic displacement by a large

effusion, pneumothorax, subphrenic abscess or large liver. The sign is impossible to demonstrate in an obese or emphysematous patient.

2. Normally the inner and lower costal margins move away from the midline on deep inspiration, but if the diaphragm is depressed for any reason (including paralysis), the movement is towards the midline. Stated differently, if one hand is laid flat over the lower chest anteriorly and the other over the epigastrium, both hands are normally lifted with each inspiration, but in diaphragmatic paralysis there is a paradoxical retraction of the epigastrium with each inspiration.

3. There may be signs of partial collapse of some basal segments produced by the high diaphragm. If the patient already has an absorption collapse of a lower lobe, the signs of this will be accentuated.

4. Tidal percussion is more valuable in this lesion than in emphysema, because diaphragmatic paralysis is nearly always unilateral and the difference between the two sides is often readily demonstrable.

Even with a great deal of practice, the above signs are very rarely conclusive and a radiograph is the only reliable evidence. Each dome of the diaphragm is seen on a sufficiently penetrated film in both the postero-anterior and the lateral view. The right dome is normally about ½ inch higher than the left. Sometimes the right dome, especially in the lateral film, appears to have in part a double contour. This is of no significance. If paralysis is present the film may show a high diaphragm, but this may be due to adhesions or merely displacement. The real test will be screening, which will demonstrate that the diaphragm moves paradoxically, that is, upwards on deep inspiration or sniffing.

Sputum: macroscopical examination

Sputum is material coughed up from trachea, bronchi and lungs. It probably always contains some saliva and is always alkaline unless contaminated, for example by vomit. The main constituent of sputum is mucus.

AMOUNT

The quantity of sputum varies considerably, but very large amounts are found with cavitation (bronchiectatic, tuberculous or lung abscess) and with acute pulmonary oedema, when it is not only copious but frothy, tenacious and often streaked with blood. A rough measurement of the amount of sputum is an important guide to the effect of therapy, medicinal or surgical, in any patient with cavitation of any type. Its volume is not always a reliable indication of the severity of the disease.

Patients with cavitation of the lung or bronchiectasis frequently describe how alteration in position produces an increase in the amount of their sputum.

CONSISTENCY

All sputum is either mucoid, mucopurulent or purulent. Each variety may, however, occur successively in the course of any one disease.

Mucoid sputum is whitish in colour and may be watery, but is usually thick and tenacious. It is found especially in acute pulmonary oedema, asthma, and virus pneumonias.

Purulent sputum contains nothing but pus and occurs when a lung abscess ruptures into a bronchus. This is the only cause of purulent sputum, but many people incorrectly use the term when, in fact, they mean mucopurulent. Sputum is often mucopurulent – that is, consisting of a mixture of mucus and pus – and almost all bacterial infections of the bronchi or lung give rise to this type of sputum. It may be nummular (like coins), the sputum if expectorated into fluid taking on the shape of flattened discs which consist of a gob of pus surrounded by a halo of mucus. Such sputum indicates cavitation of any type.

Stratification is a phenomenon which may be exhibited by mucopurulent sputum when it is placed in a conical glass. The sputum separates into three layers: (1) a small lowest layer consisting of pus and debris (because of the relative smallness of this layer, it is essential to use a conical glass like a urine glass, otherwise the amount will be too small to form a distinct layer; (2) a middle semi-opaque layer consisting of a mixture of mucus and pus which have not separated out; and (3) an uppermost layer consisting of frothy mucus. Such stratification of sputum is seen with cavitation of any type.

COLOUR

The colour of the sputum may be a useful guide. It may consist more or less entirely of blood, being then often referred to as frank haemoptysis. The commonest causes of this are pulmonary tuberculosis, mitral stenosis, bronchiectasis and carcinoma of the bronchus, but the number of possible causes is extremely large and it is foolish to attempt to memorize any long list. On the other hand, sputum may be merely bloodstained and the causes of this are, of course, the same as those of frank haemoptysis.

A 'rusty' sputum has a reddish-brown colour due to the presence of altered blood pigment, and was a frequent finding in the now comparatively rare pneumococcal pneumonia. Sometimes in this condition the sputum is thin, watery and brown ('prune juice'), and this is a bad prognostic sign. Such sputum is also seen in carcinoma of the bronchus.

Such terms as 'raspberry sputum' and 'blackcurrant sputum' have been used to indicate the presence of bloodstained lung debris, which is particularly likely to occur in carcinoma of the bronchus.

Apart from blood or altered blood pigment, an important factor influencing the colour of sputum is consistency, mucoid sputum being white and the mucopurulent type being various shades of yellow and green. Sputum of any shade of yellow or green always indicates infection of bronchus or lung. In town dwellers the sputum is frequently flecked with black owing to inhalation of carbon particles. In coal miners and people who live in coal-mining areas, this phenomenon is well marked. Sputum coughed up after rupture of an amoebic abscess of the liver through the diaphragm and the lung into the bronchus is often described as resembling anchovy sauce.

ODOUR

A very foul odour of the sputum should always be regarded as a suspicious sign of an anaerobic infection. It is very commonly found where there has been stagnation of the sputum, and this is very likely to occur in bronchiectasis or an abscess cavity of a lower lobe.

DEPOSITS

Following a paroxysm of asthma, especially in chronic cases, the patient may cough up small white bodies, usually the size of a pin-head but sometimes larger. When examined with a hand lens, these are found to consist of a centrally highly refractile wavy thread around which is coiled a network of fine fibres having a spiral arrangement, the whole being usually surrounded by mucus in which are embedded (1) numerous leucocytes, especially eosinophils, and (2) colourless pointed crystals the shape of elongated diamonds.

In people exposed to asbestos dust, regardless of whether or not they have pulmonary involvement, the sputum may contain asbestos bodies, which are elongated refractile beaded fibres with bulbous ends enclosed in a proteinaceous sheath. In the rare idiopathic condition of fibrinous bronchitis, the sputum contains mucinous casts of the bronchi which can be seen and identified as such with a hand lens.

MALIGNANT CELLS IN SPUTUM

Whenever bronchial carcinoma is suspected the sputum should be examined for malignant cells but the percentage of positive results and their reliability depends very much on the methods used and the experience and care of the pathologist. Sputum specimens obtained through a bronchoscope more often give positive results than ordinary sputum but the results are more often false than with ordinary sputum. The limitations of the technique and the harm that may be done by a wrong diagnosis of cancer based on cytology of the sputum should never be forgotten.

ORGANISMS IN SPUTUM

Organisms may not be uniformly distributed in the sputum with the result that cultures from one part of a sample may not grow all the organisms actually present and may miss even the most important. The organisms found may also vary in different samples from the same patient obtained on different days. The dominant growth reported may not be a pathogen. Even in very good laboratories, in a considerable proportion of patients with bronchial or pulmonary infection the organism actually responsible for the infection may not be discovered. In patients with pulmonary tuberculosis, especially those receiving chemotherapy, negative sputums may be reported even though the disease is still active. Any bronchial or pulmonary infection causing predominantly mucoid sputum is unlikely to respond either to sulpha drugs or to antibiotics. When making a decision as to which antibiotic to employ the clinician should never be a slave to pathologists and experience and clinical judgment are often far better guides than the results of cultures and sensitivities in determining which drug to use.

14 The Cardiovascular System

'It has been demonstrated again and again that by means of proper bedside methods in collaboration with an electro-cardiograph and postero-anterior and lateral X-rays the nature and severity of the great majority of heart diseases including congenital lesions can be established correctly.' E. N. Silber and L. N. Katz in their monumental *Heart Disease*, Collier-Macmillan, 1975.

Even with the help of the most modern investigatory techniques the good doctor must still rely on the basic skills of history-taking and careful clinical examination, and with increasing clinical experience he will come to realize more and more that with sophisticated methods he still depends on his clinical judgment for their interpretation and evaluation.

'When catheterization is even mentioned by a "modern" cardiologist a master clinician can only wonder about the physician's ability and pity the patient who is to be subjected to such an unnecessary procedure. Why are patients submitted to cardiac catheterization in order to learn, for example, if they have a cardiomyopathy? This practice is ridiculous, absurd and unnecessary. In fact that diagnosis cannot be made by catheterization. ... The abuse of cardiac catheterization needs careful study and control. Catheterization can provide only a crude record of blood flow for just a few beats, whereas there are 115, 200 beats or more per day for the average person. The information obtained is therefore extremely limited. ... The master cardiologist can determine cardiac function and the cardiac state at the bedside every time he sees his patient and at any time he wishes, and he can predict cardiac function amazingly accurately for the near and distant future and under varying circumstances. The contrast between the master cardiologist at the bedside with his stethoscope, sphygmomano-meter, flash light, tongue depressor and ophthalmoscope and the 'haemodynamist' in his cluttered 'cath. lab.' with poor recorders, bulky apparatus, several assistants, technicians, nurses, orderlies, haematostats, scalpels, drapes, dyes, contrast material, X-ray equipment, flashing lights, noisy humming and buzzing motors and TV monitors, trying to study a patient intelligently to render a supposed clinical service is striking to say the least. . . . The data are often of little clinical value, meaningless, or incorrect and often misleading. This is not the way to practice good clinical medicine. Such procedures are of value only in extremely rare and highly selected cases. . . . What is needed today is better bedside doctors, master clinicians, well trained clinicians, physicians who assume personal responsibility for their patients and do not delegate their care to interns and residents who are in training, doctors who are not too important to visit a patient in his home at 2 o'clock in the morning, doctors who also know general medicine and who will study and examine the whole patient, talk to the patient, understand the interrelationships of all the diseases of the patient, understand the patient's reaction to his disease and his surroundings and family, write orders which the patient can carry out himself, and, above all, the physician must use his five "senses" and his own computer, the greatest computer of all, the human brain. . . .

'No one can be a good clinical cardiologist if he is not first and foremost a master general internist, one who can and does take a complete history, who performs a complete examination, who knows what laboratory tests to order and does so and can interpret the significance of the results in the light of the clinical picture. Special gadgets and procedures are used only when needed (and this is rarely) and when they can definitely be helpful in clinical service to the patient.' Dr G. E. Burch, the distinguised senior cardiologist from New Orleans, in *American Heart Journal*, 1973.

The physician when talking to patients must always be firm and decisive in his statement whether or not the patient has heart disease. To miss a heart lesion is a serious error but often a more grievous and possibly more tragic fault is to diagnose or even hint at the possibility of heart disease when in fact there is no valid evidence. Any possible anxiety produced is never diminished by using vague words such as 'slight' or 'little'. Moreover the practical impact on the patient even if the verdict is later reversed is unlikely to be completely eradicated, however imposing the reputation of the cardiologist who later declares the heart to be normal. Informing a patient or his relatives that he has heart disease of any type or severity must always be based on incontrovertible evidence and when there is any doubt it is far better to inform the patient, at least initially, that his heart is normal even though subsequent events may prove this to be wrong. It is unlikely that thereby any patient will be deprived of important therapy. Iatrogenic cardiac neurosis is far too common.

A further important consideration should be that in a patient with an organic heart lesion there is frequently a psychogenic overlay, and such symptoms may dominate over those actually due to the disease and only by careful questioning and attentive listening will the physician be able to differentiate those symptoms and assess their true severity. Many patients with organic heart disease because of fear exaggerate their symptoms.

The electrocardiograph is a valuable instrument but even with the most advanced machines and methods the certain information it yields is limited. Moreover technical errors and misinterpretations are common. These strictures are accentuated when the clinician relies on reports made by others who have never seen the patient. Electrocardiographs have been a tremendous help but have also been the cause of a great deal of iatrogenic illness and thereby needless patient suffering.

Before the cardiovascular system itself is examined, the following points, which are all discussed in greater detail elsewhere, should be sought for and a quick assessment made: (1) dyspnoea at rest or produced by slight exertion—for example, that of undressing; (2) cyanosis, especially of the labial, lingual and buccal mucosae; (3) cyanosis, clubbing and arachnodactyly or other congenital abnormalities.

The pulse

It is unusual to find undergraduates or recent graduates who are able to give with confidence a correct and full opinion on any pulse. This is because they have not practised and have come to rely entirely on the sphygmomanometer. A full assessment of the pulse records tension, equality, volume (and any special details if volume is altered), rate, rhythm, state of the vessel wall, and any other features. Whenever convenient, it is better to feel the brachial artery rather than the radial because the pulse findings in the former are usually easier to assess, but most clinicians prefer palpation of the radial pulse because it is more often easily accessible. The carotid pulse is sometimes more informative than either, especially for an assessment of the form of the pulse wave, and the physician should practise its palpation as a routine procedure in all patients. Palpation of arteries should always be light and done with the palmar aspect ot the fingers held slightly flexed at the proximal interphalangeal but extended at the distal interphalangeal joints.

TENSION

The tension (systolic pressure) is determined by feeling the radial artery with three fingers—the upper one compressing the vessel from above, the middle one feeling the pulse, and the lower one obliterating the ulnar collateral vessels below. The degree of pressure necessary to obliterate the pulse as felt by the middle finger gives the estimation of the systolic pressure, and the fullness of the pulse between each systole gives a measure of the diastolic pressure. However, often a more satisfactory technique is to feel and gradually compress with the thumb of one hand the brachial artery in the region of the inner and lower aspect of the upper arm, while the radial artery is felt with the fingers of the other hand. With practice the systolic pressure can be assessed in the great majority of cases within a margin of 10 millimetres. Many clinicians wrongly do not believe this and so, misguidedly, do not advise students to practise the determination of blood pressure without using an instrument. Of course I am not advocating that the sphygmomanometer should not be used routinely.

EQUALITY

After determining the systolic pressure, the two pulses should routinely be felt simultaneously to assess whether there is any gross difference between them. The commonest cause of such an inequality is an abnormal position of the radial artery, but aortic aneurysms, and occasionally any other swelling in the superior mediastinum which compresses the subclavian or innominate artery, can produce this effect. Rarely, thrombosis or embolism of the subclavian, axillary or brachial artery may be the cause. If the radial pulses are unequal, the next immediate procedure is to feel simultaneously both brachial arteries, because if these be equal and the radials unequal, the probability is that an anatomical variation of the radial artery is present. Blood pressure recordings in each arm would be the final proof, but it is not a routine practice to record blood pressure in both arms, and this diagnostic point would be missed unless feeling both radials simultaneously first aroused suspicion.

VOLUME

Pulse pressure (pulse volume) is the degree of expansion of the artery with each pulse wave and represents the difference between the systolic and diastolic pressures. It should always be determined on palpation of the radial artery with the patient's arm horizontal, assessing the amplitude of the pulse wave. If it seems that the volume is large, the arm should be raised as high as possible. This will confirm or nullify the impression, since raising a limb lowers the diastolic pressure and therefore accentuates the pulse pressure. If, on the other hand, the suspicion is that the volume is small, then depressing the arm below the horizontal will help to resolve the doubt.

The pulse volume should be described as normal, small or large, and terms such as full, good, strong, weak and poor should be avoided. Does the term 'strong pulse' refer to systolic pressure or pulse volume? Do such terms as 'full' and 'good' refer to the normal or the abnormal? Is not the opposite of 'full' empty?

The commonest cause of a large pulse volume is hypertension, but the diastolic pressure is then also high, and this should be determinable on palpation. On the other hand, if the high pulse pressure is primarily due to a low diastolic, the systolic being normal or raised, then a collapsing pulse results. The emphasis is that a collapsing pulse and a high pulse pressure are not quite the same, since with the former but not with the latter (hypertension) there is not only a large pulse pressure but a rapid increase and a very rapid fall of pressure.

A collapsing pulse is best appreciated on raising the patient's arm as high as possible and feeling the radial artery with several

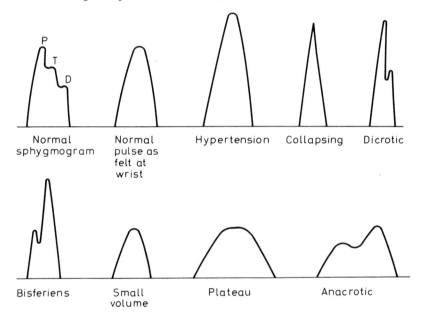

Figure 2. *Diagrammatic representation of various pulse waves. P — percussion; T — tidal; D — dicrotic*

fingers, the pulse wave being a forceful jerk which reaches the peak of its volume very rapidly, and this peak being of very brief duration so that there is also a very rapid diminution of the volume. For this reason older clinicians called it *pulsus celer* (abrupt pulse). The synonymous term 'water-hammer pulse' derives from a piece of physical apparatus consisting of an hermetically sealed tube, half filled with fluid and the other half a vacuum, so that when the tube is inverted the column of fluid, having no air resistance, plops down the tube, striking the end with a noise like a hammer blow and giving a palpable thud. Another name for this type of pulse is 'Corrigan's* pulse' after the Irish physician of that name who, in 1832, described it as 'a jerky pulse with a full expansion, followed by a sudden collapse'.

The causes of a collapsing pulse are aortic regurgitation, severe anaemia, any large arteriovenous aneurysm (including patent ductus), Paget's disease, and complete heart block.

A collapsing pulse from whatever cause may be associated with marked transmitted bilateral pulsation in the neck, better seen with the patient sitting up, and also with capillary pulsation. The latter is an alternate flushing and blanching synchronous with the heart action, blanching with each diastole and flushing with each systole. It is most readily seen on the application of steady firm pressure on the patient's nail, but it can also be observed in the lips and in the retina on ophthalmoscopy. Causes of a large volume pulse which is not collapsing other than hypertension are causes of tachycardia including anxiety, exercise, fevers and thyrotoxicosis. With fevers, but especially typhoid, the large volume pulse may be associated with a palpable extra impulse felt during the decrease of volume (dicrotic pulse).

The most important causes of a small pulse volume are aortic stenosis and shock from any cause (including myocardial infarction). Other causes are pericardial effusion, constrictive pericarditis, pure mitral stenosis and severe pulmonary stenosis, but in the last three of these the reduction in the pulse volume is difficult to appreciate on palpation because it is never of even moderate degree. In aortic stenosis the pulse may show in addition to the small volume a slow rise, a sustained volume and a slow fall — the plateau pulse or pulsus tardus (*tardus* meaning lazy, that is, slow to reach its maximum, and plateau because the sphygmogram has a plateau shape). In addition, an extra impulse may be felt during the increase of volume, and this constitutes the anacrotic pulse. To appreciate this anacrotic element with certainty on palpation is difficult even for the most experienced physician.

It is wrong to regard the terms small volume, plateau and anacrotic as synonyms, as is so often done. Each term indicates a special feature, although all three may be present at the same time. A pulse should never be described as anacrotic unless the meaning of the term is clearly understood, there is certainty of the presence of this sign, and it is realized that the term implies the diagnosis of aortic stenosis allowing of no alternative.

In cases where the patient has aortic regurgitation as well as aortic stenosis, it is unlikely that the pulse volume will be small

*Sir Dominic J. Corrigan (1802–80) described the pulse in *Edinburgh Med. and Surg. J.* 37(1832), 225. Although a graduate of Edinburgh he worked for many years in Dublin.

unless the regurgitation is very slight. With such a combination the pulse, though not of small volume, may exhibit an extra impulse during the increase of volume, giving two palpable components of the pulse with each heartbeat. This is the pulsus bisferiens, differing therefore from the anacrotic pulse in that it is unassociated with a small volume. Both the anacrotic and the disferiens types of pulse are often more readily appreciated by palpation of the carotids than at the radial pulse.

Pulsus paradoxus
In normal people deep inspiration causes an increase of pulse rate and a diminution of pulse volume. However, the latter is rarely of such a degree that it can be recognized for certainty on palpation, although it may be readily appreciated whilst recording the blood pressure instrumentally. A pulsus paradox is a readily recognizable diminution of pulse volume on deep inspiration. It is therefore an accentuation of a normal phenomenon. An arbitrary figure of less than 10 mm determined with a sphygmomanometer is usually accepted as normal. Sitting or standing often accentuates the phenomenon and therefore renders it easier to appreciate. A pulsus paradox is usually present in patients with pericardial effusion (probably in all those with tamponade). It also occurs with constrictive pericarditis but far less frequently than with effusion. It occasionally is present with obstructive airway disease. If the pulse is regular variations in volume with different beats is found with atrio-ventricular block, regular extrasystoles with artificial ventricular pacing and with a pulsus paradoxus. In patients with pulsus paradoxus alterations of volume are not affected by holding the breath. With regularly occurring extrasystoles the time intervals from larger to smaller beats is always shorter than from smaller to larger beats but this variation is not present with pulsus paradoxus.

RATE
The heart rate should always be noted and for this purpose a watch must be used, except by the more experienced who have repeatedly checked their estimated figures against actual rates counted with a watch. The words tachycardia and bradycardia are pompous ones merely indicating fast and slow rates respectively, and have no more precise meaning unless preceded by an adjective such as paroxysmal.

RHYTHM
Whether the pulse is regular or not should always be determined and, if it is irregular, the type of irregularity must be diagnosed (*see later*). It is not usual to depend on the pulse alone to determine the nature of a cardiac arrhythmia because auscultation of the heart is, in the

great majority of cases, more helpful. However, with practice the diagnosis of the rhythm can be made correctly on the pulse alone in most cases, but only with practice, and guesswork should never be indulged in.

VESSEL WALL

Whether or not the vessel wall is unduly thickened is a sign that becomes better discerned with increased experience. Many physicians find it easier for this particular purpose to palpate the brachial artery just above the inner aspect of the elbow where, if atherosclerotic, it can be seen tortuous and pulsating forcibly (locomotor brachial) and the thickening of the vessel wall can be easily appreciated. I do not think that thickening and undue tortuosity of vessels should be ignored and discounted as being of no importance, as is often done nowadays. On the other hand, the importance of these findings must not be exaggerated, since they are often present with the benign and relatively unimportant Monckeberg's degeneration of the media.

The neck vessels

The pulse having been examined carefully, attention should then be turned to the neck in search of vascular engorgement and pulsation, which may be either venous or arterial.

JUGULAR VENOUS PULSE

In regard to venous distension, attention should be focused on the internal rather than the external jugular veins, as the latter often give equivocal evidence because of their frequent constriction in normal people by the cervical fascia. Jugular vein distension is often best analysed when observed tangentially with the patient's head turned slightly. The lighting must be good and the patient should not be wearing a collar. While usually it is easy to differentiate between arterial and venous distension, occasionally difficulty arises and then the evidence must be more carefully weighed. With organic tricuspid regurgitation the jugular vein distension may be so marked as to be mistaken for carotid pulsation.

Venous pulsation and venous distension have the following characteristics:

1. They can be accentuated by the patient's lying flat, by deep expiration, by coughing and by compression of the abdomen (not necessarily in the region of the liver).
2. Although easily seen, they are usually impalpable or felt with great difficulty.

3. Venous pulsation is rarely forcible but has a gentle diffuse pattern.
4. Provided the heart is not very fast, it may be possible to see component waves with each pulsation.

The jugular venous pulsations have been described as the window of the heart. Unfortunately careful observation of them is sometimes neglected especially by those who are more interested in electro-cardiographs. If the the internal jugular veins are obviously engorged with the patient sitting upright, then the jugular venous pressure must be markedly increased and indicates a raised pressure in the right atrium (referred to as raised central venous pressure). With the patient flat or almost so, venous distension may be seen sometimes in normal people, but never higher than immediately above the inner end of the clavicle. The height of the venous column above the manubrio-sternal junction, which is roughly at the level of the right atrium, is recorded, always stating the position of the patient when the measurement was made; this is done preferably with the patient sitting roughly at an angle of 45° because in normal people in this position there is either no jugular vein distension or if present it extends at the very most to 2 cm above the clavicle. If the neck veins are distended, note should be made whether they show pulsation, because, at least theoretically, where the venous distension is due to obstruction of the superior vena cava or of the jugular veins, then no pulsation is visible, but this presupposes that the obstruction is complete.

Hepato-jugular reflux

With the patient sitting or propped up with pillows and breathing normally and not deeply, the abdomen is palpated in the right hypochondrium with gradually increasing pressure which is maintained for at least a minute. The liver need not be enlarged for this procedure and, if it is, pressure over it may cause severe discomfort and then the test can often be demonstrated equally well by pressure below the liver.

Such a procedure helps to distinguish between arterial and venous pulsation in the neck – the former being unaffected and the latter increasing with such pressure. It may also, by rendering the top of the venous column more obvious, help in studying the pattern of the venous pulse. Furthermore, it helps to differentiate between jugular distension due to cardiac failure and that secondary to venous obstruction, because the former will be aggravated and the latter unaffected by the pressure, but this differentiation presumes that the venous obstruction is complete and is not a reliable distinction. It is claimed that in a patient without obvious jugular distension a positive hepato-jugular reflux, in the absence of pericardial disease, is an early sign of right-sided cardiac failure.

Venous waves

Jugular venous tracings show that the venous pulsation is a composite affair consisting of 5 waves per cardiac cycle. These are designated the *a, x, c, v* and *y* waves, the *a, v* and *c* being crests (positive waves) and *x* and *y* troughs (negative waves). The *a* wave is presystolic as timed by the carotid — that is, it precedes the carotid pulse and coincides with the first heart sound. The *x* trough (or descent) is early in systole; it follows the *a* wave and is normally greater than the *y*. The *v* wave, which is roughly equal in amplitude to the *c*, is in early diastole. The *c* wave is transmitted from the underlying carotid and is usually not seen. The *y* trough is also not usually seen. By far the most commonly and readily seen and also the most important is the *a* wave, which corresponds to atrial systole and occurs immediately prior to and coinciding with the first heart sound.

The hepato-jugular reflux may give considerable help in recognition of the individual waves, as may also their timing by simultaneously feeling the carotid with the thumb pressed just below the angle of the jaw. The experienced physician is able to recognize these individual waves and assess whether they are normal, diminished or increased in amplitude, but others should be endowed with humility and not base their diagnosis on any spurious or imaginary findings in the neck veins. On the other hand the less experienced must always try to visualize and assess the venous waves so that perhaps after a great deal of critical experience he will also be able to analyse them accurately. But statements made after inspection, such as 'This patient cannot be fibrillating because there are *a* waves', or 'This patient has got heart block because he has cannon *a* waves', are the antithesis of humility, and all but the very experienced are usually wrong when they base their diagnosis on such findings. Analysis of the venous pulse waves is extremely difficult when the heart is fast or when the venous distention is minimal or so marked as to extend to the angle of the jaw.

Giant (very prominent) *a* waves are seen in marked pulmonary hypertension, in severe pulmonary stenosis and also in tricuspid stenosis. Cannon *a* waves, which are not only large but exhibit a very rapid rise and fall of volume, are found in complete heart block and sometimes with ventricular tachycardia. With atrial flutter and with supraventricular tachycardias rapid regular wave undulations may be visible without the possibility of recognizing the individual components. The *a* waves are absent in atrial fibrillation. In complete atrio-ventricular block, the *a* waves are dissociated — that is, independent in timing of the other waves. Prolongation of the *a-c* interval may be seen on a venous tracing from a patient with partial atrio-ventricular block, but is very unlikely to be recognized without such instrumental aid. Large *v* waves are seen in organic tricuspid regurgitation associated with atrial fibrillation. Marked *y* waves (diastolic collapse) may be seen in any patient with a very high jugular venous pressure, but are also seen with pericardial effusions producing cardiac tamponade and with constrictive pericarditis. A slow *y* descent with absence of a visible *y* trough in the presence of a markedly raised jugular venous pressure is reputed to be typical of tricuspid stenosis. Sometimes a prominent *x* descent is seen in constrictive pericarditis.

Causes of raised jugular venous pressure
The causes of venous engorgement of the neck (increased jugular venous pressure) are as follows:
Congestive cardiac failure. The raised venous pressure is then nearly always associated with liver enlargement. High jugular venous pressure without hepatic enlargement strongly favours superior vena caval obstruction rather than congestive cardiac failure; similarly, a large liver without high jugular venous pressure is extremely unlikely to be due to cardiac failure.
Obstruction of the superior vena cava or jugular veins by any neck swelling such as a large thyroid.
Organic tricuspid regurgitation.
Pericardial effusion and constructive pericarditis.
A large pleural effusion. This is a rare cause.
Increased blood volume, for example, in acute nephritis, steroid therapy and polycythaemia vera, and after large intravenous infusions.
Very slow heart rates, whether of sinus rhythm or due to block. Therefore with complete heart block, raised venous pressure is not in itself evidence of cardiac failure.
Severe physical effort. This and conditions which raise the intra-thoracic or intra-abdominal pressure, such as coughing and tight garments, are only temporary. However, more persistent causes of raised intra-abdominal pressure such as ascites may also raise the jugular venous pressure.
High cardiac output, due to thyrotoxicosis, severe anaemia, high fever, pregnancy, Paget's disease and arteriovenous fistulae – may cause a minor rise in jugular venous pressure.

Valsalva manoeuvre
This is done by raising the intrathoracic pressure by means of forced expiration against a closed glottis (mouth closed tightly and nose squeezed). It is best accomplished by the patient, whose nose is squeezed with a nose clip, blowing into a mouthpiece connected with an aneroid or mercury manometer and maintaining a pressure of 40 mm for 10 seconds. This results in an increase of pulse volume and rate during the strain of blowing which is followed on release of the strain by an abrupt diminution of volume and rate. There may be a second increase of pulse volume before the rate gradually returns to normal.

These separate phases can be recognized and assessed critically only with instrumental aid.

The essential feature produced by this manoeuvre in a normal person is a diminution in the pulse pressure and an alteration of pulse rate and systolic pressure, which are less important. In heart failure (even in its earliest stage), in constrictive pericarditis and with large left-to-right shunts the manoeuvre fails to produce any alteration in the pulse volume. It is also claimed that with pathological sinus bradycardia due to sino-atrial disease, which is a very rare condition but may cause syncopal attacks, the responses are considerably reduced. In contrast with these conditions, extensive pulmonary disease such as emphysema causes an exaggeration of the normal response.

Superior vena caval obstruction

'Superior vena caval obstruction' is a far better term than the vaguer and less precise 'superior mediastinal obstruction'. The manifestations of this syndrome are (1) non-pulsatile distension of the jugular veins with little or no increase of the distension on abdominal compression; (2) oedema of the head, the neck and sometimes the upper limbs; (3) cyanosis of the head and neck; and (4) collateral veins over the upper chest. All the above signs may be accentuated by getting the patient to lean forward. Two other very rare accompaniments are bilateral exophthalmos and papilloedema.

Not all the signs need be present before a diagnosis of superior vena cava obstruction is considered. If only one sign is present, then such a contingency is merely possible; if two signs are present, the diagnosis is a probable one; while if three or four are demonstrable, the diagnosis is a certainty.

The causes of superior vena caval obstruction should be considered primarily on an anatomical basis under the headings of (1) enlarged nodes from whatever cause; (2) cardiovascular lesions (aneurysm, constrictive pericarditis, large pericardial effusion, and rarely a huge left atrium); (3) enlargement of the thyroid or thymus, or a dermoid or any other mass in this site.

ARTERIAL PULSATION IN THE NECK

Arterial pulsation in the neck is better observed with the patient sitting up with his chin elevated slightly. When palpating a carotid it is advisable to do so in the lower half of the neck so as to avoid compression of the carotid sinus. The physician may find it preferable to use his thumb rather than one or two fingers. Such pulsation may be transmitted or expansile. If it is transmitted, it will look like a piston working up and down on either side of the neck; it is then always bilateral, and is seen in any condition in which there is a collapsing pulse. Any supposed minor differences between the strengths of palpation on the two sides should be ignored.

Expansile arterial pulsation may be seen on the right side of the neck or in the suprasternal notch; it is very rare on the left side of the neck, and therefore is very seldom bilateral. It is seen not only as an up-and-down movement but as a movement in all planes. Often, however, an easier differentiation lies in the fact that it may be felt as a swelling around which the fingers can be cupped, a technique never possible with transmitted pulsation.

Expansile pulsation is seen with an aneurysm or with a kinked carotid. The latter condition is brought about by an anatomically abnormal disposition of the great vessels and is due to uncoiling of the aorta; it is present with hypertension, usually associated with marked atherosclerosis, but with coarctation, for example, it occurs without atherosclerosis.

The heart

INSPECTION AND PALPATION

On inspection of the heart it is necessary to look for the following characteristics:

1. The position and character of the apex beat. This is best ascertained with the patient lying flat or sitting upright and with the physician on the patient's right side and looking tangentially across the praecordium. Any leaning or turning to either side may alter the position of the apex beat.
2. Abnormal pulsation.
3. Prominence of the praecordium (which may indicate a very long-standing cardiac enlargement). The praecordium is the area of the chest wall which overlies the heart.
4. Other deformity of the chest, often secondary to spinal deformities, which may cause alteration of the position of the heart, occasionally a systolic bruit and, rarely, right-sided cardiac involvement.
5. Systolic retraction.

Apex beat

The size of the heart is assessed clinically by noting the position of the apex beat, and in this context palpation is more important than inspection. This is usually regarded as the position of outermost impulse, although some clinicians favour its description as the position of maximum impulse. Thus, concerning such an elementary point as what constitutes the apex beat, leading cardiologists themselves are not in agreement and hence students are confused.

Regarding the mode of description of the position of the apex beat there is also a lack of uniformity. The usual techniques are those of describing its position in terms of distance from the midline, or in relationship to the mid-clavicular line or, in men only, relative to the nipple line. The first technique is the most usual, but has the obvious drawback that in some degree the measurement depends upon the size of the chest. This can be partially overcome by measuring from the midline tangentially instead of circumferentially, but this is not a common practice. Many claim that measurement from the mid-clavicular line is the most accurate, but this feigns a precision which does not exist, the exact mid-clavicular point never having been actually determined.

When feeling for the apex beat, one or two flexed fingers should be used and not the palm of the hand, as this is too large to localize a circumscribed area which normally is less than one inch in diameter, is confined to the fifth space and does not visibly lift the palpating fingers.

Systolic retraction of the intercostal muscles in the region of the apex beat is seen with any enlarged heart but especially if this is mainly right ventricular. Occasionally it is seen in very thin people who do not have cardiac enlargement. It is considered by some clinicians to be an important sign of adherent pericardium and then will involve the ribs as well as the intercostal muscles and will be seen over a much larger area, including the scapular region. The retraction is followed by a discernible outward movement. Systolic retraction is best sought for with the patient sitting upright with his hands on his head and holding his breath after a deep inspiration. Good lighting is essential. It is only when there is a localized thrust that the position of the apex beat is a completely reliable guide to cardiac size. Clinically it is desirable to talk in terms of cardiac enlargement and not to attempt the virtual impossibility of distinguishing between hypertrophy and dilatation or the assessment of the relative degree of each. The presence of gross chest deformity, including scoliosis, makes the position of the apex beat unreliable evidence of cardiac size. In an adult, cardiac enlargement must be suspected if the apex beat is more than 10 cm from the midline, is lateral to the mid-clavicular line or is below the fifth intercostal space, provided that the heart is not displaced by a right pleural effusion or pneumothorax, or by fibrosis or by collapse of the left lower lobe, or by chest deformities or if the diaphragm is markedly pushed up, for example by a late stage pregnancy.

Character of beat

It is fashionable to use various terms such as diffuse, slapping, thrusting, heaving and tapping to describe the different features of the apex beat in different conditions. Unfortunately no unanimity exists about these terms and there is always the danger that their use will engender the crime of Procrustes, the apex beat described not as it actually is but so as to fit in with a preconceived diagnosis. The normal apex beat is localized to a fairly small area and is of brief duration. Sometimes it is described as a visible and palpable thrust, a thrusting apex beat being then regarded as a normal phenomenon. However, most clinicians use the term 'thrusting' as synonymous with 'forcible' and of brief duration. Some pedants maintain that an apex is technically a point and that therefore the term 'diffuse apex' is illogical; but by the same criterion, so is the term 'heaving', because a point has position but no magnitude.

With enlargement of the left ventricle the apex beat is usually forceful, lifting the palpating fingers with each systole, and it is difficult to diminish its intensity by digital pressure. A heaving apex beat is one with not only an increase of amplitude but also a prolonged (sustained) amplitude and it is typically found in uncomplicated aortic stenosis. While it is true that it is sometimes difficult to determine the heart size clinically and that an X-ray is a more reliable indicator, yet it cannot be stressed too often that the difficulties have been grossly exaggerated and with careful critical and continued practice a doctor can improve this clinical ability. If the physician ignores this advice he will be at a complete loss when confronted with a common situation of not having X-rays immediately available, or if the patient is too ill to obtain films satisfactory for this purpose. On X-ray the maximum width of the heart on a postero-anterior film should not exceed 50 per cent of the chest cage measured inside the rib at the same level as the cardiac measurement. Even X-rays are not always a definite answer to the determination of heart size because this becomes difficult in the presence of a large effusion, gross thoracic cage deformity, especially deformed sternum or marked scoliosis, or a large mediastinal opacity of any nature. Also it must never be forgotten that serious heart disease may be present with a heart size which clinically and radiologically is normal.

Right ventricular enlargement
When the apex beat is formed by an enlarged right ventricle, it is often difficult to see and feel, and may have a diffuse sharp tapping quality which is sometimes more marked in the left parasternal region than the apical area. Systolic retraction may be evidence of right ventricular enlargement and has been described previously. With right ventricular enlargement there may also be a parasternal lift (heave) which is a visible and palpable impulse along the left sternal border and which is often more forcible than the actual apical impulse. Because a large right ventricle is often associated with pulmonary hypertension pulsation in the second and third left interspaces close to the sternal border it is often visible and there may also be epigastric pulsation which is very tender on pressure but this is not pathognomonic as it is commonly seen in normal thin people and

those with organic tricuspid regurgitation and also with aneurysms of the abdominal aorta. In the last named condition the epigastric pulsation will be expansile and not transmitted.

A right ventricular type of apex beat and the associated findings described above are best seen in a patient who has right ventricular enlargement with little or no left-sided enlargement, such as occurs in pure mitral stenosis, cor pulmonale, atrial septal defect and patent ductus.

It must again be emphasized that in conditions where it is known that an enlarged right ventricle occurs, such as mitral stenosis and many of the congenital heart lesions, it is essential to avoid automatically diagnosing parasternal heaves and tapping apex beats unless it is beyond doubt that they are present. It is useless to hoodwink oneself into imagining these physical signs when in actual fact they are not detectable.

In the presence of a ventricular aneurysm due to previous myocardial infarction an added impulse is often visible and palpable, independent and above and internal to the apex beat.

Absent apex beat
If the apex beat is not visible or palpable, or is so only with great difficulty, then the reasons for this should be immediately sought before proceeding further. The cause is rarely in the heart itself. Obesity, well developed pectoral muscles, and emphysema are the usual explanations, but should be accepted only if in fact the patient has evidence of these. Gross displacement of the heart, particularly to the right may be due to a congenital or acquired dextrocardia. Pericardial effusions and weakness of the cardiac musculature are possible but unusual causes of a poor cardiac impulse.

Thrills
Thrills should be regarded as palpable bruits and described as a feature of bruits and never independently.

Following determination of the size of the heart, thrills should be sought for over the whole of the praecordium. They are best felt with the palm of the hand. Except in mitral stenosis it is exceptional for a thrill to be localized to a small area. Thrills occur only when the bruit is loud and if a bruit is soft any apparent thrill is almost certainly a wrong interpretation of the sensation felt. The common reasons for missing thrills are that:

1. They are not felt for as a routine.
2. The patient is not positioned, as thrills at the base are often felt better when the patient is sitting up and leaning forward and at the apex when the patient turns on his left side.
3. The hand is pressed too heavily against the chest because of the desire not to miss any thrills, which may have the effect of actually abolishing the thrill.

Thrills always indicate an organic disease and the cause must be found. Diastolic thrills in the region of the apex are almost always due to mitral stenosis. Diastolic thrills at the base are unusual and, when present, are nearly always due to aortic regurgitation. Rarely there may be a diastolic element in the thrill accompanying the continuous murmur of a patent ductus.

The commonest cause of a systolic thrill at the apex area is a ventricular septal defect, a far less common cause being mitral regurgitation. A systolic thrill at the base, if maximal on the right side and especially if also felt in the right side of the neck, is most often due to aortic stenosis but may be caused by an aneurysm. A thrill over the carotid may occasionally be felt with carotid obstruction. A systolic thrill at the base, if maximal on the left side and especially if also felt in the left side of the neck, is most likely to be due to a congenital heart lesion.

PERCUSSION

Percussion of the heart is not always done as a routine, and it is far better either to do this properly or not to do it at all. The size of the area of cardiac dullness is influenced not only by the patient's position but also by the shape of the chest and the position of the diaphragm. Any distinction between superficial (relative) and deep (absolute) cardiac dullness is impractical and should not be attempted. However, although percussion of the heart is of no value in the majority of cases, it can be of the greatest importance diagnostically in the following circumstances:

1. In cases of aneurysm of the ascending aorta and of the arch.
2. In the diagnosis of pericardial effusion.
3. Where there is a huge right or left atrium, when dullness continuous with the cardiac dullness may be detectable well to the right of the sternum.
4. Gross diminution of cardiac dullness is important evidence of emphysema.
5. Percussion would be the only indication of the size of the heart in a patient in whom the apex beat was not visible or palpable (for example, due to emphysema or obesity) when radiology is not available.

When percussing the cardiac borders, it is very important that the percussion should be light and that the fundamental rules of percussion should always be observed. The pleximeter finger must be parallel to the percussed border. Percussion should always be from resonant to dull — that is, from axilla to mid-sternum — and along an axis at right angles to the border percussed. The right border of the heart is normally beneath the sternum and is therefore not definable by percussion except when the right side of the heart or the left atrium is grossly enlarged or a pericardial effusion is present.

AUSCULTATION

When buying a stethoscope, it is mandatory to be discriminating in your choice and not to buy a model that has no other virtue than that of being fashionable. The earpieces must fit without the slightest discomfort, and the rubber tubing should be thick with a bore of about three-sixteenths of an inch and a length of six to ten inches. A diaphragm as well as a bell is essential. The earpieces, bell and diaphragm must all be intact and should be discarded as soon as they show any sign of being chipped, cracked or damaged in any way. A modern stethoscope in good condition is a prerequisite for satisfactory auscultation.

On auscultation, attention should be concerned separately with the rhythm, the heart sounds and the bruits. Concentration should be given to each of these separately, because if an attempt is made to determine two points such as rhythm and bruits at the same time, it is very easy to make mistakes. Concentrated listening, attempting to be certain of one feature at a time before being concerned with any other feature, is a necessary requisite of successful auscultation. Concentrated listening demands peace and quiet. The Austrian author Stephan Zweig (1881–1942) in his *World of Yesterdays* wrote: 'The eternal secret of all great art, indeed of every mortal achievement, is concentration.' The German author and politician Ferdinand Lassalle (1825–64) wrote in 1863: 'The whole art of practical success is concentrating all effort at all time upon a single point.' Silber and Katz wrote in *Heart Disease*: 'Without unusual talent or especially acute hearing the physician by virtue of good methods and reasonable experience can develop his auscultatory skill to a level compatible with the sensitivity of the finest phonocardiographic equipment.'

Anybody who is not deaf can hear a heart but meaningful listening is more than that and is a constant awareness of, analysis and correlation of all that is heard. Successful ausculation depends on concentration together with a good auditory memory backed up by sound experience. Moreover, although auscultation is a very important aspect of cardiac examination it should never be the only technique performed with any thoroughness, dismissing inspection, palpation and percussion in a perfunctory manner or even omitting any of them, as is too often done.

Unfortunately some auscultators are persistent missers, while others are persistent fakers or sufferers from auditory hallucinations. The defect of the first group, the missers, may be due to defective hearing, poor auditory memory or a bad stethoscope, but is most often due to lack of concentration. The second and third groups of auscultators too often become consultant cardiologists, infecting their students with the malignant disease of guessing.

Rhythm

Abnormal rhythms are due either to impulses arising from a site other than the sino-atrial node or to interference with conduction.

Determination of the rhythm should be considered as an exercise in logic, in deductive reasoning from accepted premises. For example, 'Is this rhythm normal or abnormal'? should always be the first question to pose; the answer nearly always being very obvious, because an abnormal rhythm must show itself by either irregularity or a gross abnormality of rate, or both.

If the rhythm is abnormal, the cause must be one of the following: sinus arrhythmia, extrasystoles, atrial fibrillation, heart block, atrial flutter, or paroxysmal tachycardia. The second stage diagnosis is to decide which abnormalities it could possibly be (which usually reduces the problem to consideration of two or three arrhythmias). The final diagnosis is to determine exactiy which arrhythmia is present.

Very fast hearts

If the heart rate is about 120 or more per minute then, provided that the patient is not pyrexial or thyrotoxic or has not very recently carried out some strenuous exercise, then the strong probability is that an abnormal rhythm is present. The possibilities are atrial fibrillation, atrial flutter, or paroxysmal tachycardia. A history of previous attacks of sudden onset and sudden cessation strongly favours the diagnosis of paroxysmal tachycardia. If it can be confidently established that the heart is irregular, then atrial fibrillation is the probable cause and flutter with varying block is far less likely. Often mention is made of varying block causing cardiac irregularity but although this does happen it is unlikely to do so during the comparatively short time of listening. It must be appreciated that with a marked increase of rate it can be extremely difficult to be certain that it is irregular.

If there were a gross difference between a fast venous rate in the neck and the heart rate this would indicate that the patient had some degree of atrio-ventricular block and should lead to a definite diagnosis of atrial flutter. But as a practical point it must be emphasized that in this condition, even though the neck veins are engorged (which they are not necessarily), counting the venous rate in the neck is frequently impossible. In atrial flutter the atrial rate, and therefore theoretically the jugular venous rate, is over 300 beats per minute and nobody can even approximately count rates above 200 beats per minute. Therefore, in such a patient if it is possible to count the rate with reasonable accuracy (but it is emphasized again that this is frequently impossible) the diagnosis may be made if, with a heart rate of about 150 beats per minute, the venous rate is obviously well above this figure. The venous pulse wave may show very large *a* waves which are two, three or four times as frequent as the *v* waves.

Atrial flutter is nearly always associated with organic heart disease, usually hypertension, or coronary thrombosis, and only very rarely with mitral stenosis, thyrotoxicosis, pulmonary embolism or chest injuries.

Carotid sinus compression may, on occasion, be an important clue in the differentiation, because in atrial fibrillation such a procedure will have no effect whatsoever on the rate or rhythm. In atrial flutter, on the other hand, it will always increase the block and therefore reduce the ventricular rate, but only while the compression occurs, so that the heart abruptly reverts to its previous rate as soon as the pressure is removed. In supraventricular paroxysmal tachycardia such pressure may slow the heart, but if it does so it cures the condition so that the heart remains slowed even after the compression is removed. With sinus bradycardia any slowing produced by carotid compression is gradual and a return to normal after release of the pressure is also gradual. Carotid compression in the elderly should always be done on one side at a time and for less than a minute otherwise cerebral anaemia with unpleasant consequences may occur.

Ventricular paroxysmal tachycardia is rarer than the supraventricular type and, unlike the latter, is usually seen in patients with hypertensive, coronary or aortic heart disease. It very rarely responds to carotid compression and is often followed by congestive cardiac failure. An interesting feature of paroxysmal tachycardias is that they may be accompanied or followed by polyuria. Supraventricular tachycardia is only rarely associated with organic heart disease but does sometimes occur with mitral stenosis or coronary thrombosis. It may be due to digoxin therapy especially if there is hypokalaemia and with tricyclic antidepressants and monoamine-oxide inhibitors especially when taken with foods rich in tyramine.

Irregular hearts
If the heart is irregular, then the stage 1 diagnosis is that this patient must have an arrhythmia. Stage 2 considers the possibilities, which are sinus arrhythmia, extrasystoles, atrial fibrillation and partial atrial ventricular heart block. The commonest cause by far of a fast irregular heart is atrial fibrillation. The differentiation between these four conditions can be made with a very high degree of accuracy provided that a basic and routine approach is used. The pulse rate, the heart rate and, if possible, the jugular venous rate are all counted and any difference between them is noted, but only gross differences are significant. The heart is then carefully auscultated, a distinctive pattern being listened for. Finally, provided it is certain that the patient is fit enough, he should be exercised or given an injection of atropine or an inhalation of amyl nitrite.

Sinus arrhythmia can be easily recognized and dismissed by noting that the arrhythmia varies grossly with depth and rate of inspiration. It is of no significance.

Extrasystoles. In extrasystoles there is frequently, but not always, a pulse deficit (heart rate greater than the pulse rate) because the premature contractions are often too weak to produce a palpable pulse wave. On auscultation, runs of normal beats are usually heard which are then followed by the irregularity, such a state of affairs never being found with the other two arrhythmias. However, when there are very many extrasystoles or when they occur regularly, it may be very difficult or impossible to come to a decision on this basis. In any case, it should always be noted that with extrasystoles long pauses are always followed by strong beats and short pauses by weak ones. On exercise the irregularity will become less, although it may not disappear completely unless the exercise has been fairly vigorous.

The terms extrasystoles, ectopic beats and premature beats should be regarded as synonyms. All are premature beats usually instead of, and not in addition to, the normal beats, and the word 'extrasystoles' should be taken to indicate an extra (ectopic) focus of origin of the beat and not necessarily an extra heart beat. The differentiation between atrial, nodal and ventricular extrasystoles cannot be made for certain except by electrocardiography, and such accuracy has no clinical value. Extrasystoles are very common in normal people. Excess of stimulants, digoxin and emotional disturbances predispose to them. On the other hand extrasystoles may occur in patients with organic heart disease, especially coronary thrombosis, and they may be the forerunner of a serious arrythmia including ventricular tachycardia and ventricular fibrillation. The recognition of multiple extrasystoles by ECG monitoring has resulted in the more aggressive and sometimes successful therapy of coronary thrombosis.

Fibrillation. In atrial fibrillation there is usually, though not always, a pulse deficit, but the venous rate in the neck cannot be counted. On auscultation an irregular irregularity is heard, by which is meant that the beats are irregular in both times and force. The phrase 'irregularity in time' requires no explanation. 'Irregularity in force' means that, in contrast to extrasystoles, there is no correlation between the strength of a beat and the length of the preceding pause; the long pauses are frequently followed by small beats and vice versa, so that on auscultation, unlike the situation with extrasystoles, the strength of the next beat cannot be predicted. Finally, and this is often a most important diagnostic point, the irregularity is accentuated by exercise.

The common associations of atrial fibrillation are as follows:
1. Mitral stenosis.
2. Thyrotoxicosis — remember that in a elderly patient atrial fibrillation may be the first and only obvious manifestation of this condition, so the neck must always be examined in any patient who is fibrillating, although the absence of thyroid enlargement does not exclude the possibility.

3. Atherosclerosis of coronary vessels, with or without hypertension.

Heart block. With partial atrio-ventricular heart block, often simply referred to as partial block, there is never a pulse deficit and, if it is possible to count the venous rate in the neck, this will be observed to be far greater than the heart rate. On auscultation there will be grouped beats — *x* beats followed by a long pause, then *x* beats again, and so on. Such a finding, however, is not pathognomonic, because regularly occurring extrasystoles will produce the same auscultatory findings but with heart block following exercise, though the ventricular rate will be increased, the arrhythmia will still persist and *x* beats will still always be followed by long pauses. From the above considerations it will be seen that, in fact, a certain diagnosis of partial heart block is often a very easy one provided that the possibility is considered and the above procedures are methodically carried out.

Heart block is classified anatomically as sino-atrial, atrio-ventricular, and right bundle or left bundle branch block and hemiblocks. Sino-atrial block is usually secondary to digitalis or quinidine intoxication and cannot be diagnosed clinically. In itself it is of no clinical importance. Atrio-ventricular block is subdivided according to degrees. The first degree is a lengthened P-R interval (normally 0.12—0.22 second) as shown on ECG. Many regard it as evidence of a latent or potential rather than an actual block. The second degree is increasing length of the P-R interval with each succeeding beat until a beat is dropped (this is always a very transient state of affairs) and is called the Wenkebach phenomenon. The third degree is partial block in which every second or third or fourth or fifth beat, and so on, is dropped in regular sequence. Complete block is where no impulses from the atrium get through to the ventricle, which then assumes a regular rhythm of its own (idio-ventricular) with a rate of usually about 36—44 beats per minute. A heart block does not necessarily go through these phases of progression and may be complete from the start. It is extremely doubtful whether the first two degrees of atrio-ventricular heart block or a bundle branch block can be diagnosed with certainty or even probability except with an electrocardiogram. As is discussed later, their presence may be suspected by heart sounds, paradoxical splitting of the pulmonary second in left bundle branch block and non-fixed splitting in right bundle branch block.

The diagnosis of third-degree block has been discussed previously. Complete block can be diagnosed clinically with certainty if the patient has a heart rate of 36—44 beats per minute which does not increase with exercise. Confirmatory evidence will be provided if the venous rate in the neck is about 72 beats per minute compared with the ventricular rate of 36—44 beats per minute. The presence of visible cannon *a* waves in the neck, the varying intensity of the mitral first sound, and the hearing of independent atrial sounds are all comparatively unimportant additional clinical findings of which it is extremely difficult for even the expert to be certain. Patients with complete heart block often have a high pulse pressure. The vast majority of them have left ventricular enlargement, but this often precedes the heart block and is not a consequence of it and the large left ventricle may be associated with a functional mitral regurgitation. In elderly patients with complete block a degenerative aortic stenosis is fairly common.

The commonest causes of atrio-ventricular block are hypertension, coronary disease, as a complication of cardiac surgery, syphilis, rheumatic fever and diphtheria. In the last two conditions the block is nearly always of a minor degree. The commonest causes of left bundle branch block are atherosclerosis, hypertension, coronary disease and aortic stenosis. The commonest causes of right bundle branch block are mitral stenosis, atrial-septal defect and pulmonary embolism. Transient bundle branch block may occur with severe infections, during cardiac surgery, and with digoxin, quinidine and procainamide therapy. Right bundle branch block is very occasionally seen in normal children and young adults.

The attempt has been made to persuade the reader that with practice he can diagnose the exact nature of any arrythmia other than bundle branch blocks. Unfortunately many young doctors having found early in their careers that they cannot do so and consequently never make any genuine effort to acquire the ability, but such a nihilistic attitude usually indicates a complete reliance on ECGs.

Bruits

Having determined the rhythm, it is advisable next to concentrate on the presence of any bruits and to leave the consideration of heart sounds till later. It is important to develop the habit of describing all bruits in full detail and not dismissing them merely as systolic or diastolic. It is essential that all the following features of any bruit must be carefully sought, namely timing, duration, quality, area of maximum intensity, conduction, presence or not of a thrill, and alterations with exercise, posture and respiration. The terms 'bruit' and 'murmur' should be regarded as synonymous.

Timing

The technique of commencing auscultation at the aortic area, where usually it is easier than at the apex to differentiate between the first and second sounds, often helps to time murmurs, and this order of procedure may be found useful.

The usual way to time bruits is to place a finger on the point of maximum cardiac impulse and thus recognize the first sound, which is synchronous with it. If the cardiac impulse is forceful, it may lift the bell of the stethoscope with each systole, thus giving the timing of the first sound and so of any bruit. An alternative method, especially when the apex beat is feeble, is to feel the carotid pulse, because this immediately follows the first sound. A technique occasionally found useful when timing is difficult is to place the flat hand over the point of maximum cardiac impulse and to listen with the stethoscope between abducted fingers. The recognition as to which is the first heart sound and which the second and therefore the correct timing of a bruit can be made without any detailed evaluation of those heart sounds by noting that the first heart sound is synchronous with the apical or carotid impulse. Many undergraduates, inexperienced postgraduates and others similarly lacking in confidence, are often over-concerned with their difficulty in timing bruits. This undoubtedly does need diligent practice but it should be recognized that experience will also bring the reward of being able to distinguish each bruit by its own distinctive quality, which can come to be as readily recognized as can the opening chords of some familiar music without any recognition or analysis of the individual notes forming those chords.

It must be emphasized that to describe a murmur as an aortic or a mitral one is begging the question and is usually quite unwarranted. The division into aortic and mitral areas is conventional and does not mean that any sounds heard in either area necessarily come from that particular valve. Far better, for example, to speak of a systolic bruit in the aortic area rather than an aortic systolic bruit. It is an Irishism to talk of an aortic diastolic bruit as being due to pulmonary regurgitation, or a mitral systolic bruit as being due to ventricular septal defect. It is very important, moreover, that auscultation should never be restricted to these conventional areas. These are very elementary points, but frequently forgotten when describing and discussing bruits.

Diastolic bruits must be differentiated from other sounds which may occupy diastole, namely a split second sound, a third or fourth heart sound, triple rhythms, and an opening snap.

Duration
The duration of a murmur, especially if systolic, is very important. The typical bruit of mitral regurgitation (functional or organic) is pansystolic — that is, occupying the whole of systole. The typical bruit of aortic or pulmonary stenosis does not last throughout systole and is heard mainly or entirely in mid-systole. The distinction between a bruit that is truly pansystolic and one that occupies the greater part of systole is extremely difficult, especially if the heart is fast. Try to make such a distinction, but beware of the crime of Procrustes. The frequently expressed viewpoint that pansystolic bruits always and without exception indicate regurgitation lesions and short crescendo-dimuendo bruits stenotic lesion is not true.

Diastolic bruits are often of comparatively short duration: the only common exception to this is the bruit of mitral stenosis, which may, in the absence of fibrillation, be heard throughout mid and late diastole right up to the first sound.

Quality
When describing the quality of a murmur, the conventional epithets loud, soft, rough, blowing and rumbling should be used. Attempts to describe bruits in terms of either musical notation or a jargon derived from physics are strongly deprecated, because either vocabulary is meaningless to most doctors. Any romantic description using epithets or metaphors drawn from obscure sounds is likely to lead to confusion and not to further understanding. The author advises against the use of romantic terms such as groaning, vibratory, diamond, dovecot or seagull bruit, and also deprecates terms derived from the jargon of rheology which concerns the measurement of the flow of liquids, such as ejection and flow, with its subdivisions of turbulence, laminar and jet. The use of such terms is too often a conceit implying a certainty concerning the physical mechanisms responsible for them; their use may have the virtue of brevity but this is often at the expense of detailed observation and true understanding.

It is impossible to put into words an accurate description of anything heard. One recognizes somebody's voice on the telephone or the bark of one's own dog, but it would defy the analysis of all but the very few to explain to anybody else why that particular voice or that particular bark is recognizable. A bruit is a noise, and must be described in the terms which would be used to describe any other noises and in a language as standardized and as simple as possible. Hence the suggestion above that, save perhaps in the exceptional case, only words such as soft, loud, blowing, rough, and rumbling be used. What is one man's musical bruit is another man's squeak or even rasp.

Loudness
The method commonly practised of describing a systolic murmur in terms of grades, numbered according to loudness, is not advised because it presumes an accuracy which is in fact impossible and makes no allowance for observer error, because what appears to one observer to be a grade 1 murmur may be regarded as a grade 2 murmur by somebody else equally competent. Moreover, without scientific instruments to measure the degree of loudness of the sound, how can the correctness of either viewpoint be logically assumed? Also, one does not know that the loud bruit was always loud. Does a soft bruit, which would be dismissed as having no significance because of its lack of volume, ever become loud and therefore important? A faint (soft) systolic bruit, especially of short duration and localized to a small area, is extremely unlikely to be of significance

except very rarely in congenital heart lesions. A special feature of the loudness of a bruit is whether or not it is equally loud throughout as typically is the systolic bruit of mitral regurgitation, or crescendo as is often the diastolic bruit of mitral stenosis, or crescendo-diminuendo as is the bruit of aortic stenosis, or diminuendo as is usually the diastolic bruit of aortic regurgitation.

Maximum intensity
The position of maximum intensity need not, and usually cannot, be pin-pointed to some very small area such as that immediately above a particular rib. The danger of doing this is that incorrect inferences are likely to be drawn from a premise which, at best, is frequently uncertain. Generally one should be content to state, for example, that the murmur is maximal to the left or right of the sternum and over the upper or lower part of the sternum, being more precise only when one is absolutely certain.

Conduction
Conduction (propagation) of a bruit, especially systolic, can be important, because a significant systolic bruit at the apex is likely to be conducted to the axilla and one in the aortic region to the right side of the neck. Conduction of a systolic murmur into the right side of the neck is frequently missed because the observer has listened too high and too laterally above the clavicle. If a systolic murmur is heard at the base, it is advisable to listen immediately above the inner end of the clavicle; if that murmur be heard there, then regardless of whether it is loud or soft, it must be deemed that the murmur is conducted into the neck. As a general rule, a systolic bruit which is loudest at the base and is conducted to the left side of the neck is much more likely to be due to a congenital than to an acquired lesion.

Thrills
Thrills have been discussed previously. They must always be regarded as a feature of a bruit and not described independently, as is so often done. The presence or absence of a thrill depends mainly upon the loudness of the bruit.

Effects of exercise, positioning and respiration
The heart should never be regarded as normal until auscultation has been carried out after exercise and positioning. One must always listen for bruits with the patient in three different positions — lying flat, lying on his left side, and sitting up leaning forward. The patient must sit up and breathe deeply for about three times and then hold his breath at the completion of the third respiration before listening for the blowing diastolic bruit of aortic regurgitation. He must be exercised and turned on his left side before listening for the rumbling

diastolic bruit of mitral stenosis. A bruit arising from the right side of the heart is louder during inspiration, while one from the left side of the heart is not altered, but this differentiation is neither important nor wholly reliable.

The blowing diastolic murmur of aortic regurgitation is likely to be missed because it is high-pitched and most people have greater difficulty in hearing high-pitched sounds, and it is here that the diaphragm is essential. The rumbling diastolic murmur of mitral stenosis is frequently missed because it is usually heard over a small area only, and unless the stethoscope bell is placed over this spot the murmur will not be heard.

Significance

All diastolic murmurs should be considered significant and an explanation for them sought. A systolic murmur may or may not be significant, but such a bruit must be regarded as having significance only after the probable and possible significances have been fully considered and dismissed for good reasons. A systolic bruit associated with a thrill is always a significant one.

When discussing the possible significance of a systolic bruit, a tidy method must be used and on the evidence a decision must be made whether such a murmur is more likely to be due to a congenital or to an acquired lesion. Whichever group is favoured, that must be discussed completely before the other group is considered. Thus, the congenital and acquired lesions must be discussed separately and probabilities must always be considered before possibilities. A systolic bruit not occupying the whole of systole and heard over a wide area at the base is common in severe anaemia, in thyrotoxicosis and in high fever from any cause. When a systolic murmur is present as the only positive physical sign and no radiographs are available, it is very rarely possible for a certain diagnosis to be made and such a case must be considered as a logical exercise, weighing up the pros and cons of each possible lesion.

There are no criteria for distinguishing with certainty a systolic bruit which is significant from one which is not. It is better to avoid the terms 'innocent', 'functional' and 'organic' when describing bruits. But this difficulty does not justify complex invasive investigations in an attempt to solve the problem. Undoubtedly the risk of complications and even of iatrogenic heart disease by such techniques is far greater than any problematical risk by failing to diagnose with precision a heart lesion. In hearts as elsewhere investigatory prudence is a sign of clinical wisdom.

Extra-cardiac bruits

Extra-cardiac bruits are those which are heard at a site other than over the praecordium and are not conducted from the heart. The following are some extra-cardiac bruits:

1. A systolic bruit may be heard over any part of the body which
   has become pathologically very vascular. This is seen over the
   thyroid in the presence of thyrotoxicosis. In Paget's disease
   of bone because of the vascularity it causes it may rarely
   exhibit a bruit over the affected bones.
2. A systolic bruit may be heard over a large artery if it is
   obstructed, such as the carotid, femoral, brachial or renal.
   Such a bruit over the carotids however is not proof of stenosis,
   neither does absence of such a bruit exclude stenosis. Sometimes
   a bruit is heard over the opposite carotid to the one obstructed,
   and that is impossible to explain. A systolic bruit over a main
   artery is more likely to be significant if it is heard only with
   light pressure of the stethoscope and is constantly present on
   different days.

Venous hum. This is sometimes called a *bruit de diable* from a
supposed resemblance to the noise made by a diabolo (a toy). It is a
loud pansystolic bruit, occasionally extending into diastole, heard in
children above either clavicle. It is abolished or greatly lessened by
lying down or by stethoscope pressure or Valsalva* manoeuvre. It is
heard in healthy children and is of no significance, its only importance
being that it should not be mistaken for a significant bruit.

Heart sounds

Critical discussion
Having noted any bruits which are present and having determined the
detailed features of those bruits, then and then only should you give
special consideration to heart sounds. Some cardiologists, especially
when teaching, attach far too much importance to heart sounds.
Every student must make sure that he can appreicate, recognize and
discuss all the points concerning rhythms and bruits before indulging
in abstruse auscultatory findings such as paradoxical splitting,
summation gallops, and loud third heart sounds. He must always
have his feet firmly on the ground, and avoid the romances of
auscultation and the Procrustean crime of inventing the findings to
fit in with an assumed diagnosis. Especially in regard to hearing,
suggestibility is a potent source of error, and some persuasive doctor
can make the less experienced and uncritical hear anything that he
wishes him to hear. The Hans Andersen story, 'The Emperor's
Clothes', should be compulsory reading for all students. The subjects of the naked Emperor were afraid to admit that they could not
see his beautiful clothes, so enthusiastically described by the charlatan
tailors. Many students can be shamed into saying that they hear anything, being afraid lest they be deemed either deaf or daft.
   A great deal of the modern confusion on auscultation with
special reference to heart sounds is based on phonocardiography.

*Antonio Maria Valsalva (1666–1723), Bologna Surgeon.

It is assumed that because a graphic record displays for example, seven sounds within the cardiac cycle, the auscultator not only should but must hear that number of sounds. That phonographic and stethoscopic findings are strictly comparable is extremely doubtful. When a phonocardiograph shows some sound that has not been heard, the truth may be that the sound is an artefact, existing in the machine but not in the patient's heart. Too many clinicians are too readily prepared to doubt their hearing ability or the precision of their stethoscopes after they have studied a phonocardiograph. The essential value of phonocardiography is in timing sounds, and the other characteristics such as quality and duration can be greatly altered by technical factors concerning the machine itself. But apparently with increasing years, and even sometimes with increasing deafness, some cardiologists hear many more things than they could in their prime. Perhaps they also have become as stupid as the Emperor's subjects.

It is correct to say that the cardiologist can so attune his hearing that he can appreciate points previously not recognized, but the wisdom of attempting to teach such refinements to beginners is extremely doubtful. Furthermore, it is not generally appreciated that there is great dispute among experts themselves, not only concerning the interpretation of their phonocardiographs (and such disputes are surely beyond the scope of any but the specialists), but also concerning the interpretation of auscultatory findings. Conclusions drawn from the heart sounds are often based on poor foundations.

One author has described how in cases of mitral stenosis with regurgitation he often hears systolic and diastolic murmurs, an accentuated first sound and a split second sound, an opening snap, a third heart sound and a triple rhythm all in the region of the apex, and that these eight sounds, which all occur during a fraction of a second, he can not only time accurately but also recognize and label individually. In truth the phonocardiogram may show such an orchestra of sound, but the ability to sort out the components on auscultation and describe them in detail must be vouchsafed to the very few. Imaginative listening is to be strongly deprecated.

A further important point is that what was said about the artificiality of the conventional descriptive localization of bruits also applies to heart sounds. The heart sounds have a common origin regardless of their position of maximum intensity. When, for example, the mitral first or the aortic second sound is discussed, the first and second heart sounds are described as they are heard in the conventional mitral and aortic areas; the terms 'mitral' and 'aortic' sound are employed as useful and accepted abbreviations, instead of saying in full 'the second heart sound as heard in the aortic area' and so on. It will be appreciated that to talk, as some cardiologists do, of a split pulmonary second heard in the mitral area, is indeed heaping confusion upon confusion. Over the whole of the praecordium two heart sounds are usually heard, and usually we should be content to hear only two and not overstretch our auditory imagination.

The two sounds are commonly represented phonetically by *lub dup*. The first heart sound is normally louder at the apex, and the second at the base. The second sound is higher-pitched, more abrupt and shorter than the first. The pause preceding the first sound (diastole) is longer than that following it (systole). The recognition of the individual heart sounds can be learnt only by diligent practice. The term 'quiet heart' used by some, and which is apparently meant to indicate that the heart is normal, is better avoided. The antonym of 'quiet' is 'noisy', but what is a 'noisy heart'?

Both heart sounds, especially in the mitral area, are likely to be diminished by obesity, emphysema or pericardial effusion. They are both likely to be accentuated in any condition causing a marked increase in heart rate, but in either group of conditions, although both heart sounds are diminished or accentuated, they will still retain their own distinctive qualities.

First heart sound

The first heart sound indicates the onset of ventricular systole and is associated with closure of the mitral and tricuspid valves, although other factors about which there is much controversy play a part. It is nearly always best heard over the mitral area. Although theoretically it has two components, these cannot normally be heard independently. A loud first heart sound heard in the mitral area is found in tachycardia from any cause, and in mitral stenosis unless it is associated with marked mitral regurgitation or valve calcification. A diminished mitral first may indicate an early stage of atrio-ventricular block or other myocardial involvement, especially when due to infarction, but it is a very unreliable criterion of either of these conditions. The first heart sound may be diminished or absent in a rapidly progressive aortic regurgitation especially when associated with rupture or bacterial endocarditis of the valve. The mitral first is often masked if there is a loud pansystolic bruit in the area. Variations in intensity of the first heart sound occur in atrial fibrillation, complete atrio-ventricular block and ventricular tachycardia especially at the apex or lower left sternal border.

Splitting of any sound was in the past often described as reduplication. It is claimed that with practice it is possible to appreciate two closely spaced sounds as two different sounds when the interval between them is as short as 0.02 second. When listening for a split sound in any area, it is important that the patient should breathe quietly and not deeply and should not hold his breath. A split mitral first sound must not be mistaken for a presystolic bruit, which has an entirely different quality. A split mitral first may be heard with a right bundle branch block and will then be associated with a widely split pulmonary second sound. Splitting of the second heart sound usually refers only to auscultation at the base.

Second heart sound
The second heart sound is best heard at the base, where it is usually louder than the first heart sound. It is due to closure of both the aortic and the pulmonary valve and therefore has two components, an aortic (best heard in the aortic area) and a pulmonary (best heard in the pulmonary area). Except in infants and children, the pulmonary component is normally softer than the aortic. The aortic component may be widely conducted, but the pulmonary one is nearly always localized and cannot be heard at the apex. The physician should always concentrate on the relative loudness of the two components of the second sound in each of the aortic and pulmonary areas independently. Most physicians claim that in the majority of patients they can hear only a single heart sound at the base. Occasionally, even in healthy people (nearly always children and young adults) both the aortic and the pulmonary component can be distinctly heard on deep inspiration but the two components on expiration coalesce to form a single sound. A loud pulmonary second sound without any other cardiac or pulmonary abnormality is of no significance.

A split pulmonary component is far commoner than a split aortic component. Three different types of pulmonary splitting have been described:
1. A non-fixed splitting in which the two components are heard both in inspiration and expiration, and during inspiration the interval between them is reputed to be less than 0.02 second. It is usually described as a feature of right bundle branch block and of pulmonary stenosis, but some claim that it is most often heard with aortic stenosis and with left bundle branch block and with hypertension.
2. A wide splitting which varies only slightly with respiration is the so-called fixed splitting, the most important cause of which is a large atrial septal defect.
3. A splitting which increases or appears only on expiration is called a reversed or paradoxical splitting. This may be heard in pulmonary stenosis, patent ductus, large left-to-right shunts, left bundle branch block and aortic stenosis.

In pulmonary stenosis and also in aortic stenosis, the associated diminution of the second heart sound may render the certain recognition of splitting extremely difficult.

A loud pulmonary component is heard in patients with pulmonary hypertension from whatever cause. With pulmonary stenosis and with Fallot's tetralogy the pulmonary component is diminished.

A loud aortic component of the second heart sound is heard in systemic hypertension and also with an aortic aneurysm. In the

H

latter condition the sound may have a resonant tambour quality, often described as ringing. A diminution of the aortic second sound is a feature of aortic stenosis, and also of hypotension from whatever cause. Alteration of the first heart sound heard at the base (aortic first or pulmonary first sound) is of very doubtful significance.

Third and fourth heart sounds

Phonocardiography shows a third heart sound in a large number of normal people, especially children and young adults, the actual percentage being a matter of dispute. Such a sound is in diastole, is always localized to the region of the apex or xiphisternum, and is often palpable. It is soft and low-pitched and never rough or rumbling, and is accentuated by the patient lying flat and by exercise and deep inspiration. The bell and not the diaphragm must be used for its recognition. It is the sum total of these features which allows the differentiation of this sound from either a bruit or a split sound.

The general consensus of opinion is that the presence of a third sound in infants, children and young adults, especially if the heart rate is fast, is of no significance unless it is very loud and the heart is slow. It nearly always (possibly always) is important in those aged over about 40 years. It may be heard in mitral regurgitation in the absence of gross mitral stenosis; in constrictive pericarditis (some dispute that then it is really a third heart sound, being earlier and higher-pitched); in septal defects, in patent ductus, in cardiomyopathies and in cardiac failure (but the hearing of a third heart sound, even if certain, must be regarded as the flimsiest reason for such a diagnosis). Some cardiologists maintain that they can hear a third heart sound in a variety of other conditions.

Even if it is true that a fourth heart sound is often seen on phonocardiographs of normal people, it is certainly rarely heard. It is low-pitched and in late diastole just before the first sound, and it is best heard over the apical or xiphoid area. It is reputed to be an atrial sound, and in young people is of no significance. Some claim that a fourth heart sound is significant if it can also be felt. When heard in older people it will be extremely difficult to differentiate from either a third heart sound or a split first heart sound. It is reputed to be heard in atrio-ventricular block, cardiac failure, systemic and pulmonary hypertension and stenosis at any valve. Probably discussion of the fourth heart sound is better left to real experts and to the smart Alecks who pretend to be.

Triple and gallop rhythms

A triple rhythm is the presence of an extra sound which is not a bruit, an opening snap, or a splitting of the first or second heart sounds. If such an extra sound is in systole, it is of no significance and will not be discussed further.

The extra sound in diastole is always low-pitched but never rough or rumbling, is often palpable, and is best heard with a bell and not a diaphragm and with the patient lying down. It is localized to the region of the apex or to the fourth or fifth interspace near the left sternal margin, or to the epigastrium just below the xiphisternum. Its description is identical with a third and also a fourth heart sound, and the orthodox view is that the extra sound heard in a triple rhythm is actually either a third or a fourth heart sound or a coalescence (summation) of both. A difficulty of definition is that a third heart sound may be heard in several different conditions. Should the definition of triple rhythm include the reservation that those conditions have been excluded?

The extra sound is reputed always to be due to ventricular filling as a result of atrial contraction. It never occurs in the presence of atrial fibrillation. The three heart sounds, not being equally accentuated or spaced, have a special cadence which can be imitated by enunciation of the word Těnněs-sēē. When the heart is fast the cadence (the timing and accentuation of the sounds) may resemble the sound of galloping horses, and then the term 'gallop rhythm' may be used. A gallop rhythm is thus a triple rhythm with a fast rate. Obviously it is an Irishism to use the term 'slow gallop'. However, a fast rate is not an essential feature of a triple rhythm, although in fact the rate is nearly always above ninety.

Three types of triple rhythm have been described:

1. Diastolic gallop (triple) rhythm, when the extra sound is in early or mid diastole. It is sometimes called a protodiastolic or ventricular gallop. The extra sound is reputed to be a third heart sound.
2. Presystolic gallop (triple) rhythm, when the extra sound is in late diastole. It is otherwise known as an atrial gallop. It is reputed to be due to a loud fourth heart sound and must be distinguished from a split first sound.
3. Summation gallop, when the extra sound is very loud and is heard throughout the greater part of diastole. It occurs only when the heart rate is over about one hundred. It is reputed to be due to the coalescence of a third and fourth heart sound.

The importance of a triple rhythm, whether it sounds like galloping horses or not, is that it indicates a myocardial involvement otherwise perhaps diagnosable only by means of an electrocardiogram. It is reputed to be the earliest manifestation of heart failure in a patient who is not fibrillating and is especially likely to be heard in the presence of hypertension, coronary disease, aortic regurgitation or stenosis.

An atrial (presystolic) triple rhythm may be heard in any patient with a large left ventricle or pulmonary hypertension from any cause or pulmonary stenosis. A ventricular (diastolic) triple rhythm is an early sign of congestive cardiac failure and indicates a grave prognosis. It may also be heard with thyrotoxicosis and left to right shunts but in these two conditions the finding does not imply a bad prognosis. Rarely it occurs with pulmonary hypertension. A summation gallop is most often heard in patients with systemic hypertension who later develop congestive cardiac failure and thereby a superadded ventricular triple rhythm and the two becoming fused.

In my long experience as a teacher of clinical medicine, I have found that it is far commoner for the inexperienced to diagnose triple rhythms when they are not present than to miss them, even mistaking the rumbling diastolic bruit of mitral stenosis for a triple rhythm.

Valvular disease

There must be a routine and methodical way of discussing the diagnosis of valvular lesions. The following technique, in the order given, is advised:

1. *The cardinal sign.* This is always a particular kind of bruit which, though in itself not pathognomonic, is essential for the diagnosis of a lesion and only rarely occurs with any other condition. The diagnosis of any particular valvular disease in the absence of the characteristic bruit should not be made by anybody except perhaps the most experienced.
2. *Confirmatory evidence.* This is often found in the pulse, but the size of the heart and aspects outside the heart, such as facies and later radiographs and electrocardiograms, should be discussed.
3. *Any other bruits.* These may be heard in the particular condition or may be due to another lesion; they should be mentioned, and a full discussion of their probable and possible significance considered.
4. *The aetiology.*
5. *Cardiac failure.* Is this present?
6. *Treatment and prognosis.*

In discussing a patient with more than one valvular disease the main lesion should always be considered first and then the other murmurs described. Their probable and possible significance should be discussed later, always discoursing on diastolic before systolic murmurs. The main lesion can usually be determined easily; for example, in a case of mitral stenosis plus aortic regurgitation, if the patient is fibrillating it is almost certain that the mitral stenosis is the definite and dominant lesion, and the probability of the additional presence of aortic regurgitation should then be considered. On the other hand, if fibrillation is not present and there is a high pulse pressure, aortic regurgitation should be considered to be the definite and main lesion, and the probability of mitral stenosis also being present should then be discussed. In a patient with diastolic and systolic bruits at the base, although the diagnosis of aortic stenosis and regurgitation may be the correct one, these conditions must be considered separately; the dominant lesion can usually be easily decided by the pulse pressure, and then the presence or absence of the other lesion can be reviewed. In this way a necessary manoeuvrability is attained, because it must always be remembered that there are at least two ways of interpreting any particular bruit.

The various valvular lesions are considered below under the relevant headings.

AORTIC STENOSIS
Cardinal sign
The cardinal sign is a systolic bruit loudest at the base, which is conducted to the right side of the neck and may be heard over the whole of the praecordium. It is usually loud, high-pitched and rough, and may have a harsh rasping quality. The loudness increases towards and reaches a maximum about mid-systole and then gradually diminishes, ending appreciably before the second sound, but this last point may be difficult to appreciate if the second sound is grossly diminished. Expressed differently, the bruit is not pansystolic and has a gradual *crescendo* followed by a gradual *diminuendo* intensity. It is often absurdly referred to as a 'diamond murmur' because the phonocardiographic tracing has the shape of a diamond, and by others is conceitedly designated an ejection bruit. Very rarely the bruit is loudest down the left sternal border. It may be accompanied by a thrill, which is sometimes felt best in the right side of the neck and is often felt only if the patient sits or stands leaning forward and holds his breath in expiration.

These features of the bruit are not pathognomonic even if all of them are present. Aortic aneurysm, hypertension and sclerosis of the aortic valve may all cause an exactly similar bruit, except that only with an aneurysm and in aortic stenosis itself may the murmur be accompanied by a thrill. With congenital heart lesions a bruit of a similar character may be heard but, except in coarctation, the position of its maximal intensity is to the left of the sternum, and conduction to the right side of the neck is very unlikely.

Is it possible to have aortic stenosis without a thrill? The answer to this frequently posed question is yes, provided that:
1. The bruit has the qualities described above. The diagnosis of aortic stenosis when the systolic bruit is not as described — for example, if the murmur is maximal at or confined to the left side of the sternum, or is not *crescendo-diminuendo* with the maximum in mid-systole — may be correct but more often is proved to be wrong.

2. There is no suspicion that the heart lesion is syphilitic. Such suspicion may, for example, be aroused by the presence of pupillary abnormalities, optic atrophy or leucoplakia. Aortic stenosis is never syphilitic, and the coincidental presence of aortic stenosis and syphilis is an extremely rare one.
3. The patient is not hypertensive. Coexistence of hypertension and aortic stenosis, although it occasionally does occur, is so unusual that the problem must always be reconsidered before diagnosing such a coincidence.

Confirmatory evidence

The confirmatory evidence is given mainly by the pulse, which has a small volume and may also be plateau, occasionally anacrotic and, if the stenosis is associated with regurgitation, bisferiens.

A diminished aortic second sound is often regarded as important confirmatory evidence, but the negative aspect of this is perhaps more important, namely that a well marked aortic second sound should make one hesitate to diagnose aortic stenosis because it suggests either aneurysm or hypertension. Moreover, a normal aortic second sound does not rule out aortic stenosis.

The heart is enlarged, often considerably so, the apex beat being displaced outwards and downwards and exhibiting not only a forceful but also a sustained impulse. This enlargement can be confirmed radiologically, and the radiograph may also show calcification of the aortic valve. The latter finding has often been interpreted as indicating an atherosclerotic aetiology of the lesion. Calcified aortic stenosis is not a specific entity, and the term gives no clue to the aetiology because the valve is often calcified with increasing duration of the disease and ageing of the patient, regardless of the primary cause of the valve lesion, which may even be — though it very rarely is — a congenital anomaly of the cusps.

Other bruits

The only other murmur found in a patient with pure aortic stenosis is a systolic murmur at the apex which is conducted to the axilla. If the bruit is pansystolic, it indicates a functional mitral regurgitation due to a stretching of the mitral ring because of enlargement of the left ventricle; but if it has more or less the same features as the basal systolic murmur, it is due to conduction of the aortic stenotic murmur. If the systolic murmur is conducted not only to the axilla but also to the left scapular region, then it must come from the mitral valve and not be merely a conduction of the aortic stenotic murmur itself.

Aetiology

The only common causes of aortic stenosis are congenital, rheumatic and atherosclerotic. The aetiology favoured depends upon the age of the patient and the presence or absence of other valvular lesions.

If aortic stenosis is the sole lesion in any patient under the age of about forty years, then a congenital aetiology is the likely one. On the other hand, if it is the sole lesion in an older patient, the likely aetiological factor is atherosclerosis. If the lesion is associated with a definite mitral stenosis, then it must be rheumatic. The combination of aortic stenosis and aortic regurgitation is nearly always rheumatic, and this is the probable aetiology even in an older patient, but the possibility of an atherosclerotic cause should also be considered. Remember that complete heart block and bundle branch block are very commonly associated with aortic stenosis, especially in the elderly. In such a patient the pulse volume may not be small but may be large and even collapsing.

AORTIC SCLEROSIS

In some quarters aortic sclerosis has become a fashionable diagnosis although there is not agreement as to its precise meaning. The term is generally used to indicate a thickening of the aortic cusps which does not produce any significant obstruction to outflow of blood from the left ventricle − that is, there is no aortic valve stenosis.

Aortic sclerosis will give rise to a systolic bruit at the base which has all or most of the features of the aortic stenotic bruit but is never associated with a thrill. However, the pulse volume will be normal and neither anacrotic nor plateau. It is sometimes claimed that the condition may produce enlargement of the left ventricle, but it is difficult to explain this in view of the absence of any obstruction to the outflow of blood.

AORTIC REGURGITATION

Cardinal sign

The cardinal sign of aortic regurgitation (incompetence) is a blowing decrescendo diastolic bruit at the base, conducted down the left border of the sternum, where it is often best heard. The murmur is often described as being of a high pitch, but unfortunately many cannot appreciate pitch or do not really understand what the term means. The bruit can be imitated by whispering the word 'awe' during inspiration and is often best described as a 'whiff'. High-pitched bruits are difficult to hear unless a diaphragm is used. Added difficulties are that the bruit is often soft and short or may be localized to the second or third interspace on the right, or to the fourth interspace near the sternal edge on the left, or it may be heard only down the right sternal edge, or only when the patient sits up and holds his breath at the height of expiration. For all these reasons, it is frequently the most idfficult of all bruits to hear: indeed, there may well be disagreements, even between experts, as to whether such a murmur is present.

Phonocardiograms have demonstrated that this bruit is always early in diastole, and this point is frequently emphasized by the auscultator. However, the importance of such a distinction is obscure, and one must beware of the automatic emphasis that such a bruit is early in diastole whether or not one has truly been able to verify this nuance.

Rarely the bruit is accompanied by a diastolic thrill, and this is reputed to be commoner in syphilitic cases. The loudness and the duration of the bruit are extremely variable and are in themselves of no significance. When listening for this bruit it is essential for a diaphragm to be pressed firmly against the chest and for the patient to be sitting up and holding his breath at the height of expiration.

Such a bruit is not pathognomonic of aortic regurgitation, although it indicates that lesion in the great majority of cases, because pulmonary regurgitation also gives rise to the same type of bruit.

Confirmatory evidence

The best confirmatory evidence is the finding of a collapsing pulse with its associated features. The absence of a collapsing pulse does not exclude aortic regurgitation, but would indicate either that the lesion was only slight or that there was an additional significant degree of stenosis. With the patient sitting or standing, the carotid arteries may show a visible abrupt rise to a high amplitude and a quick fall in volume.

Further confirmatory evidence is cardiac enlargement, which, in uncomplicated aortic regurgitation, is caused solely by enlargement of the left ventricle. The radiograph may also show calcification of the aorta. If this is of the ascending aorta, it favours a diagnosis of syphilitic aortitis, whereas calcification of the arch or of the descending aorta is nearly always atherosclerotic. Electrocardiography will show left axis deviation.

Other bruits

A rough rumbling diastolic bruit, localized to the mitral area and called an 'Austin Flint* murmur', is sometimes found. Such a bruit has the features of a mitral stenotic bruit, and although subtle differential points are described, such as its not being quite as loud or quite as rough, such nuances are incapable of appreciation by the great majority of physicians. The bruit is not accompanied by an opening snap (described later). Should an Austin Flint murmur ever be diagnosed? Yes, if there is good reason to suspect that the aetiology of the aortic regurgitation is syphilitic, because then mitral stenosis must not be diagnosed; but apart from this contingency, such a murmur should always be considered as due to mitral stenosis. In the presence of atrial fibrillation the Austin Flint murmur should never even be considered as a possibility.

*An American physician who wrote in 1862.

In the great majority of cases of aortic regurgitation, the blowing diastolic murmur is accompanied by a systolic murmur. The features of this should be noted in the particular patient to whom you have listened, as these details give an important clue to the likely cause of that murmur. A commonly used phrase, 'to-and-fro murmur', to describe the combination of diastolic and systolic murmurs has the great disadvantage that it automatically ascribes one cause, aortic regurgitation, to both murmurs and does not make one consider other possibilities for the systolic element. The popular term 'flow murmur' is pompous and should not be used. This systolic murmur may be due to aortic stenosis provided that the requirements described above are complied with. Aneurysm (*see* below) must always be considered. Aortic sclerosis must be considered in any patient who has no evidence in the pulse supporting the diagnosis of aortic stenosis.

The systolic murmur may be due to a coincidental hypertension, and the presence of aortic regurgitation with hypertension in a person under the age of about 40 years should make one think of the possibility of coarctation and search for its confirmatory signs. Such consideration is frequently missed because of the oft-repeated misleading statement that with uncomplicated aortic regurgitation the systolic pressure is frequently high. Only after the above four conditions have been carefully considered and discarded as unlikely should the murmur be dismissed as of no significance. The patient may also have a systolic murmur at the apex conducted to the axilla, and this either indicates a functional mitral regurgitation or has no significance. A short booming sound synchronous with the pulse, referred to as a 'pistol shot', is often heard over the femoral artery, and sometimes over the same site a combination of systolic and diastolic bruits is heard if the pressure with the stethoscope is only slight.

Aetiology

There are only two common aetiologies of aortic regurgitation, namely rheumatic fever and syphilis (the valvular lesions being then always secondary to an aortitis), and these should always be considered before other possibilities are even mentioned.

Syphilis does not affect the valve cusps, therefore the resultant regurgitation is not complicated by stenosis. The presence of pupillary changes, optic atrophy, or leucoplakia of the tongue is a frequent indication of the possibility of syphilis, and after diagnosing an aortic lesion one should always examine the eyes and tongue, although of course cardiovascular syphilis can occur without other syphilitic lesions. A syphilitic aetiology should be considered when the aortic regurgitation is the sole lesion, especially in a patient over 40 years of age.

Rarer causes are ankylosing spondylitis, rheumatoid arthritis, non-specific urethritis, atherosclerosis, bicuspid aortic valve (which is a congenital anomaly and may be associated with other congenital anomalies and may form part of the Marfan syndrome), ruptured aortic cusp, dissecting aneurysms of the ascending aorta, bacterial endocarditis and following aortic valve surgery.

AORTIC ANEURYSM

The only pathognomonic sign of an aneurysm is an expansile pulsation in the second or third right interspace. If the patient is lying flat, this is best seen with the observer's eyes at the same horizontal level as the patient's sternum — that is, tangentially. An expansile pulsation in the right side of the neck or the suprasternal notch is suspicious but not pathognomonic, being more frequently caused by a kinked carotid. Dullness to the right of the sternum should be sought, and there may be exquisite tenderness in the region because of bone erosion by the aneurysm, which usually distends in a forward direction. There is nearly always a loud rough systolic bruit at the base, often conducted to the right side of the neck and usually associated with a thrill. The second sound in the aortic area is loud, often being described as ringing or metallic or of a tambour-like quality. Manifestations of compression of the trachea, the superior vena cava, the cervical sympathetic or recurrent laryngeal nerve, the main bronchus, or the innominate or subclavian artery (shown by pulse inequality), should be looked for.

The absence of any, or even all, of these signs does not exclude the presence of aneurysm. It is an aneurysm of the ascending aorta which is more likely to give rise to signs (aortic regurgitation and expansile pulsation to the right of the sternum). Aneurysms of the arch or the descending aorta are more likely to give rise to compression symptoms.

A tracheal tug is elicited with the patient sitting up, with his mouth closed and his head extended. The physician should stand behind him and grasp the cricoid cartilage between finger and thumb, maintaining a steady upward pressure. A pull or tug downwards is felt. This sign is important because it is often positive when the aneurysm extends backwards and does not cause a visible expansile pulsation.

MITRAL STENOSIS

Cardinal sign

The cardinal sign is a rough rumbling low-pitched diastolic murmur, localized to the mitral area and accentuated by exercise and turning the patient on to his left side. Nobody should make a diagnosis of mitral stenosis unless he has heard such a bruit. The bell and not the diaphragm must be used. Attention must be concentrated, and the importance of positioning and exercise cannot be over-emphasized.

The bell must be applied firmly, but the pressure against the skin should be gradually relaxed while listening, as the bruit may be rendered audible by alteration of stethoscope pressure. The only other such murmur is the Austin Flint murmur diagnosed with certainty only in the presence of a syphilitic aortic regurgitation.

Other features of the bruit which may be present are its accompaniment by a diastolic thrill and a presystolic accentuation. The older cardiologists used to boast that whereas the tyro could hear only one bruit in mitral stenosis, they could often hear two separate bruits, mid-diastolic and presystolic. However, since the introduction of phonocardiography and the demonstration that two such bruits are indeed extremely exceptional, it is no longer fashionable for cardiologists to hear them and the phrase 'mid-diastolic with presystolic accentuation' is now the popular one. If the patient fibrillates the murmur loses its presystolic accentuation, but when one is considering whether or not a patient with mitral stenosis is fibrillating, the presence or absence of presystolic accentuation should not influence one's opinion.

In the presence of cardiac failure, especially in elderly people, the characteristic bruit of mitral stenosis may be difficult to hear. The effect of valvotomy on the bruit is extremely variable; it may even be rendered more obvious, and its loudness is of no value in the assessment of the operative result. The duration of the bruit is a guide, but an unreliable one, to the degree of the stenosis. Its loudness is certainly no criterion.

Confirmatory evidence
In regard to the confirmatory evidence, the pulse in an uncomplicated mitral stenosis is frequently referred to as being of small volume, but in a case of pure mitral stenosis it is very likely to be normal. Although in severe cases there may be some diminution of pulse volume, this is of such minor degree as rarely to be recognizable on palpation, even though instrumental aids may show it. The negative aspect of this fact is more important, namely that if a patient with mitral stenosis has a large-volume pulse, then he must have some additional lesion.

The size of the heart, as judged clinically by the position of the apex beat, is not increased in an uncomplicated mitral stenosis. Although it is true that there is enlargement of the right side of the heart and the left atrium, which can be seen radiologically and verified *post mortem*, this is rarely of such a degree as to be diagnosable clinically. Moreover, enlargement of these chambers does not, save in very exceptional circumstances, cause any downward and outward displacement of the apex beat. Enlargement of the right chamber of the heart and the left atrium may be recognized, when extreme, by dullness to the right of the sternum, but not by displacement of the apex beat.

If a patient with mitral stenosis has an increase in the size of the heart, some additional lesion must always be sought for. He may have another valvular lesion. He may have coincidental hypertension, and with the increasing recognition of mitral stenosis in the older age groups, such a coincidence is now fairly commonly found. He may have an adherent pericardium. Cardiac failure in itself should never be regarded as a satisfactory explanation of a clinically enlarged heart in a patient with apparently pure mitral stenosis.

The mitral facies, with dilated capillaries and venules on the cheeks, is neither pathognomonic of, nor always seen in, mitral stenosis. It is sometimes seen in patients with pulmonary hypertension from other causes. Its presence should be regarded as an incentive to examine the patient carefully for the possibility of a mitral stenosis. The term 'malar flush', sometimes used, is unsatisfactory because this indicates a transitory and not a permanent phenomenon.

Auscultation

In mitral stenosis frequently the presystolic murmur ends in a loud first sound, often described as slapping. But the presence of this sound is in itself poor confirmatory evidence, and the hearing of it, especially in the absence of tachycardia, should be regarded as a finding which draws one's attention to the possibility of mitral stenosis and demands that its murmur be sought for after exercise and posturing of the patient. On the other hand, if the patient definitely has got mitral stenosis, a diminished mitral first sound suggests but does not prove that the lesion is only of mild degree, or that there is a dominant mitral regurgitation, or that the valve is calcified. A loud slapping first sound is nor proof that the mitral valve is pliant and therefore likely to respond well to surgery.

An opening snap is a short sharp high-pitched sound immediately following the second sound. It is best heard just internal to the apex beat, usually being localized to that region; it is heard better with the diaphragm, and is not altered by deep inspiration. There is only a very short interval between the opening snap and the diastolic bruit. It is sometimes claimed that the shorter the interval between the second heart sound and the opening snap and the longer the duration of the diastolic bruit the more marked the stenosis, but few honest cardiologists would claim to be able to make this assessment with certainty. When there is a rumbling mid-diastolic bruit and also an opening snap and a loud first heart sound the result can be represented phonetically by rhoo-phfoot-tata (rhoo representing the rumbling diastolic, phoo its presystolic accentuation ending in the first sound, and tata the second heart sound followed closely by the opening snap). The significance of hearing an opening snap in a patient with mitral stenosis is that the patient is unlikely to have a significant degree of associated mitral regurgitation. It is a less reliable indication that the valve cusp is pliant (mobile) and not calcified. Subtle differentiations between an opening snap and a split second sound heard at the apex, are that an opening snap occurs later in diastole, and that the Valsalva manoeuvre will delay an opening snap but will have no effect on splitting, but neither point has much practical value.

The opening snap also very closely resembles a third heart sound, the points of differentiation being that the former is closer to the second sound; is clicking, higher-pitched and shorter; is often heard over a wider area, and is usually also palpable – all of which can also be very subtle and difficult points of differentiation. But an opening snap may be considered important in a patient with combined mitral stenosis and regurgitation because an opening snap would suggest dominance of the stenosis and a third heart sound would suggest dominance of the regurgitation.

Once again it is necessary to emphasize the difficulties and lack of reliability of such differentiations and therefore the danger of basing opinions on the flimsy evidence of imaginative listening. Mitral stenosis can be diagnosed with certainty although an opening snap has not been heard.

Other bruits
The only other bruit commonly heard in cases of mitral stenosis is a systolic bruit at the mitral area conducted to the axilla, and such a murmur either means a mitral regurgitation, or has no significance.

In mitral stenosis, in addition to the characteristic murmur, there may be a blowing diastolic murmur down the left border of the sternum. This should always make one think first of aortic regurgitation, but where there are no peripheral signs of this condition and one feels confident that the pulmonary second is increased, the possibility should always be considered of pulmonary regurgitation secondary to pulmonary hypertension ('Graham Steell* murmur'). An opening snap should not be confused with the Graham Steell murmur.

From the above descriptions it will be realized that the following diastolic bruits may be heard at the mitral area: the mitral stenotic bruit, the Austin Flint bruit, the aortic regurgitation bruit and the pulmonary regurgitation bruit. There is also the Carey Coombs† murmur, which is a low-pitched, relatively short *diminuendo* diastolic bruit. Heard in the apical region during an attack of acute rheumatic fever, it commonly comes and goes. The absurdity of talking about mitral diastolic bruits, instead of speaking of a diastolic bruit in the mitral area and giving a full and detailed description of the bruit, is thus further emphasized.

---

*Graham Steell (1851–1942), a British surgeon who wrote his account in 1888.
†A British physician who wrote his account in 1924.

Radiography

In minor degrees of pure mitral stenosis, the cardiac outline seen radiologically is often normal. In more severe lesions the postero-anterior view shows a normal aorta, an enlarged pulmonary conus (pulmonary artery and its left main branch), a normal left ventricle, and an enlarged right atrium; if there is considerable enlargement of the hilar pulmonary vessels, it will be due mainly to venous and not arterial enlargement and therefore probably will be associated with congestive changes at the bases. Stated differently, hilar enlargement – especially on the right side – is never marked in pure mitral stenosis unless failure is present, and this will be shown radiologically by bilateral basal lung changes and possibly by pleural effusion. This cardiac silhouette is not pathognomonic of mitral stenosis because a cor pulmonale will give the same picture, but in the latter case the pulmonary lesion will be recognized readily except when it is caused by emphysema. A similar cardiac outline can also be caused by a patent septum or patent ductus, but then there will be obvious enlargement of hilar arteries, and the lung bases are likely to be clear.

Occasionally, enlargement of the right ventricle and/or of the left atrium may be demonstrable on the postero-anterior view; the latter may appear as a hump below the pulmonary arc on the left border or above the right atrium on the right, or its curved right border may be seen through the heart shadow. Often the enlarged left atrium is concealed by the dilated main pulmonary artery and its left branch. Very dense, well-defined, usually small shadows may be seen scattered throughout both lung fields, but especially the mid and lower zones. They are due to haemosiderosis (deposition of iron); and they are probably due to minute organized and calcified haemorrhages secondary to pulmonary hypertension. Sometimes the lung fields show well-defined horizontal parallel linear shadows at the bases and in the region of the horizontal fissure, usually just above the diaphragm; these are commonly regarded as being due to dilated septal lymphatics. Calcification of the valve may be seen. The X-ray may exhibit a diversion of the blood into the upper lobes which then appear more vascular than the lower.

In mitral stenosis a right anterior oblique view will show enlargement of the left atrium, and this does not occur with either cor pulmonale or congenital heart lesions. A barium swallow in this oblique position may show a marked concavity and backward displacement of its lower portion due to the enlargement of the left auricle.

Aetiology

The aetiology of mitral stenosis should always be considered as rheumatic, even though there be no definite history of rheumatic fever or chorea, unless some extremely unusual associated features outside the heart make one think of some comparatively rare cause such as systemic lupus erythematosus.

MITRAL REGURGITATION

Types

Mitral regurgitation may be either functional or organic. The former type, seen whenever there is marked enlargement of the left ventricle, is therefore found especially in hypertension and aortic disease. It follows that the diagnosis of functional mitral regurgitation should never be made unless one can definitely demonstrate left ventricular enlargement and a cause for it. Organic mitral regurgitation is due to a valvulitis and in the great majority of cases is associated with mitral stenosis and without it the diagnosis of organic mitral regurgitation should not be made without great hesitation, especially in a middle-aged or older person.

Rupture of the chordae tendinae or the papillary muscle which is usually due to coronary thrombosis, have been described as a cause of mitral incompetence, or an explanation of identical signs, and very dubious claims have been made that such lesions can be diagnosed on auscultation. But although many patients with coronary thrombosis have the murmur of mitral incompetence, this may well have been present prior to the coronary thrombosis and not caused by it.

Cardinal sign

The characteristic bruit is systolic, usually loud and always long, occupying the whole (pansystolic) or at least the greater part of systole. Commonly it is of the same intensity throughout its duration. It is usually high-pitched and blowing, but may be harsh and medium-pitched. It is maximal in the region of the apex beat and conducted to the axilla; its loudness is not a reliable indication of its severity.

It is important to realize that absence of any of the above features of the bruit makes the diagnosis of mitral regurgitation a possibility rather than a probability. The diagnosis is far too often made on insufficient evidence and turns out to be incorrect.

It is unusual for this murmur to be conducted upwards, and if a systolic murmur is heard down either side of the sternum and also in the axilla, then, regardless of where it is considered to be maximal, either the patient has mitral regurgitation (functional or organic) plus some other lesion (acquired, such as aortic stenosis, or congenital, such as septal defect) or the case is not one of mitral regurgitation. Stated differently, it is very common for a basal systolic bruit to be conducted to the apex, but unusual for an apical systolic bruit to be conducted up towards the base. It is unusual for the murmur of mitral regurgitation to be accompanied by a thrill, and systolic thrills in this area are much more likely to be due to a septal defect.

Confirmatory evidence

The confirmatory evidence is enlargement of the left ventricle. The presence of an opening snap means that a significant degree of mitral regurgitation is unlikely, but the absence of an opening snap should not be regarded as confirmatory evidence of mitral regurgitation. The presence of a well-marked third heart sound in a patient with mitral stenosis is evidence of an associated significant degree of regurgitation. With a pure mitral regurgitation the mitral first sound is likely to be diminished, but if it is associated with stenosis the sound will be normal or increased, the loudness of the first sound being inversely proportional to the severity of the regurgitation. This, however, is not completely reliable evidence.

The radiograph will show, in addition to the features of the mitral stenosis, an enlargement of the left ventricle. Expansile pulsation of the left atrium, seen on screening, is considered to be a more important diagnostic sign, but the appreciation of this is extremely difficult and many authorities even deny the pathognomonic nature of this sign.

Whether a patient with mitral stenosis also has a significant degree of mitral regurgitation has now, because of consideration of surgery, become an important assessment, but there is no infallible guide, and reliance on even a combination of the above signs gives an accuracy short of 100 per cent.

PULMONARY REGURGITATION

Pulmonary regurgitation is always functional except when due to damage to a congenital stenotic valve as a result of either surgery or infective endocarditis. The cardinal sign is a blowing diastolic bruit down the left border of the sternum in the absence of peripheral evidence of aortic regurgitation, but invariably associated with a loud pulmonary second sound except in the post-operative cases. Such a diagnosis cannot usually be made clinically with certainty, but can merely be considered as probable or possible. The condition occurs in mitral stenosis and patent septum (especially atrial).

TRICUSPID REGURGITATION

Tricuspid regurgitation may be either functional or organic. When functional, it is due to a stretching of the ring because of enlargement of the right ventricle associated with congestive cardiac failure or cor pulmonale.

Organic tricuspid regurgitation is due to a valvulitis and is rarely seen except in association with mitral stenosis. Very rarely it is caused by bacterial endocarditis or systemic lupus erythematosus or associated with a carcinoid tumour.

The diagnosis of tricuspid regurgitation can be made with certainty in a patient with mitral stenosis if he has an expansile pulsation of the liver and/or varicose veins of the lower limbs which exhibit expansile pulsation – a rare phenomenon. Because of its diagnostic implication, an expansile pulsation of the liver should never be diagnosed unless one is certain that it is expansile and not merely transmitted. If the liver pulsation is timed with the carotid, it may be found to be later in systole than the carotid pulsation, and this is strong evidence that it is an expansile and not a transmitted hepatic pulsation. The only other cause of this sign is a large angioma of the liver, which is extremely rare. On the other hand, in a patient with mitral stenosis the condition of organic tricuspid regurgitation should be considered as a probability if the patient has (1) raised jugular pressure which increases on pressure below the right costal margin, especially if associated with marked pulsation in which one is certain that one can see large *a* waves (in the absence of fibrillation), and (2) an enlarged liver without other commensurate evidence of cardiac failure. Hepatomegaly is a constant finding in tricuspid regurgitation, whatever its type or its aetiology. Ascites and/or pleural effusion are common with tricuspid valve lesions of all types.

Tricuspid regurgitation, either functional or organic, causes a systolic bruit which in the vast majority of cases is impossible to differentiate from the bruit of mitral regurgitation especially because tricuspid regurgitation and mitral regurgitation often occur together and the bruit of each is virtually indistinguishable. An unreliable distinction is that in mitral regurgitation the bruit is maximum near the apex and in tricuspid regurgitation it is maximum near the xiphoid. A distinction that is perhaps more valuable is that on doing the Valsalva manoeuvre in tricuspid regurgitation the bruit promptly increases in intensity whereas in mitral regurgitation the bruit may not increase in intensity and if it does it does so only slowly.

TRICUSPID STENOSIS

This is a rare acquired lesion and, when it occurs, is nearly always associated with a rheumatic mitral stenosis and often with aortic valve disease as well and an isolated lesion is very rare. It causes a rumbling diastolic bruit, sometimes with pre-systolic accentuation, localized to the region of the xiphoid or to the right of the sternum. The loudness of this may be increased on deep inspiration, which has no effect on the mitral stenotic bruit. Jugular venous pulsation, if present, may show a very large *a* wave and a diminution of the *y* descent. In actual fact this bruit cannot be distinguished with certainty from the murmur of mitral stenosis, and it is very doubtful if the diagnosis can be made with certainty on clinical grounds.

Pericarditis

Pericarditis is rarely an entity on its own and is more often a localized manifestation of a generalized disease. The types of pericarditis are (1) dry, (2) with effusion, (3) adherent, and (4) constrictive.

DRY PERICARDITIS

In dry pericarditis the cardinal sign is the hearing of a rub which has usually a scratching quality but has been variously described as rasping, scraping, grating, rustling or crackling or the crunching sound made by walking over freshly fallen snow and it may even, like the pleural rub, resemble the creaking of new leather, but its character varies not only in different patients but at different times in the same patient.

The rub is present during systole and diastole but is often of inconstant timing and rarely may occur only in systole. It is usually localized to a comparatively small area, most often in the third and fourth interspace immediately to the left of the sternal edge; it is increased by pressure of the stethoscope and may be altered by change of posture, generally being increased when the patient is leaning forward or sometimes by holding the breath at the end of expiration. An important feature is that it is transient. Sometimes a pericardial rub can be felt as well as heard especially if the patient is sitting up and leaning forward. Any dry pericarditis may later be complicated by an effusion, but two common causal conditions in which this rarely occurs are cardiac infarction and uraemia. Pain is a common symptom of pericarditis but it has no special features, its site, quality and intensity differ considerably in different patients and it may mimic any pathology in the chest or abdomen.

PERICARDIAL EFFUSION

With a pericardial effusion the patient is often restless, looks anxious, and occasionally is cyanosed. He is often most comfortable leaning as far forward as possible. The apex beat will be seen with difficulty. In children, particularly if the effusion has been present for a long time, there may be bulging of the praecordium. The apex beat may not be palpable even with the patient leaning forward and, if it is felt, it may be possible to demonstrate that its position is internal to the left cardiac border as assessed by percussion.

Especially in acute pericardial effusions, cardiac tamponade may develop. By this is meant a cardiac compression due to the pericardial effusion which is of such a degree as seriously to interfere with diastolic filling and to a lesser degree the contraction of the ventricles. It causes a marked rise in the jugular venous pressure and a marked fall of the systemic blood pressure. The jugular vein distension will be considerably accentuated by deep inspiration. A pulse paradox is nearly always present.

On percussion there will be an increase in cardiac dullness to the right and left, and this impairment of percussion note will be marked because it is due to fluid. It may be possible to demonstrate that the shape of this dullness alters with the position of the patient, being globular when he is lying down and pear-shaped with the stalk uppermost when he is sitting up. However, it is easier to demonstrate, especially in fat people, that there is dullness in the second left interspace immediately to the left of the sternum which is present when the patient lies down, disappearing when he sits up. If the effusion is fairly large, there may be a moderate impairment of percussion note over the left lower lobe of the lung, associated sometimes with bronchial breath sounds, signs which are not due either to consolidation or collapse of the lower lobe. A described sign, rarely demonstrable, is dullness in the fifth right interspace immediately to the right of the sternum, sometimes described as demonstrating that the cardio-hepatic angle, which is normally acute, has become obtuse. Some radiologists report an equivalent sign, the cardio-phrenic angle becoming obtuse instead of the normal acute angle, but this also is unreliable because the commonest cause of alteration of the angle is normal pericardial fat.

On auscultation, frequently a pericardial rub can still be heard even though the effusion be fairly large. The cardiac sounds will be distant and faint but will have their normal accentuation. In subacute or chronic pericardial effusion hepatomegaly and ascites with a minor degree of peripheral oedema are common.

If the effusion is less than about 200 ml the X-ray silhouette will be normal. Larger effusions will show a generalized increase of the cardiac shadow with, later, a loss of the normal convexities, especially on the left border, which becomes straight. If the patient is fit enough, alteration in the shape of the opacity can be demonstrated radiologically with the patient lying down and sitting up. On screening, a comparative lack of pulsation of the enlarged heart may be a distinctive feature but, surprisingly, this expected sign is often absent. A rapidly increasing generalized cardiac enlargement shown on serial X-rays is virtually pathognomonic of pericardial effusion.

CONSTRICTIVE PERICARDITIS

It is usual although controversial to differentiate between constrictive pericarditis and adherent pericardium. Constrictive pericarditis is caused by extensive adhesions between the two pericardial layers, is usually seen in young people, and is most often the end result of a tuberculous lesion. Rarely other organisms including viruses, are the cause. The condition is never due to rheumatic fever. It interferes with normal cardiac diastolic relaxation, and this impairs the venous inflow into the right ventricle. It is now considered that neither superior nor inferior vena caval obstruction is a factor in the production of the circulatory disturbances.

The neck veins are engorged and show pulsation, in which it may be possible to observe a diminution of the venous distension with each diastole (diastolic collapse) and an increase with deep inspiration. Marked and sharp x and y descents may be discernible. In about half the cases a pulsus paradoxus is present.

The apical impulse is often difficult to see and feel. In the majority of cases there is no cardiac enlargement. This statement assumes that adherent pericardium is regarded as a different condition. There may be a systolic retraction of the interspaces and ribs, but when present indicates an associated adherent pericardium rather than constrictive pericarditis. Usually in the region of the apex, but sometimes over a wider area, an extra impulse may be felt during diastole which is described as a tap, a knock or a palpable shock, and this is synchronous with an extra sound which has been variously interpreted and labelled, but is usually described as a loud third heart sound. The rhythm is nearly always normal, but may rarely show atrial fibrillation. Ascites with little or no peripheral oedema is often a comparatively early sign, usually being associated with a palpable liver and occasionally also with a palpable spleen. A pleural effusion unassociated with cardiac failure is fairly common.

A radiograph will nearly always show no cardiac enlargement in the absence of an adherent pericardium but usually shows linear calcification along the cardiac border, often along the diaphragmatic border or in the atrio-ventricular groove. This is often best seen in lateral and oblique views. Its absence does not exclude the diagnosis. A calcified pericardium may occur without causing any symptoms or clinical signs whatsoever.

ADHERENT PERICARDIUM

The physical signs of an adherent pericardium, which is due to adhesions between the parietal pericardium, chest wall, pleura and diaphragm, are (1) cardiac enlargement; (2) systolic retraction, especially over the scapular region; (3) fixity of the apex beat.

The condition can never be diagnosed with certainty, but should be considered in any patient with an enlarged heart for no apparent reason. Some deny that it ever causes either cardiac enlargement or serious impairment of the circulation. It may be associated with a constrictive pericarditis, and some cardiologists do not make any distinction between adherent and constrictive pericarditis.

Rheumatic fever

In the wealthier countries of the world the clinical picture of rheumatic fever has altered considerably during the past few decades and, especially in adults, the symptoms are often atypical and vague with an insidious onset. The classical clinical picture, which is still frequently seen in the poorer countries, can be remembered by the mnemonic CANT CHAPS, the letters standing for carditis, arthritis, nodes, tonsillitis, chorea, hyperpyrexia, anaemia, pleurisy and pneumonia, and skin lesions.

CARDITIS

The carditis is a pancarditis and is the most important manifestation of the rheumatic process. How can one, during or soon after a rheumatic infection, know whether or not the heart is involved? If the patient has a pericarditis, either dry or with effusion, this is certain proof. Pericarditis developing early in the disease is not a bad prognostic sign, but it becomes so if it occurs after about the eighth week from the commencement of the illness. The development of fibrillation, flutter or paroxysmal ventricular tachycardia would also be incontrovertible evidence. However, apart from the development of a first degree atrio-ventricular heart block, recognizable on electrocardiography as a prolonged P-R interval, such arrhythmias are unusual, and while atrio-ventricular block is strong suspicion of heart involvement it is not certain proof because it may be transient without further evidence of heart involvement ever developing. The atrio-ventricular block very rarely progresses beyond the first degree.

Cardiac enlargement is very difficult to assess in its minor degrees clinically and radiologically, even presuming that the patient is fit for such an investigation (portable films not being satisfactory to assess cardiac size). The increase in heart size shown by standard and uniform radiological techniques must be at least 10 per cent to be significant. Moreover, cardiac enlargement is a late sign. Frequently in children there is a transient enlargement during the course of any acute infection, but this is rarely followed by permanent cardiac damage. Thus any cardiac enlargement in rheumatic fever, even if it can be demonstrated, does not necessarily prove that the heart has been affected.

Assessment of the cardiac sounds as an indication of myocardial damage is a pastime which has been critically discussed previously and inferences drawn from such findings are rarely justifiable. The hearing of any diastolic bruit should always be regarded as evidence of valvular involvement. However, it takes several years for the characteristic mitral stenotic bruit to develop because the stenosis of the valve is a very gradual process, and therefore the absence of such a murmur does not exclude mitral valvular disease. A Carey Coombs bruit should always give rise to suspicion of mitral valvulitis. A systolic murmur anywhere over the praecordium, whatever its quality or degree of loudness, is almost invariably present when cardiac involvement occurs during an acute attack. However, such a bruit, whatever its loudness or length, does not prove cardiac involvement but should arouse suspicion, especially if it is pansystolic and conducted to the axilla. Even then however, it may subsequently disappear without a mitral valve lesion ever appearing. It is rarely justifiable to prolong extensively the child's bed rest and perhaps even cause the patient to be regarded as a permanent invalid on the basis of such a systolic murmur.

It will be seen from the above that the assessment of cardiac involvement, in the absence of the more obvious signs of cardiac failure, can be extremely difficult if not impossible. Certain points outside the heart should always be considered. The presence of continued fever or the recurrence of fever after previous subsidence, in spite of adequate salicylate therapy, should always draw attention to the possibility either that the diagnosis is wrong or that, if it is correct, cardiac involvement is present. A persistently high pulse rate, especially during sleep, which is out of all proportion to the temperature should also arouse suspicion but is an unusual finding. Remember that anxiety is the commonest cause of a rapid pulse, and moreover many patients with carditis do not have tachycardia. Rheumatic nodules are rarely seen except in severe rheumatic infections and, therefore, their presence usually indicates cardiac involvement. A persistently high sedimentation rate is good evidence of continued activity of the rheumatic process and should always lead to a suspicion that the heart is involved.

ARTHRITIS

The arthritic manifestations of rheumatic fever are classically characterized by effusions into large joints, the condition flitting from joint to joint, with usually only one or two severely involved at the same time. Involvement of the small joints, such as those of the hand, is most unusual. The above type of arthritic involvement is more likely to be seen in young adults. The joint lesions invariably clear up completely without residual damage.

In children, instead of joint involvement there is often pain in muscles and in the structures around the joints without actual swelling. These symptoms are often dismissed as 'growing pains', but their occurrence should always arouse suspicion of the possibility of rheumatic fever. However, many children with such pains never develop any evidence of rheumatic complications. The pains are therefore not in themselves pathognomonic and, unless some other manifestation such as unexplained anaemia or pyrexia is present, it is doubtful whether the diagnosis of rheumatic infection is justifiable by their presence alone.

RHEUMATIC NODULES

Rheumatic nodules lie in the subcutaneous tissues and are unattached to the skin, which is not reddened and can be moved over them, but they are often attached to tendon sheaths, ligaments or other periarticular tissues. They are painless and usually symmetrically distributed, especially in the region of bony prominences such as the spine, scapulae, elbows and knees. Histologically they consist of a conglomeration of Aschoff's* nodules, which are the basic histological element of the rheumatic fever process. They rarely occur before weeks or months after the onset of the acute infection. They are seen only in severe rheumatic infections and are therefore very likely to be associated with cardiac involvement. They are unusual in adults.

TONSILLITIS

Tonsillitis due to a Group A streptococcus is a frequent precursor of rheumatic fever, and many regard such an infection as the real *fons et origo* of the condition. Some adults with established valvular heart disease of rheumatic pattern give a history of recurrent tonsillitis in childhood without a history of any other manifestations of rheumatic fever. On the other hand, recurrent tonsillitis is very common but comparatively few cases are complicated by rheumatic disease, and therefore it must be difficult to assess whether or not such a history is in fact significant. There is usually an interval of one to four weeks between the initial tonsillitis and the development of other rheumatic symptoms, and this is difficult to explain satisfactorily.

CHOREA

Chorea (rheumatic chorea, Sydenham's† chorea) is characterized by choreiform movement (*see* chapter 16), clumsiness of movements, muscle weakness, psychological disturbance and fever.

The choreiform movements are always bilateral but may be grossly asymmetrical. They are often most marked and commence in the face, varying in degree from a simple twitch of the eyelids or lips to the most complicated grimaces. In severe cases the limbs, especially the upper limbs, are suddenly agitated. The trunk is often involved, with writhing movements which may be so violent as to throw the patient out of bed. All movements cease during sleep and are aggravated by observation and emotion. Fever is often absent when the dominant manifestation of the rheumatic process is chorea.

Thomas Sydenham of England, in his famous description of the condition, wrote in 1726: 'The hand cannot be steady for a moment. It passes from one position to another by a convulsive movement however much the patient may strive to the contrary. Before he can raise a cup to his lips he makes as many gesticulations as a mountebank.' The term chorea derives from the Greek *choros*, meaning a group of dancers, musicians or singers. An alternative name is St

*L. Aschoff was a nineteenth-century German pathologist.
†T. Sydenham (1624–89), English physician.

Vitus's dance. St Vitus was a Sicilian youth who was martyred in 303 during the Diocletian persecution of the Christians. He was canonized and later a shrine was erected in Zebern (Czechoslovakia). During the Middle Ages pilgrims came to the shrine to seek a cure for diseases reputed to be due to demonic possession. In 1374 an epidemic started and rapidly spread throughout Europe which was called the Dancing Mania. This lasted to well into the fifteenth century and was certainly mass hysteria and St Vitus's shrine was the popular place to seek a cure. The great Sydenham himself confused the condition with rheumatic chorea.

The clumsiness of movement is in some measure itself due to the choreiform movements, but it may actually precede them and is frequently marked when they are slight. It is particularly observed in the upper limbs, where all movements are seen to lack precision. Dysarthria is frequent, speech being slow, slurred and usually mono-syllabic, and itself can be regarded as an ataxia of speech. The tongue, when protruded at the request of the examiner, darts in and out like a jack-in-the-box. Rarely, deglutition may be affected. Involvement of the lower limbs will render the gait clumsy and unsteady, and in severe cases walking is impossible.

The muscle weakness is shown by undue fatigability and has no relationship to the severity of the movements. It is never complete, and slight choreiform movements persist in the partially paralysed limb. These motor changes are associated with hypotonicity of the limbs, which may be demonstrated by difficulty in maintaining a posture of the outstretched upper limbs. When the hypotonicity and weakness are comparatively marked, the condition is some-times referred to as chorea mollis because of the flaccidity of the muscles. Neither marked weakness nor marked hypotonicity is in itself a bad prognostic sign.

Psychological disturbances are always present in some degree, a child being nervous, excitable and restless, often with disturbance of sleep. Occasionally there are more severe symptoms, varying from a mild delirium to acute mania, and these are more likely to occur in older patients, especially if pregnant. The prognosis of the mental condition is always good.

The severity of choreiform movements is always inversely propor-tional to the joint involvement, and patients with rheumatic chorea do not usually have any other rheumatic manifestations apart from cardiac involvement.

HYPERPYREXIA

Hyperpyrexia is very unusual, and when it does occur the patients are nearly always adults. It is often associated with delirium.

ANAEMIA
Anaemia, the cause of which is obscure, is an extremely frequent concomitant of rheumatic infection. It is usually associated with a mild leucocytosis of 10,000–16,000 cells per cubic millimetre.

PLEURISY AND PNEUMONIA
Pain of a pleural type (rarely followed by effusion) and pulmonary infection are fairly common. When the evidence for the latter is radiological and not entirely clinical, some authorities have recorded an incidence of over 10 per cent.

A point which is still controversial is whether or not there is a specific rheumatic pneumonia. The commonest manifestations of such a pneumonia are dyspnoea, increase of pulse rate and fever, which, in a child with rheumatic fever, would make one think of cardiac rather than pulmonary involvement. The presence of pleural pain would support the latter diagnosis, but if pain is present with pericarditis it may simulate pleurisy. Cough is frequently absent and the physical signs in the lungs, if any at all, are crepitations; however, if these are confined to the lower lobes they could reasonably be regarded as due to pulmonary oedema secondary to myocardial involvement or pulmonary infarction. There is no distinctive X-ray picture, but lung opacities, especially of the upper and mid zones, in the absence of any clinical evidence of cardiac failure are very suggestive.

SKIN LESIONS
The rashes which have been described as part of the rheumatic infection are many and varied. Formerly the commonest were sudaminal (sweat) and toxic (due to salicylates), but nowadays the most important consists of pink or pale red well-defined round, oval or crescentic macules which rapidly spread over the trunk and the proximal part of the limbs, always affecting the former more than the latter. Their centres rapidly fade, leaving a red rim with a faintly brownish centre. The individual lesions disappear in 1–3 days but reappear in fresh crops. The circles or segments of circles often coalesce and intersect to form complex patterns. The rash which is sometimes described as erythema multiforme occurs in only a small minority of cases.

Erythema nodosum – characterized by red nodules, often painful and tender, especially over the legs but occasionally on the thighs and rarely on the upper limbs – in a minority of cases, usually children, is a rheumatic manifestation.

An unanswered problem is whether such skin lesions can be the sole evidence of rheumatic infection, especially when they follow tonsillitis. Should such a child automatically be presumed to have a rheumatic infection and be treated accordingly? No satisfactory answer has been given to this important question.

Congestive cardiac failure

Congestive cardiac failure is characterized by a variety of symptoms and signs none of which individually is distinctive. Yet the condition can be readily recognized at the bedside without any instrumental, biochemical or radiological investigations. Some cardiologists restrict the term to those patients with heart disease who develop a raised jugular venous pressure but this will exclude acute left ventricular failure in which condition neither is usually a feature. Other cardiologists avoid the term altogether claiming that its use adds confusion and is not helpful.

There are many unsolved questions with regard to congestive cardiac failure. What is the precise mechanism producing both the dyspnoea and the oedema? What are the minimum manifestations necessary before making the diagnosis correctly? Are the mechanisms of acute and chronic failure identical? At what discernible point does a diseased heart with adequate function become one with congestive cardiac failure? Has the division of cardiac failure into forward with low cardiac output and backward with high cardiac output any real practical value?

The manifestations of cardiac failure, at least theoretically, are many because every part of the body depends for its proper functioning on being supplied with a sufficiency of oxygenated blood pumped by the heart. But different organs have different degrees of vulnerability to oxygen lack and as a consequence the prominence or vagueness and the severity or mildness of the symptoms arising from each part of the body varies enormously.

The main manifestations are as follows:

1. *Dyspnoea* is an entirely subjective phenomenon and is no different from that which may occur in healthy people when performing strenuous or unfamilar exertion. It is discussed in more detail later.

2. *Oedema* of various parts of the body is one of the most frequent signs and its commonest site is in the lower limbs. It pits on pressure, is bilateral but sometimes not symmetrical, is aggravated by exertion or standing and is less marked or even disappears after adequate rest. However, slight pitting oedema of the lower limbs does sometimes occur in healthy people especially in hot climates. In patients who have been confined to bed for some time sacral oedema may be more prominent than of the limbs. In severe cases the pitting oedema may spread up the legs to thighs and abdominal wall and genitalia.

   Acute or chronic pulmonary oedema is probably an invariable feature of congestive cardiac failure although its presence may be difficult to diagnose clinically, its main sign being crepitations at both lung bases. For reasons not properly understood pleural effusions due to heart failure are often unilateral and are more frequently right sided and may be localized in an interlobar fissure.

3. *Cyanosis* has been discussed previously. It is of the peripheral type and is not associated with clubbing unless the patient also has infective endocarditis or lung disease. Cyanosis is not an essential feature of congestive cardiac failure.

4. *Raised jugular venous pressure* has been discussed previously.

5. *Gastro-intestinal and hepatic manifestations* are common. Tender hepatomegaly may precede any oedema. Jaundice is a late sign and if the failure has been of long standing splenomegaly may develop. Anorexia, nausea, vomiting, flatulence and postprandial distension are all common symptoms which may occur, but they are all non-specific.

6. *Cerebral symptoms* such as failing memory and insomnia are often troublesome at an early stage. In severe cases delirium and drowsiness often develop.

7. *Oliguria and nocturia* are the commonest manifestation of renal involvement with cardiac failure. The urine is of high specific gravity, acid, and contains many urates which precipitate out as a pinkish deposit when the urine cools. Proteinuria, usually less than 1 g per day, with a few red cells and hyaline casts is a usual finding.

8. *Cardiac enlargement* is nearly always demonstrable and there may or may not be an arrhythmia.

9. The supposed value of assessing the heart sounds as a guide to cardiac function has been described previously.

When discussing cardiac failure it is always important to be precise about grammatical tense, so that when a patient is said to have cardiac failure the present time is meant and any evidence, for example, of a previous history of swelling of the legs is not acceptable. Stated differently, the patient could have had cardiac failure in the past without necessarily having it at present.

LEFT VENTRICULAR FAILURE

It is sometimes useful to consider the differentiation between right and left ventricular failure, but examples of each must be carefully chosen. As a general rule, the heart fails as a whole. In so far as there is such a thing as pure left failure, the best examples of it are hypertension, aortic valvular disease and acute myocardial infarction. The best example of a pure right failure is cor pulmonale, a condition characterized by cardiac involvement secondary to disease of the lungs or pulmonary vessels.

The special manifestations peculiar to pure acute left failure as opposed to right are as follows:

1. *Paroxysmal dyspnoea,* often occurs at night, and because it is paroxysmal and is accompanied by wheezing it is sometimes

described as 'cardiac asthma', but unlike the dyspnoea and wheezing of bronchospasm it is mainly inspiratory.

2. *Acute pulmonary oedema,* which is a sudden massive transudation of fluid into alveoli which were previously unaffected. This definition excludes, for example, the acute exacerbations of chronic pulmonary oedema frequently seen in mitral stenosis. Acute pulmonary oedema is often preceded on the previous nights by paroxysmal dyspnoea, but this must be considered as a different manifestation. Acute pulmonary oedema causes severe dyspnoea and the coughing up of large amounts of frothy, tenacious, mucoid, usually bloodstained sputum.

3. *Pulsus alternans,* which is a regular alternation of small and large beats. This is a phenomenon rarely recognizable on palpation but better appreciated on auscultation over the brachial artery during blood pressure recordings, the lowering of the pressure causing an apparent sudden doubling of the rate. Pulsus alternans cannot be appreciated, and therefore should never be diagnosed, in the presence of fibrillation. In order that it should not be confused with a pulsus paradoxus, the patient should be asked to hold his breath.

4. *Triple rhythm,* described previously.

RIGHT VENTRICULAR FAILURE

Pure right failure is extremely difficult to recognize clinically. It causes jugular venous engorgement with peripheral oedema and sometimes ascites. The occurrence of these without commensurate dyspnoea may be a clue, but the signs are far from pathognomonic. Most commonly right-sided failure is a consequence of progressive left-sided failure, but pure right failure may occur as a result of (1) cor pulmonale, (2) congenital heart lesions with shunts, (3) peripheral arterio-venous aneurysm effects, or (4) gross deformities of the thoracic cage. Right-sided failure in all these conditions is often precipitated by bronchial or pulmonary infection.

Cor pulmonale

Cor pulmonale is cardiac involvement, always right-sided, secondary to disease of the lungs or pulmonary vessels. Acute cor pulmonale is synonymous with massive pulmonary embolism. Chronic cor pulmonale is a consequence of marked pulmonary hypertension secondary to extensive lung disease, especially emphysema and bilateral fibrosis from any cause. Pulmonary hypertension secondary to a primary lesion which is not in the lung parenchyma or arteries, for example, mitral stenosis, congenital heart lesions with shunts, and paralysis of the respiratory muscles, should never be included as a cause of chronic cor pulmonale although any of them may cause pulmonary hypertension.

A point of considerable importance is that although the commonest cause of cor pulmonale is emphysema, the latter is often seen in patients who also have a coincidental systemic hypertension which produces left-sided cardiac involvement. The term 'cor pulmonale' should not be restricted to those who have pure right-sided involvement without any coincidental left-sided enlargement. Moreover, it is illogical to ascribe any dyspnoea which may be present in such a patient to the cor pulmonale when much of the dyspnoea may actually be caused by the left-sided involvement due to the systemic hypertension.

Pulmonary artery occlusion (embolism or thrombosis) produces an acute cor pulmonale. There is a rare chronic type of cor pulmonale, due either to widespread sclerosis or emboli of unknown aetiology, affecting the small pulmonary vessels and called primary pulmonary hypertension or primary vascular sclerosis or endarteritis. This rare condition should be considered only after all other possible causes have been excluded and it cannot be diagnosed for certainty without special investigations.

Symptoms due to chronic cor pulmonale are dyspnoea on exertion and rarely at rest unless there is either bronchospasm or pulmonary infection, effort syncope, epigastric discomfort, headache and, in severe cases, mild delirium due to carbon dioxide retention. Acute cor pulmonary causes severe chest pain and dypsnoea and may be difficult to distinguish from coronary thrombosis if a cause for pulmonary embolism is not obvious.

Signs of chronic cor pulmonale are always modified and often completely masked by the causal condition. The self-critical physician will realize that it is extremely difficult and often impossible to be certain of its presence on clinical grounds alone. There are no pathognomonic signs, only hints and suggestion to be interpreted with due care and circumspection.

Briefly the signs are:
1. Cyanosis of the central type, which may be very slight or marked and is often exacerbated by bronchial or pulmonary infection.
2. Distended and pulsatile neck veins,in which giant *a* waves may be visible.
3. The signs in the heart of right-sided enlargement and pulmonary hypertension, which include parasternal heave, an accentuated pulmonary second sound, and a systolic and very rarely a blowing diastolic bruit down the left sternal margin. Atrial fibrillation is a rare finding.

4. The radiograph will show a large pulmonary conus and right atrium with prominent hilar arteries. Unless the condition is complicated by cardiac failure, the lung bases are clear, showing normal or even diminished vessel markings. Pleural effusion is an extremely rare complication of a chronic cor pulmonale even in the presence of cardiac failure but is fairly common with acute cor pulmonale, when it may be bloodstained.

Cardiogenic shock

Cardiogenic shock has many possible causes, including severe myocardial infarction, acute pericardial tamponade, a long sustained very fast ventricular rate, ruptured chorda tendinae or papillary muscle, perforation of a valve cusp, severe stenotic valve lesions especially aortic, ball valve thrombus or myxoma of the atrium, and massive pulmonary embolism and tension pneumothorax.

Cardiogenic shock is associated with an abrupt fall of blood pressure which triggers off various haemostatic mechanisms in an attempt to restore the cardiac output and those reflex effects often modify the clinical picture considerably. The jugular venous pressure is usually but not always raised.

Dyspnoea

The best definition of dyspnoea, in spite of protests that the phrase is unscientific, is shortness of breath or breathlessness, or when breathing becomes a laboured conscious effort. It is not synonymous with an increase in respiratory rate (tachypnoea) and many clinicians would also exclude from the definition an increase in the depth of respiration (hyperventilation) and either of these may be voluntary, hysterical or due to organic disease.

Dyspnoea may be present either only on exertion or also at rest (orthopnoea). The former occurs not only with cardiac disease but with pulmonary and pleural lesions and with anaemia. Marked abdominal distension and paralysis of the respiratory muscles and abnormalities of the thorax, including spondylitis, are also causes of dyspnoea. For reasons not understood, it occurs in obesity without apparent cardiac involvement and in healthy people, especially if sedentary and middle-aged or older, when they are engaged in what for them has become an unusual exertion. Anxiety is another common cause of dyspnoea, especially these days when the mention of coronary heart disease by newspapers and television and radio are so frequent. Dyspnoea on effort is not peculiar to heart or lung disease.

Some physicians use the term 'dyspnoea' only if actual disease is present. Any severely dyspnoeic patient may be seen to use involuntarily his accessory muscles of respiration, the scalenes, sternomastoids, trapezius, serratus anterior and pectorals. Dyspnoea at rest is seen with cardiac involvement (but only when severe). It is rare in pulmonary disease unless there is extensive pneumonia or tracheal, laryngeal or bronchial obstruction (including spasm). It is most unusual in anaemia except when extreme. Other causes are described below. Special types are the following:

Asthma. This is paroxysmal dyspnoea and is described in Chapter 14.

Stridor. This is a high-pitched, harsh, whistling, crowing or vibrating noise, especially accompanying inspiration, and indicates laryngeal or tracheal obstruction. When due to tracheal obstruction, it is often accentuated by hyperextension of the head.

Cheyne–Stokes* respiration. This is characterized by periods of apnoea, followed by a gradual increase in the depth of respiration without increase in rate until the patient breathes normally, and then there is a gradually decreasing depth until apnoea recurs. The periods of apnoea last 10–60 seconds. It was graphically described by Hippocrates as 'like a man recollecting himself'. Each cycle, which is repeated every half to two minutes, is accompanied by periodicity of blood pressure and pulse rate, both – except if cardiac failure is present – rising in the hyperpnoeic phase. The condition is found in severe left ventricular cardiac failure (especially in elderly patients who have had barbiturates or opiates). It also occurs in renal disease and in the terminal phases of raised intracranial tension from whatever cause. Cheyne–Stokes respiration indicates a grave prognosis, whatever the cause. It may be followed by paroxysmal dyspnoea.

Biot† breathing. This is characterized by short periods of irregular breathing, varying in depth and rate, followed by periods of apnoea but lacking the waxing and waning and periodic features of Cheyne–Stokes. It is the fibrillation of respiration, the physician not being able to predict the rate or depth of successive respirations. It is seen in meningitis and is due to gross depression of the respiratory centre.

Kussmaul‡ breathing. This is an acyanotic, low, deep, sighing inspiration and expiration. The respiratory amplitude is often markedly increased, and expiration is accompanied by a hissing noise. Kussmaul breathing is associated with a low arterial pH. It often begins while the patient sleeps, and is classically seen in ketosis and acidosis due to diabetes, uraemia or drug intoxication.

Hysterical dyspnoea. This usually consists of deep breathing with a sudden holding of the breath after about every sixth breath, as if the patient had been doused with cold water. Sometimes the deep

---

*George Cheyne (1671–1743) was a Scot who worked in Dublin; William Stokes (1804–78) was a Dublin physician.
†Camille Biot (1878–   ), a French physician.
‡Adolf Kussmaul (1822–1902), a German physician.

breathing is so marked a feature that hyperventilation produces tetany.

Stertorous breathing. This is a noisy breathing heard in some comatose patients and is due to vibration of the soft tissues of the nasopharynx, larynx and cheeks. In dying patients it is often accompanied by bubbling sounds produced by mucus in the air passages which would normally have been expelled by coughing.

Asphyxia (suffocation). This may be due to strangulation, drowning, paralysis of the respiratory muscles, acute pulmonary oedema, laryngeal or tracheal obstruction, or very rarely severe asthma. The primary fault is a ventilatory one, with a rising blood carbon dioxide and falling oxygen and a rapidly developing cyanosis. Stridor is a common association.

Bacterial endocarditis

The term bacterial (infective) endocarditis is used in distinction from the more usual rheumatic, syphilitic, atherosclerotic and congenital varieties of valve involvement. It is divided into two types, acute and subacute, but there is much overlapping between them, each sometimes having some of the features which are usually considered to be the differentiating points from the other.

In the pre-antibiotic era, two distinct types of bacterial endocarditis — acute and subacute — were readily distinguishable. The subacute variety was nearly always due to non-pyogenic organisms of low virulence, of which by far the commonest was a non-haemolytic streptococcus. This infection of the valves was superimposed on a previously damaged valve due to some congenital or acquired (most often rheumatic) lesion.

The condition is characterized by:
1. A pre-existent cardiac lesion and the development of new ones.
2. Septicaemia, by which is meant organisms living and thriving in the bloodstream, and all its consequent manifestations.
3. Emboli with resultant infarcts which, not being due to pyogenic organisms, do not form abscesses.

Subacute bacterial endocarditis often follows a minor infection or a minor operation. In the acute disease, a previously normal heart becomes involved during the course of some pyogenic coccal infection such as a pneumococcal pneumonia or puerpural sepsis, with a resultant pyaemia. By this is meant the carriage of pus in the bloodstream from one site to another with resultant emboli which, being associated with pyogenic organisms, causes abscesses in the various organs involved.

Of recent years the two types have been far less distinctive. Also the main age incidence has shifted from the young to the middle-aged and even elderly and, very significantly, staphylococci and various Gram-negative bacilli have become common causes. The injudicious use of antibiotics may be an important factor in this altered clinical picture. Cardiac surgery may be complicated by infective endocarditis.

The clinical signs of infective endocarditis are as follows:

1. Pyrexia may be of varying and various degrees and of any type, but is usually remittent. It may, however, be continued and, especially if due to pyogenic organisms, is likely to be intermittent and accompanied by rigors. Any of the symptoms and signs which are common to any fever, such as headaches, sweating, anorexia and loss of weight, may be present. Spontaneous remissions may occur, but during these periods the temperature never returns completely to normal, although it may show a substantial reduction.

2. Signs of a congenital or acquired heart lesion will be present from the commencement of the illness in the subacute forms of the disease, but will occur comparatively late in the acute forms. Atrial fibrillation is very rare. Cardiac failure is a late complication, and it is most unusual for the disease to start when the heart is already failing.

3. There may be emboli, especially in the kidneys, spleen, brain, intestine and main peripheral arteries, and rarely in other sites.

4. Clubbing and often also splinter haemorrhages may develop.

5. Skin changes include pallor (due to an associated anaemia) which often has a café-au-lait tint. Purpura is frequent and usually presents as crops of petechiae which, with a hand lens, may be seen to have distinctive yellowish-grey pale centres. Petechiae in the conjunctivae and in the hard and soft palates are common. Purpuric lesions may occur in the retina (Roth's spots). Osler's nodes are raised, very tender, painful reddish-blue lesions of a size varying from pinhead to pea. These occur especially on the thenar and hypothenar eminences; they last for only short periods of a few hours to at most three or four days before they disappear completely, but may be followed by new lesions. Similar but non-painful lesions may occur on the palms and soles.

The majority of cases of infective endocarditis involve the left side of the heart. Gonorrhoea and infection secondary to non-sterile intravenous injections (usually in drug addicts) may cause a right-sided endocarditis, and this may also be a complication of right-sided congenital heart lesions.

Positive blood cultures are more likely to be obtainable in cases of left-sided involvement and septicaemia than in those involving the right side of the heart or in those with pyaemia. A moderate degree of polymorph leucocytosis is nearly always present in any type of infective endocarditis.

I

Congenital heart disease

In any patient the likelihood of congenital rather than acquired heart disease should be considered:

1. If the patient has any other obvious congenital abnormality, such as mongolism or arachnodactyly.
2. If cyanosis and clubbing have been present since an early age.
3. Where the patient is below the age of about 8 years. In this connection it must be remembered that congenital heart lesions do occur in older people, even in the elderly, and acquired heart lesions in early adolescence.
4. Where the systolic bruit has some distinctive characteristics, the most usual of which are its position of maximal intensity in the region of the left border of the sternum and the fact that it is not conducted to the right side of the neck.

CLASSIFICATION

Congenital heart lesions should be considered under three groups: cyanotic right to left shunt (venous to arterial), non-cyanotic (mainly obstructive malformations), and potentially cyanotic left to right shunt (arterial to venous), but many other classifications have been suggested. The main objection to the above classification is that when any patient is seen for the first time he is either cyanosed or not, and lacking prophetic wisdom one cannot state whether cyanosis will develop or not at a later date.

CYANOTIC GROUP

Cyanotic congenital heart disease is always associated with clubbing. The patient is frequently dwarfed and may have infantilism. A secondary polycythaemia is usually present, and the blood has a low oxygen and high carbon dioxide content. Children with this condition find that their most comfortable position is one of squatting, sitting on their haunches. Except in transposition of the great vessels cyanosis is always greater in the lower than upper limbs.

Tetralogy of Fallot

The commonest cyanotic congenital heart lesion, if the infant was born cyanosed and remained cyanosed, is the tetralogy of Fallot. In any cyanosed and clubbed infant this condition should be excluded only for a very good reason and auscultatory romance in the pulmonary area is rarely acceptable as such evidence.

The tetralogy of Fallot consists of pulmonary stenosis, dextroposition of the aorta so that part of its orifice is in the right ventricle, right-sided cardiac enlargement and a patent ventricular septum. Cyanosis (which is usually marked) is always present. The heart is not enlarged clinically, and the apex beat is often very difficult to locate. There is a systolic murmur down the left border of the sternum: this is usually but not necessarily maximal in the third left interspace (it may be in the second or even the fourth), is usually loud but sometimes faint, is often conducted to the left side of the neck, and may be accompanied by a thrill. The pulmonary second sound is diminished.

These are not in themselves pathognomonic findings, but in the great majority of cases the cardiac silhouette is. This shows a normal aortic knuckle with a concavity where the pulmonary conus should be and an upturning of the lowest part of the left border, so that the silhouette comes to resemble a clog (*coeur en sabot*), with its upturned toe in contradistinction to the boot-shaped heart produced by a large left ventricle. This clog appearance is due to the fact that the lowest part of the border is formed by the right ventricle and not by the left, but of course oblique views would be necessary to establish this. Moreover, there is also enlargement of the right atrium, and there may be prominence of the aortic shadow above this due to the dextroposition of the aorta. An essential finding is that the pulmonary arteries at the hilum and in the lung fields are poorly shown. Without such a cardiac silhouette associated with clear lung fields, the diagnosis of tetralogy of Fallot cannot be made with certainty.

Pulmonary stenosis
Pulmonary stenosis may be associated with a septal defect or form part of a more complex congenital lesion, but it may be the sole lesion. Patients with pure pulmonary stenosis may be cyanosed or not, although the reasons for this are controversial. All degrees of severity of pulmonary stenosis are encountered, with a correspondingly wide variation in the magnitude of symptoms and signs, some achieving adolesence or even adult life without symptoms while others exhibit a severe disability in infancy. A rare form of pulmonary stenosis which is probably acquired is that associated with a carcinoid tumour of the small bowel.

If the patient is cyanosed, then he will have clubbing, but unlike in the tetralogy of Fallot this is often much less than would be expected from the degree of cyanosis present. If he is not cyanosed, he will not have clubbing unless there is a complicating infective endocarditis or a coincidental pulmonary infection.

The cardinal sign is a systolic bruit, which is usually loud and rough and of a *crescendo-diminuendo* type but may be soft. It does not occupy the whole of systole, is usually maximal in the second left interspace, and is propagated down the left border of the sternum, occasionally into the left side of the neck, and is often accompanied by a thrill. Prominent '*a*' waves may be visible in the jugular veins. The apex beat is typically diffuse and tapping and difficult to feel. The pulmonary second sound is diminished but widely split (rarely paradoxical). The splitting is difficult to appreciate either because of the softness of the pulmonary component or the replacement of the aortic component by the bruit.

With mild degrees of pulmonary stenosis the X-ray appearance of the heart may be normal, but in other cases the postero-anterior view will show a normal aortic knob with a normal or enlarged pulmonary conus (due to post-stenotic dilatation of the pulmonary artery), a normal left ventricle, a large right atrium and hilar, pulmonary arteries and diminished arterial vasculature of the periphery of the lung fields. Post-stenotic dilatation occurs only in valvular stenosis (which is the far commoner type) and not in infundibular stenosis.

The important complication apart from cardiac failure is the occurrence of infective endocarditis, and this has two unusual features: (1) the emboli are entirely pulmonary and not systemic; (2) positive blood cultures are unusual.

Eisenmenger* complex
Since Eisenmenger's original description in 1897 when there was very little known or interest taken in either cardiac embryology or congenital heart lesions, there has been controversy concerning the precise definition of the complex. He himself described a single infant who had been cyanosed since infancy but yet had been able to lead a fairly normal life before dying at thirty-two. Postmortem showed a huge right ventricle and a large ventricular septal defect, dextroposition, and pulmonary infarction due to a pulmonary artery occlusion and atherosclerosis of the pulmonary arteries. This last finding was not emphasized by either Eisenmenger himself or subsequent writers until the 1940s, when it was first suggested that the pulmonary vessel disease is an early and important lesion causing marked resistance to blood flow in the lungs and thus producing marked pulmonary hypertension. It was not till later still that it became generally accepted that the right to left component of a bidirectional shunt was the sole cause of the cyanosis. This syndrome has been broadened by some to include lesions other than a ventricular septal defect as the cause of the shunt.

Progressive cyanosis, clubbing and polycythaemia are present since early or late infancy or childhood. If the infant survives to adult life syncope, haemoptysis and angina may become prominent features. Most die before the age of forty. A systolic bruit without any distinctive features is present down the left sternal border, which may be soft or loud, long or short. Very occasionally the blowing diastolic bruit of a functional pulmonary regurgitation may be heard. An X-ray will show marked enlargement of the

*Victor Eisenmenger (fl. 1897), a German physician.

pulmonary conus and the main branches of the pulmonary arteries in the hilar region but grossly diminished vascularization in the periphery of the lungs, and the resultant appearance of the pulmonary vessels resembles a tree in winter. In this condition surgery is contra-indicated.

Transposition of the great vessels
Another rare cyanotic congenital heart lesion is transposition of the great vessels, the aorta arising from the right ventricle and the pulmonary artery from the left ventricle. This condition affects boys twice to three times as often as girls. Without surgery, survival beyond early infancy is extremely unlikely unless a shunt is also present so that blood can flow between the two currents. Those children who do survive are markedly cyanosed, with a systolic bruit down the left sternal border which is accentuated by crying. If the condition is associated with a patent ductus, the cyanosis is more marked in the upper than in the lower half of the body. Clubbing is present. The radiograph shows an enlargement of the left ventricle and right atrium, with prominent pulmonary vessels and often a narrow arterial pedicle due to overlapping of the pulmonary artery and aorta.

Tricuspid atresia
Congenital tricuspid atresia is a rare cyanotic congenital heart lesion. Survival is impossible unless a shunt is present. The condition produces cyanosis with clubbing and a systolic bruit down the left sternal border. The radiograph shows a hypoplasia of the pulmonary artery, enlargement of the right atrium and left ventricle, and clear lung fields. The electrocardiograph shows gross left axis deviation. Most cases die in infancy.

NON-CYANOTIC GROUP
Pulmonary stenosis has already been described above, and again it must be emphasized that this condition must always be considered, regardless of whether the patient is cyanosed or not.

Dextrocardia
Dextrocardia may be congenital or acquired. The latter is seen with conditions of marked collapse or fibrosis of the right lower lobe, or rarely with a very large left pleural effusion or pneumothorax. Congenital dextrocardia may be found as an isolated phenomenon, but is more commonly associated with transposition of the viscera (*situs inversus*), and this can be easily demonstrated by noting dullness over the left lower ribs anteriorly and tympany over the right lower ribs anteriorly. A large percentage of cases of congenital dextrocardia are also associated with basal bronchiectasis and malformation of the frontal sinuses.

The diagnosis is made clinically by finding the apex beat to the right of the sternum instead of in its usual position. Such an observation is usually very easy in a thin person, but in a fat person it can be very difficult, especially if the patient has large breasts. X-ray screening will confirm the diagnosis, and an electrocardiograph is pathognomonic because it shows an inversion of all the complexes in lead 1. It is true that the complexes in leads 2 and 3 are transposed, but this is not easily recognizable and thus it will be seen that the real clue is given by lead 1. Similar changes may be produced in normal people by accidental reversal of the right and left upper limb leads. The chest leads often show inversion of the QRS complexes.

Bicuspid aortic valve
A bicuspid aortic valve is a congenital anomaly which may be important either because it may be complicated by infective endocarditis or because, rarely, such a valve may not function properly.

Aortic stenosis
Congenital aortic stenosis produces the same physical signs as the acquired variety. It may be valvular, caused by the fusion of the cusps, or, less commonly, subaortic, caused by defective absorption of the primitive bulbus cordis. The prognosis is very much better than that of the acquired lesion, and the diagnosis should be considered whenever the lesion is the sole one in a patient below the age of about forty years. The condition may be complicated by calcification of the valve. The physical signs are identical with those of the acquired lesion although the pulse changes are usually less marked. As in acquired aortic stenosis angina and syncope are common symptoms.

Coarctation of the aorta
Coarctation means a congenital constriction of the aorta. This may be either the adult type, where the constriction is localized to a site at or near the insertion of the ductus, or the infantile type, which is an extensive constriction from the insertion of the ductus to the origin of the left subclavian artery. However the subdivision is not clearcut and some experts ignore it. Coarctation is unusual in so far as, unlike the majority of congenital heart lesions, it is four to five times commoner in boys than in girls. Even though it is a severe lesion, dwarfism and infantilism are exceptional, the patients often being tall and thin and may exhibit features of the Marfan syndrome. In girls the condition may be associated with Turner syndrome. The commonest association outside the heart is an aneurysm of the circle of Willis, and the possibility of a leak from such an aneurysm should always be considered in a patient with coarctation who develops intracranial signs, although, of course, such signs may be secondary to the associated hypertension.

Coarctation is often associated with a bicuspid aortic valve which may be incompetent and medial degeneration of the aorta, and as a result aortic dissection may occur. The most important sign is the presence of hypertension in the upper limbs and normal or low pressure in the lower limbs as judged by palpation of the femoral arteries, the pulsation there being assessed as less than one would expect knowing the blood pressure in the upper limbs. It is most unusual for femoral pulsation to be actually absent. Because of the circuitous course of the blood flow, the femoral pulsation is delayed as well as diminished (normally the femoral pulse slightly precedes the radial), but it may be extremely difficult to be certain of this without instrumental aids. The blood pressure in the lower limbs can be gauged roughly by wrapping the sphygmomanometer cuff around the thigh and listening over the popliteal artery, or with the cuff around the leg and palpating the posterior tibial artery. The possibility of coarctation should be considered in any patient under the age of about forty years who is hypertensive.

The next important group of signs is due to the development of collateral arteries, which may be seen anywhere over the front or back of the thorax. Sometimes getting the patient to lean forward, touching his toes, may bring out dilated scapular arteries previously not observed. Often, however, these vessels can be felt rather than seen. Most commonly they are neither seen nor felt, and the presence of a systolic bruit in the area gives the clue. This bruit, which may be heard over any part of the praecordium, is usually louder over the upper part of the chest, is present more often on the left than on the right, and may be conducted to either the right or the left carotid or both. It is usually loudest in late systole, but may be a *crescendo-diminuendo* type. The finding of a systolic bruit which is much louder at the left scapular or posterior axillary region than at the cardiac apex is nearly always due to either coarctation or a pulmonary arteriovenous aneurysm, but in the latter condition cyanosis usually occurs and will be a differentiating point.

An expansile pulsation in the right side of the neck or the supra-sternal notch due to a kinked carotid may be present, and such a finding in a patient under the age of forty years should always turn one's thoughts to the possibility of coarctation. More often there is marked bilateral supraclavicular pulsation due to dilatation of both subclavian arteries. Occasionally an expansile pulsation is visible in the second or third right interspace due to the aortic dilation. The heart is usually enlarged clinically and a systolic murmur is heard over the praecordium but, as indicated above, the loudness of this, its maximal intensity and its conduction vary considerably from case to case. Sometimes the blowing diastolic bruit of aortic regurgitation is found. This is due to the presence of either a bicuspid aortic valve or an actual aneurysmal dilatation of the ascending aorta between the constriction and the heart, with a resultant dilatation of the aortic ring.

The radiograph will show a poorly developed and elongated aortic knuckle with enlargement of the left ventricle (usually slight), and there may also be prominence of the ascending aorta. Such a radiograph is not distinctive, but it becomes so if there is also notching (a smooth, localized triangular bite) of the lower border of especially the middle ribs, which is best seen 2–3 inches lateral to the spine. The normal narrowed appearance of ribs at their neck must not be mistaken for notching, which is due to gross enlargement of the intercostal vessels. Notching is not always seen and it may be unilateral and even confined to a single rib; it is rarely distinctive before the age of ten years. The first and second ribs are not affected because their intercostal arteries arise from the subclavian above the constriction. By far the commonest cause of rib notching is coarctation. Much rarer causes are (1) arteriovenous fistula of an intercostal artery and vein secondary to injury, (2) venous distension of an intercostal vein due to subclavian, superior vena cava or innominate vein occlusion, and (3) neurofibromas. Hyperparathyroidism, when it causes rib erosion, may simulate rib notching.

The complications of adult coarctation are infective endocarditis, cardiac failure, rupture of the aorta, and cerebral haemorrhage. Arterial thrombosis, cerebral or coronary, is rare because the hypertension is unassociated with atherosclerosis. Renal involvement is most unusual.

Infantile coarctation is so called because the great majority of cases die in early infancy. In fact, there is no possibility of an infant's surviving without surgery unless the ductus remains patent, which, in the great majority of cases, it does not. If it does remain patent, then the infant has a chance, although a precarious one, of surviving. The dominant physical signs will then be those of a patent ductus because the hypertension and the collateral arteries usually associated with coarctation take several years to develop, rarely being seen before the age of ten years. Extremely few children survive until adult life, and such rare cases will have the manifestations of a patent ductus plus the classical signs of coaractation.

POTENTIALLY CYANOTIC GROUP

The potentially cyanotic congenital heart lesions are those in which the prime lesion is a shunt, namely a patent septum or patent ductus. An important consideration in order to understand this group correctly is to appreciate that the potentially cyanosed becomes cyanosed only (1) if cardiac failure is present; (2) if there is extensive pulmonary infection; (3) following marked exercise. These are three conditions which it is extremely easy to rule out, and if all of them have been excluded, the explanation of any patient's cyanosis as being due to a congenital heart lesion of this group with reversal of flow in the shunt is likely to be wrong.

Patent ductus arteriosus

The ductus arteriosus is an embryonic structure connecting the pulmonary artery with the aorta. It normally closes in early childhood, but if it does not, the condition is known as a patent ductus. Recurrent respiratory infections is a common complication in childhood but they may remain symptomless until well into adult life. Such patients are not cyanosed unless one of the above three complications is present, and are not clubbed unless they have infective endocarditis or a coincidental pulmonary infection. Patent ductus is often the sole lesion but when it occurs with other anomalies of the heart it may lessen the undesirable haemodynamic effects of the other lesions.

The pathognomonic sign is a 'machinery', 'train in tunnel' or 'humming-top' murmur, a continuous rumbling murmur occupying the whole of systole and diastole, with a systolic accentuation of greatest intensity just before the second sound. This is often accompanied by a thrill, which is usually confined to systole. It is best heard in the comparatively small area extending from the left border of the sternum in the second interspace to below the outer part of the clavicle; in fact, the murmur may be heard only within a part of this area. Frequently the loud, long systolic element, which is usually conducted over the whole of the praecordium and into the left side of the neck, is mistaken for the machinery murmur.

Any other anteriovenous communication may also produce such a bruit: for example, pulmonary arteriovenous fistulae (aneurysm or angioma); arteriovenous anastomoses of the intercostal vessels following fractured ribs; broncho-pulmonary artery anastomotic communication; perforation of an aortic sinus into the pulmonary artery or a cardiac chamber; and coronary arteriovenous fistulae. In these conditions the position of the bruit is not likely to be the same as that found with a patent ductus. In valvular disease of the heart − for example, aortic regurgitation − it is very common to find systolic and diastolic bruits in the same area, but in such a case the two bruits are not continuous, each element being distinctive and also usually being separated by short intervals from the heart sounds themselves. Rarely with a patent ductus only a rough, long systolic bruit is present, and this is most likely in the presence of cardiac failure or gross pulmonary hypertension but not otherwise. However, without a machinery murmur the diagnosis can never be made with certainty on examination alone.

Confirmatory evidence is sometimes provided by the presence of a high pulse pressure with its associated signs. Accentuation or paradoxical splitting of the pulmonary second sound is often mentioned, but the heart sounds are usually very difficult to elucidate because they are dominated by the bruit. The radiograph of the heart shows a normal aortic knob with a large pulmonary conus, usually a normal left ventricle, an enlarged right atrium, and very prominent hilar vessels owing to enlargement of the pulmonary arteries. On screening, these arteries may exhibit gross pulsation (the 'hilar dance'). An electrocardiograph is usually normal, but may show right axis deviation. The important complications of this lesion are infective endocarditis and cardiac failure.

Atrial septal defect
Atrial septal defect, occurring as the sole lesion, is common, but it may be associated with other congenital heart defects. Its peculiarities compared with other congenital heart lesions are as follows: (1) infective endocarditis does not occur; (2) atrial fibrillation is a fairly common complication in older patients; (3) it is the only congenital heart lesion in which a superadded acquired lesion may be present. The most frequently associated lesion outside the heart is arachnodactyly which may form part of Marfan syndrome.

In the embryo, the two atria are separated by a crescentic septum which is fused with the atrio-ventricular rings. There is a gap between the two limbs of the crescent, and this hole is the ostium primum, which normally closes before or soon after birth. But a second gap appears in the upper part of the embryonic septum, called the ostium secundum, and this also normally closes before or soon after birth.

An ostium primum defect is usually in the lower part of the septum and may be associated with an endocardial cushion, a deformity of the mitral and tricuspid valves, which are often incompetent. An ostium secundum defect is the commoner type of defect and is usually central and high up, and may be large, its effects being dependent mainly on its size. Anomalies of the pulmonary veins are common with secundum defects. Both types of defects may be present in the same patient. The condition may be symptomless for many years but they are very liable to recurrent pulmonary infections.

The clinical signs of the lesion are the absence of cyanosis and clubbing, a diffuse tapping apex beat, a parasternal lift, often marked pulsation in the second left interspace, and a systolic murmur down the left sternal border. The murmur is maximal in the third space; it is usually mid-systolic, of a *crescendo-diminuendo* type with secundum defects, but may be pansystolic with primum defects, and then it may also be conducted into the axilla, indicating an associated mitral incompetence. With secundum rather than primum defects, occasionally there is a blowing diastolic bruit down the left sternal border due to functional pulmonary regurgitation secondary to the pulmonary hypertension. The pulmonary second sound shows fixed wide splitting, and this should be sought for with the patient both sitting and lying.

The radiograph shows a small aortic knob with a very large pulmonary conus, a prominent right atrium and very large hilar arteries. With a secundum defect the left ventricle is normal, but it may be slightly or moderately enlarged with a primum lesion. The silhouette is thus exactly the same as that of a patent ductus and differs from it merely in the greater degree of the changes present. The distinction between these two conditions obviously cannot be made with certainty on a radiograph, the stethoscope here being a superior weapon.

When the lesion is associated with a mitral stenosis, the condition is known as Lutembacher's* complex. The consensus of opinion is that the mitral stenosis is rheumatic and not congenital, the association being merely coincidental. The interesting features of this condition are that the prognosis is usually better than with a pure mitral stenosis and the left atrium is rarely so grossly enlarged, and perhaps it is this removal of part of the strain on that chamber which is the cause of the better prognosis.

Ventricular septal defect

Ventricular septal defect is a condition often seen with other congenital heart lesions, but may occur as the sole lesion, when it is sometimes called *maladie de Roger*.†

The positive physical signs are a systolic murmur, usually loud and long, down the left border of the sternum, maximal in the fourth space and unlike the systolic bruit due to an atrial septal defect it is often accompanied by a thrill. Rarely, and then usually when there is a considerable degree of pulmonary hypertension, the bruit may be *crescendo-diminuendo* and not occupying the whole of systole. It is very unusual for the bruit of a ventricular septal defect to be conducted to either side of the neck. Its loudness and length are often inversely proportional to the size of the defect. The second heart sound in the pulmonary area is often normal but may be accentuated or split, the splitting increasing with inspiration. There may be a parasternal heave and when there is a large left to right shunt the left ventricle may also be enlarged. As the condition progresses cyanosis occurs and the systolic bruit may become progressively shorter and softer and the bruit of functional pulmonary regurgitation may develop. However many patients remain symptomless until their third or fourth decade. Infective endocarditis is a common complication.

* René Lutembacher (1884–   ), a French physician who wrote his paper in 1916.

†Henri L. Roger (1811–91), a French physician who wrote his paper in 1879.

Peripheral vascular disease

The clue to the presence of peripheral vascular disease is often given by the finding of discoloration (various shades of red and blue or marked pallor), especially at the ends of the digits and on the heels. Such discoloration is always associated with coldness of the affected parts. In severe cases the discoloration becomes progressively darker as gangrene develops. Other changes which may be present in any type of peripheral vascular disease are gangrene; atrophic changes in the skin, which becomes shiny, tightly drawn and often ulcerated; liability to infection, particularly with fungi; and brittleness and deformity of the nails and loss of hair in the affected areas. A minor degree of pitting oedema of the feet often develops and distended veins appear on the dorsum of the feet.

Having recognized the presence of peripheral vascular disease, one's next immediate task must be to distinguish the type, that is, obstructive or non-obstructive. It is important to appreciate that none of the above signs will help in this differentiation: they may all occur with either type. Furthermore, the distinction between these two groups remains valid and valuable, even though in obstructive cases there may be an element of spasm and in the non-obstructive group there may be organic changes in the terminal branches of the digital arteries in long-standing cases.

OBSTRUCTIVE TYPE

The obstructive type (also called organic) is associated with recognizable pathology of the vessels themselves, atherosclerosis (including diabetes), thrombo-angiitis obliterans, polyarteritis or embolism, and has the following characteristics.

1. Intermittent claudication is present. This is pain in limbs — usually in the calf or occasionally in the buttock, and in the case of the upper limbs usually in the forearm, which comes on only with exertion and is quickly relieved by rest. Indeed, the pain frequently forces the patient to rest. With actual or incipient gangrene, in addition to the pain of intermittent claudication there may be severe rest pain in the part most affected.

2. Pulsation in the limb is grossly diminished. In the lower limbs, pulsation should be sought for in the dorsalis pedis, tibial and popliteal arteries.

   A good technique to localize the dorsalis pedis artery is to slide the tips of the fingers between the first and second metatarsals towards the ankle and immediately lateral to the extensor longus hallucis tendon but the exact position of the vessel is subject to great variation.

The posterior tibial artery is best felt posterior to the internal malleolus, with gentle pressure against the bone underneath.

A quick feel behind the knees is of no value in assessing popliteal pulsation, because this can be done with accuracy only by careful attention to technique, constant practice and self-criticism. The popliteal artery is best felt with the patient lying prone on his abdomen, with the knees fully extended, and palpating the whole length of the popliteal fossae with the tips of the fingers. Another commonly used method, which is not so satisfactory, is to have the patient lying on his back with knees slightly flexed, and to grip the upper end of each tibia in turn with both hands with the thumbs in front and all other fingers behind.

Feeling pulsation, especially in smaller vessels, is frequently very difficult even in normal people, usually owing to an aberrant position of the vessels or obesity or oedema of the lower limbs. In all other people pulsation in these vessels should always be demonstrable, unless there is obstructive vascular disease, if it is diligently and methodically sought for. Do not lament about observer error nullifying the value of the tests, but instead practise their performance until observer error is removed. When feeling for arterial pulsation do not press too hard or pulsation in your own finger tips may be confused with that in the patient's vessels.

Special instruments (oscillometers) of various types have been devised to record more accurately the amount of pulsation in a limb. The oscillometric record is taken in the mid-thigh, around the calf and above the ankle; thus used, it may also help to localize the obstruction. An oscillometer can be improvised by wrapping the sphygmomanometer cuff around the leg, pumping it up to a pressure between the systolic and diastolic readings, and noting the oscillation of the mercury column or the swing of the aneroid needle which normally occurs but will be absent, or almost so, if there is organic vascular disease. This will be easier to demonstrate by comparison if the change is much more marked in one limb than in the other.

3. Raising the limb well above horizontal with the patient recumbent, the patient meanwhile rapidly moving his toes and ankle, will produce marked pallor if there is organic vascular disease, and the rapidity and extent of this development will give a clue to the severity of the lesion. In normal persons any pallor produced by simultaneous elevation and exercise is always very minimal and in the vast majority no colour change is produced. Furthermore, if the limbs be then placed in a dependent position, a marked bluish-red colour instead of the normal pinkish colour develops (reactionary rubor), accompanied by

dilatation of the superficial veins over the dorsum of the foot. It normally takes 6–10 seconds for these veins to refill if the limb is kept dependent and 15–20 seconds if it is kept horizontal, but refilling will take appreciably longer if there is circulatory insufficiency.

4. With obstruction of a large artery, there may be a loud systolic bruit over that artery.

An important point to realize is that the presence of any one of the above findings immediately places the patient within the category of organic (obstructive) peripheral vascular disease, and more than one of these manifestations is not necessary. Discoloration, nail changes, coldness, and loss of local hair do not help in the differentiation between obstructive and non-obstructive vascular disease because they are all common to both.

Causes of obstructive arterial disease

Atherosclerosis is the commonest cause of obstructive arterial disease. The term arteriosclerosis was first used in 1833 and for many years was regarded as purely an ageing process causing a fibrinous deposit on the intima. The British pathologist Duguid in 1946 and 1953 pointed out that the fibrinous deposit is an organized mural thombus and that cells which are circulating in the arterial blood and which are laden with cholesterol adhere to the vessel walls and together with platelets and fibrin become incorporated into the intima, narrowing the vessel lumen, and this is the basis of the atherosclersis lesion. Crawford and Charles Levene of London in 1952 showed that the thickened intima with its rich blood supply tears and this leads to intimal haemorrhages and release of cholesterol which is deposited on the intima.

Many patients with hypertension have atherosclerosis but the two are different conditions and the reason for this common but frequently occurring association is the subject of much speculation. Atherosclerosis, including the diabetic variety, which is probably not a different condition, causes very gradual symptoms and signs of obstruction to the peripheral arteries. The pathology also affects the upper limbs as well as the lower, but severe involvement sufficient to cause gangrene is unusual because of the extensive collateral circulation of the upper limbs. The association of unilateral gangrene of some fingers together with wasting of the small muscles of the same hand points to a lesion of the thoracic outlet such as a peripheral cancer of the lung.

Embolism

Arterial embolism is usually secondary to atrial fibrillation, infective endocarditis or a previous myocardial infarct. It causes sudden arterial occlusion with dramatic signs and symptoms due to that, the severity and the extent of which depend on the size of the artery occluded.

If the bifurcation of the abdominal aorta is affected there will be the signs of bilateral obstructive disease in the lower limbs, with intermittent claudication, especially if the patient is ambulant, and the pain may be in both buttocks. Lower motor neurone lesions, bladder disturbance and impotence are commonly present and are due to cutting off of the blood supply of the cauda equina.

Thrombo-angiitis obliterans

Thrombo-angiitis obliterans was first described by Buerger* in 1908. Some deny that this condition is a clinical entity and regard it as a variety of atherosclerosis. I consider this viewpoint to be misguided and misleading. The lesions are segmental with normal arteries between the affected parts and is almost entirely confined to men; the first symptoms occur in the forties. Nearly all Buerger's original cases were Jews but this is not surprising as he worked in a dominantly Jewish area of New York. Cigarette-smoking is probably an aetiological factor. The condition follows a relapsing course and fresh episodes of arterial occlusion at different sites are followed by periods of quiescence during which an adequate collateral circulation may develop in the affected part. It involves the upper as well as the lower limbs and may cause gangrene of the upper far more often than atherosclerosis does. Involvement of the coronary, renal and cerebral arteries is fairly common. Phlebitis, often of a migratory type is very common and may be the initial manifestation of the disease.

Monckeberg sclerosis

The essential feature of Monckeberg sclerosis is calcification of the media of large arteries such as the popliteal. Some regard it as a clinical entity, pointing out that the calcification is compatible with an adequate and symptom-free circulation. However, some regard it as a variant of atherosclerosis.

Diabetes

When a patient is found to have organic vascular disease, the first investigation should always be examination of the urine for sugar. Vascular involvement is the basic cause of many of the complications of diabetes. The vessels are affected in three ways: (1) by atheroma – which in every respect resembles that seen in non-diabetics; (2) by hypertensive arteriolar disease, probably often secondary to renal disease, especially pyelonephritis, which is very common in diabetics; (3) by changes in the retinal and glomerular vessels, producing in the former small haemorrhages, exudates and micro-aneurysms, and in the latter the histological changes described as intracapillary glomerulofibrosis. It is these changes in the retinal and kidney vessels which are often regarded as peculiar to diabetics.

*Leo Buerger (1879–1943), a New York surgeon.

In any patient with obstructive arterial disease, evidence of peripheral neuritis must be sought for diligently, and any positive findings such as sluggishness of any of the tendon reflexes must not be ignored or dismissed for some facile reason such as old age. The association of peripheral neuritis, especially of a sensory type, with organic arterial disease is often due to diabetes.

NON-OBSTRUCTIVE TYPE

The nomenclature of the non-obstructive group is exceedingly confused. Commonly used alternative generic names are functional, spasmodic, vasomotor or trophic vascular disease. The group includes pernio (chilblains), Raynaud's disease and syndrome (*see below*), frostbite, trench foot, immersion foot, and erythromelalgia (excessive and unpleasant dilation of peripheral vessels in response to warmth). The common practice of introducing yet further terms merely adds further confusion.

Raynaud's disease

The main difficulty resolves itself around the eponymous description of Raynaud's disease. Its author wrote in 1862 a thesis for his M.D. (Paris) entitled 'Local asphyxia and symmetrical gangrene of the extremities', in which he described records of twenty-five cases, and published in 1874 a further monograph describing sixteen other cases. Incidentally, in view of the above title it is absurd to state, as many authors do, that the term 'Raynaud's disease' excludes the occurrence of gangrene. However, it is true that in this condition gangrene occurs only after the disease has been present for several years.

Raynaud in his description insisted on the following criteria:

1. That there are paroxysms of discoloration, usually produced by cold.
2. That such discoloration always goes through three phases. In the first there is local syncope with the production of pallor (dead fingers), often preceded by pain and paraesthesia, this stage lasting from several minutes to about two hours. The second phase consists of local asphyxia with cyanosis of the part, and lasts a very variable time. This latter stage either develops into an 'active hyperaemia' with a resultant redness, or the cyanosis persists with the development of necrosis of soft tissues and gangrene. The colour changes thus pass through the sequence (*a*) white, then blue and then red with recovery, or (*b*) white, then blue followed by gangrene.
3. That the lesions are bilateral and roughly symmetrical.
4. That there are no demonstrable signs of organic vascular disease. Raynaud emphasized that in all his cases pulsation was palpable in the peripheral vessels.

Right from the original description of this condition there was bound to be confusion because some, although a minority, of Raynaud's own cases did not comply with the above criteria, a fact which he appreciated himself. If the description is strictly complied with, then Raynaud's disease is a comparatively rare condition and is confined almost entirely to women.

Normally, vessels contract in response to cold with resultant colour changes in the part supplied, but in Raynaud's disease the vessels contract excessively until there may even be obliteration of their lumen. Raynaud wrote: 'I propose to demonstrate that there exists a variety of dry non-infected gangrene affecting the extremities which is impossible to explain by a vascular obstruction – a variety characterized especially by a remarkable tendency to symmetry ... I hope to prove that this kind of gangrene has its cause in a vice of innervation of the capillary vessels.' Later, he described the condition as being due to 'impediment of the arterio-capillary circulation determined by some permanent affectation of the vasomotor nerves'.

Raynaud's syndrome

The term Raynaud's syndrome or Raynaud's phenomenon refers to a functional vascular disturbance affecting principally or entirely the peripheral limb arteries and differing from Raynaud's disease essentially in the fact that there is an attributable cause. This disorder may occur with cervical rib and related conditions; with neurological lesions, especially syringomyelia, peripheral neuritis, tabes dorsalis and poliomyelitis; with paroxysmal haemoglobinuria in the cold; with sclerodactyly (the vascular changes may precede the skin changes); with ergot poisoning (especially mentioned by Raynaud himself); with systemic lupus erythematosus, and in occupations such as the use of pneumatic drills. It will be seen when reviewing these conditions individually that in most of them, all Raynaud's own criteria are not present. 'Raynaud's syndrome' is sometimes used loosely as a generic term synonymous with non-organic peripheral vascular disease. As mentioned above, with organic vascular disease of any type, but especially with embolism, there may be a superimposed element of spasm, but to refer to this as Raynaud's syndrome is obfuscation and not helpful.

Hypertension

Recording the blood pressure

As stated previously, an effort must be made to learn to assess the blood pressure by palpation of the radial or brachial arteries. But the estimation must be checked whenever possible with a sphygmomanometer.

The patient must be physically and if possible also emotionally relaxed and that may be helped by explaining the technique if he has not had it recorded previously, and this may be accomplished by inconsequential talk while the cuff is being adjusted. The patient should be comfortable and all clothing must be removed from the arm; rolling up a sleeve is not sufficient and such apparent time-saving is a common cause of wrong readings. With the patient either sitting or lying, the cuff with its lower margin 2–3 cm above the upper limit of the anticubital fossa, is wrapped neatly, evenly and firmly around the arm well above the elbow, which must be supported and extended. If the cuff is too loosely applied, especially in obese people, false high readings are likely. If one is in doubt whether readings in an obese patient are artificially high, the procedure should be repeated with the cuff around the forearm and auscultation should be done over the radial artery. A very thin arm may give falsely low figures when the standard cuff is used. The cuff is pumped up rapidly to over 200, the patient being warned beforehand that it will be a little uncomfortable. The brachial artery is palpated in the antecubital fossa with the thumb, and the pressure is very slowly released until pulsation is just felt. It is essential always to record the systolic pressure by palpation so as to avoid the occasional occurrence in hypertensives of a silent gap which would give a falsely low reading on auscultation alone.

The cuff is then re-inflated to above the reading recorded on palpation and the procedure is repeated, but this time the brachial artery is auscultated using the stethoscope bell and not with the diaphragm, which is too large. The stethoscope must be held firmly, but only with as much pressure as is necessary to keep it in contact with the skin, and it must not touch the cuff or the tubing. With gradual and uniform reduction of the pressure (roughly at the rate of 2 to 3 mm per second: if done much quicker a false recording is likely) below the systolic, the sounds become at first less distinct but later louder and sharper, and these louder sounds become muffled and finally disappear.

There is controversy as to whether the diastolic pressure is noted when the sounds become abruptly muffled or when they disappear completely. The former is the method recommended by the American Heart Association and is usually followed in Britain. However the difference between these two techniques is rarely significant. It is true that the term 'muffled' cannot be defined accurately. On the other hand, assessment of the exact moment of the disappearance of sounds depends very much on the physician's hearing and the efficiency of his stethoscope, whereas the recognition of the advent of muffling depends far less on either of these factors.

If there is gross cardiac irregularity, especially when due to fibrillation, the systolic pressure can be determined only roughly as the highest recorded systolic, and the diastolic pressure cannot be recorded accurately. The pulse rate must always be counted immediately before or after taking the blood pressure and it must without fail be recorded in the notes alongside the blood pressure.

If high systolic readings are recorded, it is advisable to repeat the procedure several times, preferably at five-minute intervals: the lowest figure is taken as the correct one, the higher figures being produced by emotion. Or alternatively the blood pressure is recorded about five times, the cuff being deflated completely for fifteen seconds between each estimation. But taking too long a time over the recording is very likely to produce falsely high readings.

In normal people there is no significant difference between the readings taken lying and sitting, provided that the arm is held roughly at the level of the heart. However, in patients on hypotensive drugs or with a rapid fall of blood pressure, for example due to haemorrhage, the readings taken sitting may be considerably lower than those recorded lying down. In the majority of patients it is immaterial whether the pressure is taken in the right or the left arm, but if there is a suspicion of any inequality of the brachials, readings must be taken in both. Only a difference of more than five is significant.

In patients with suspected coarctation or in those with peripheral vascular disease, assessment of any difference between the blood pressures in the upper and lower limbs may be important. It is better to put the cuff around the calf and to palpate and later auscultate over the posterior tibial artery than to wrap the cuff around the lower part of the thigh and auscultate over the popliteal, as the latter procedure often gives falsely high values. If the thigh is used it may be necessary to use a wider cuff (18 cm instead of the standard 12 cm). Normally the systolic pressure in the lower limbs is 7–10 mm higher than in the upper limbs. No attempt should be made to determine the diastolic pressure in the lower limbs.

The sphygmomanometer is one of the physician's most valuable possessions but it is also one of the most abused instruments. It is such an important measurement that its recording should never be left to nurses, orderlies, pharmacists or drug store salesmen (as has been recommended in the USA) without a physician very regularly and often checking on the accuracy of the figures. When a blood pressure is recorded in any hospital notes the name and status of the person who did it should be noted. Wide fluctuations in many people's blood pressure may be due to emotional factors entirely or the patient may have a 'labile' blood pressure, but often the real reason is careless measurement.

TYPES OF HYPERTENSION

Hypertension is classified into secondary and primary (essential). In any hypertensive patient, known causes must be eliminated, essential hypertension being diagnosed only after secondary hypertension has been excluded. The vast majority cases of hypertension are primary.

Secondary hypertension
The causes of secondary hypertension are as follows:

1. Renal disease of any type except the nephrotic syndrome, which is nearly always associated with a normal blood pressure. Of recent years the importance of chronic pyelonephritis has been stressed and comparatively rare conditions such as renal artery stenosis have received a great deal of publicity.

2. Cushing's syndrome, regardless of the primary site of its causation. This is always characterized by obesity, especially of the face, neck and trunk, in women by virilism, and in men by hyposexuality. Additional features, any or all of which may be present, are hypertension, plethoric facies, diabetes mellitus, polycythaemia, pigmented striae and osteoporosis.

3. Coarctation.

4. Phaeochromocytomas, which are tumours of chromaffin tissues secreting catecholamines. They nearly always arise from the suprarenal medulla and should be suspected in any patient who has paroxysms of hypertension with transient vasomotor features (headache, sweating, palpitations, nausea, vomiting, visual disturbances, and pain in the chest and limbs). These vasomotor disturbances often induce apprehension, and the patient may exhibit evidence of thyrotoxicosis. Occasionally diabetes mellitus is a complication. An important diagnostic feature is that the condition may be associated with skin neurofibromas with typical pleomorphic lesions and café-au-lait macules on the trunk. The more difficult cases are those with sustained hypertension. The most accurate method of establishing the diagnosis is by the demonstration of an increased secretion and excretion of catecholamines and/or their urinary metabolites (the metanephrines).

5. Rarely, polycythaemia rubra vera can itself cause hypertension. Most patients with this condition have a normal blood pressure in spite of the grossly increased blood viscosity. In those who do have hypertension, the condition is sometimes designated polycythaemia hypertonica.

6. Primary aldosteronism, which is due to a tumour (nearly always benign) of the suprarenal cortex. The commonest symptoms produced are headache, polyuria, polydipsia, muscle weakness (rarely transient paralysis), paraesthesiae and tetany. The important findings are biochemical, and probably the earliest and most important is a persistent hypernatraemia. Later, hypokalaemia and alkalosis occur. Laboratories with special facilities will be able to demonstrate an increased aldosterone secretion with a lowered plasma renin activity. Patients with gross oedema from any cause, especially if they have been treated too enthusiastically with diuretics without potassium supplements, may have the same biochemical findings apart

from an increased renin activity. The hypertension resulting from aldosteronism is always comparatively mild and never malignant.

7. Long continued liquorice ingestion and oral contraceptives can cause hypertension.

Primary hypertension

The above causes having been excluded, the hypertension is designated essential, primary or idiopathic. Most cardiologists regard this as an entity, but some dissent and consider that such patients are merely the section of the population presenting arterial pressures higher than an arbitrarily selected so-called normal. Neurogenic, renal, endocrine (especially adrenal), dietetic and genetic theories have been elaborated upon, researched and discussed *ad infinitum et nauseatum* but experts continue to disagree and probably essential hypertension is of multifactorial aetiology in all cases.

What is a normal blood pressure, and what constitutes hypertension, are two hotly debated questions. Blood pressure in normal people fluctuates, especially with emotion, but the amount of such alteration depends on the individual, some people having a very labile blood pressure which can be considerably reduced merely by mild sedation. Moreover, the personality of the physician recording the pressure and his technique are also important. Blood pressure tends to rise with age but does not always do so, and formulas such as 100 plus half the age are dangerous misconceptions. The truth is that there is no mathematical rule correlating age and blood pressure.

Furthermore, there is no precisely fixed figure at any age above which the pressure should be regarded as definitely being abnormally high. However, systolic pressures between 110 and 140 mm and diastolic pressures between 70 and 90 mm should be regarded as normal at any age, and a systolic pressure above 200 mm and a diastolic pressure above 110 mm as always abnormal. Many regard pressures of 140 systolic and 90 diastolic in anybody below the age of 40 as abnormal. In those over 40 some physicians regard a systolic of 160 or less and a diastolic of less than a 100 as normal but others demand lower readings citing 150 systolic and 95 diastolic as the maximum. The Framingham (Mass., USA) study of the blood pressures of a large number of people living in the same area over a long period is very impressive but perhaps its findings have been too readily accepted. The authors of that report disagree with the usually accepted view that the height of the diastolic pressure is more important than the systolic in the diagnosis of hypertension, and consider that hypertension should be diagnosed on the basis of raised systolic pressure even if the diastolic is normal, and they also claim that a 'labile' blood pressure should not be ignored as is usually done because they believe that it is very likely to remain permanently raised in the future unless treated. But even with figures above 200 mm, the actual height of the systolic pressure may itself be of no significance the severity of symptoms, complications and prognosis of a patient with a systolic pressure of, for example 300 mm is not necessarily worse than that of another whose systolic is 220 mm. It is the intermediate figures of 150–180 mm systolic and 90–110 mm diastolic which are often found and which give rise to controversial assessments. Perhaps physicians have been too much influenced by the actuarial figures used by life assurance companies. It is important that the height of the blood pressure should always be correlated with associated findings, especially the size of the heart and any significant abnormalities in the electrocardiograph; if both these are normal, any apparent rise in blood pressure is probably of no significance.

The relative importance of heredity in essential hypertension is controversial. Some experts maintain that usually there is only one, and at most there are two or three, distinct inherited dominant genes responsible. Other experts proclaim that, excluding secondary hypertension, blood pressure is a quantitative characteristic determined by many factors, inherited and environmental, which normally control and regulate it. The latter view implies a denial that there is ever a recognizably sharp distinction between normal and abnormal blood pressure, the various figures representing a continuous gradation from well-adapted to ill-adapted within the wide variations of so-called normal. But this controversy is essentially a statistical one and is likely to prove sterile. The truth is that we do not understand either the mode of production of the raised pressure in essential hypertension or whether any mechanism responsible for the raised pressure in any particular form of secondary hypertension, renal or endocrine, plays any part whatever in the aetiology of primary hypertension, and the only common factor may be the raised blood pressure. Moreover, the role, if any, and the relative importance of environmental factors such as over-nutrition or excessive intake of various dietary constituents — for example, salt or cholesterol compounds — is very controversial.

Essential hypertension is characteristically symptomless. Certainly the old and sometimes still quoted opinion that fatigue, headaches, dizziness and epistaxis may be early manifestations of hypertension is not true. If any symptoms are present, they are usually produced by injudicious drug therapy; or are psychogenic (often produced by the physician); or indicate the onset of cardiac, renal, retinal or cerebral complications. Moreover, many of those complications may occur without any further rise of blood pressure. It may be that the height of the pressure does not itself cause the manifestations of hypertension but that these are due to associated (possibly primary) arterial or arteriolar disease.

Malignant (accelerated) hypertension
Malignant hypertension is generally defined as hypertension complicated by hypertensive retinitis, which usually includes a mild degree
of papilloedema. It is likely to be associated with a diastolic pressure
of 140 or more; indeed, some regard this as the criterion for labelling
any hypertension as malignant. The importance of differentiating
this type of hypertension lies in its bad prognosis, hence the term
malignant. With modern drug therapy this has been much improved
and even the retinitis can be cleared, and for this reason some prefer
the name 'accelerated' instead of malignant, which is indicative of
a grave prognosis. It is not a definite entity but a severe phase of any
hypertension, secondary or primary. Moreover, in any hypertensive
it is unpredictable whether or when this complication is likely to
occur. Untreated malignant hypertension is always associated with
progressive renal impairment.

It is important to realize that only a small percentage of hypertensives ever develop a malignant phase. With the onset of that
phase, rapidly progressive renal involvement becomes evident as
shown by proteinuria, with many red cells and glomerular casts
together with a rising blood urea. Cerebral and/or cardiac complications may dominate the clinical picture.

If the blood pressure is permanently lowered by any means, it is
possible to reverse malignant hypertension to its former benign
phase.

Cardiac signs
With hypertension, the findings in the heart are as follows:
1. There may be displacement of the apex beat downward and
   outward due to left ventricular enlargement, indicating that
   the hypertension has been present for some considerable time.
   X-rays confirm the left ventricular enlargement which is
   typically 'boot shaped' because the lower left border meets the
   diaphragm at an obtuse angle. There is often bilateral enlargement of the superior mediastinum due to 'unfolding' of the
   aorta and the aortic knob may show a double contour.
2. There may be accentuation of the second sound in the aortic
   area.
3. Often there is a systolic bruit at the base, usually conducted
   into the right side of the neck but not accompanied by a thrill.
   The mechanism of its production is controversial.
4. There may be a bruit of a functional mitral regurgitation.
5. Often there is a kinked carotid.

Any arrhythmia is probably not due to the hypertension itself but
to associated coronary artery atheroma.

15 The Alimentary and Genito-urinary Systems

The mouth

THE LIPS

Pallor and also cyanosis of the labial mucosa have been described in Chapter 13.

One of the commonest lesions of the lips is herpes simplex (febrilis), producing irritable vesicles which often become pustular and scab. The vesicles may extend to other parts of the face and occasionally to the buccal mucosa. The condition is often seen with the common cold, but it may occur in any acute febrile state, especially pneumococcal pneumonia.

A large persistent painless ulcer of the lips may be a chancre. This starts as a gradually increasing papule, usually single, which later ulcerates with marked induration of the surrounding tissues and enlargement of the submandibular lymph nodes, which are firm, discrete and rubbery. It has to be differentiated from a squamous-celled carcinoma, which arises typically along the line of junction between the lip and the vermillion border. It may start as an area of leucoplakia. The lesion becomes a thickened warty crusting ulcer with everted shelving edges or a persistent indurated crack. A syphilitic gumma also may cause an ulcerated swelling on the lip.

Cheilitis, an acute inflammation of the lips, is nowadays rare and usually presents as a carbuncle. Cheilosis is a non-inflammatory involvement of the labial mucosa, which becomes thinned, cracked and often ulcerated. It is a feature of deficiency of the vitamin B complex, especially of its riboflavine component, and is then often associated with an angular stomatitis characterized by fissuring of the angles of the mouth (perlèche). In elderly patients, especially if edentulous, angular stomatitis is fairly common and is often independent of vitamin B deficiency. Small linear scars radiating from the muco-cutaneous junction at the angles of the mouth are stigmata of congenital syphilis and are called rhagades. Cracked peeling lips are often due to lipsticks. Marked sudden swelling of the lips may be a feature of angioneurotic oedema.

The Peutz-Jegher syndrome is a condition characterized by small bowel polyposis and pigmented macules resembling freckles around the mouth and involving the lips, especially near their vermilion margins but, unlike freckles the pigmented spots also occur inside the mouth and on the palms and soles. It is inherited as an autosomal dominant.

Marked prominence of the lips is a feature of both acromegaly and myxoedema.

THE GUMS

Normal gums are deep red with a smooth surface and well-defined margins. In pyorrhoea the gums become swollen and their margins retracted; often pus can be expressed from their edges and they bleed easily, either spontaneously or from such minor trauma as brushing. Chronic pyorrhoea causes loosening of the teeth.

Bleeding gums are common in uraemia and in primary blood diseases, especially acute leukaemia. Swollen, spongy, bleeding gums may occur in scurvy, but this feature is often absent. In Vincent's infection the gums are painful, swollen and bleeding with loss of interdental papillae, and well-defined ulcers covered with a greyish-white membrane which can be removed fairly easily. This infection is rarely localized to the gums, usually also involving the buccal mucosa, fauces, tonsils and soft palate. It is accompanied by a foul metallic odour of the breath. When it involves the fauces and tonsils, it may be difficult to differentiate from diphtheria, but the diphtheritic membrane is always much more difficult to remove and is associated with more marked constitutional symptoms.

Hypertrophy of the gums is a feature of phenytoin intoxication, but may also be found with amyloid involvement and occasionally in uncontrolled diabetics. Intoxication, industrial or medicinal, with the heavy metals mercury, bismuth and lead may produce a gingivostomatitis similar to Vincent's infection, later followed by a brownish-black stippled pigmentation of the gums near their margins which may be permanent, but such pigmentation may occur without other signs of gum involvement. These metallic poisonings are usually associated with marked salivation (ptyalism or sialorrhoea). Any condition causing buccal ulceration may involve the gums (*see below*).

THE TEETH

Deficient teeth and/or a poor bite may be the primary cause of dyspepsia. Caries is the commonest cause of toothache. In congenital syphilis the permanent teeth, especially the upper central incisors, have a notched cutting margin which is much narrower than the alveolar margin (described as peg-shaped because of the resemblance to a tent peg); the affected teeth (Hutchinson's* teeth) are shorter and narrower than the normal. All the teeth may be unduly widely separated, and the molars may exhibit a dome-shaped deformity of their cutting surface. The commonest causes of discoloured teeth are smoking, defective dental hygiene and pyorrhoea. Tetracycline medication during the first half of pregnancy or below the age of about eight may cause horizontal yellowish-brown or greyish bands and sometimes deformity of the deciduous or permanent canines and molars. A pinkish fluorescent discoloration of the teeth is a feature of congenital porphyria. With endemic fluorosis there may be chalky white patches or dull unglazed appearance and a brownish mottling and pitting of the enamel. In rickets and other conditions associated with vitamin D deficiency, the enamel and dentine are hypoplastic and the permanent teeth often discoloured and deformed. In many congenital diseases, such as mongolism, dental maldevelopments are common.

HALITOSIS

Halitosis (foulness of the breath) is most often due to lack of dental hygiene, but may be caused by infection of the gums or tonsils. Heavy smoking imparts a persistent aroma to the breath. Recent alcoholic consumption gives the breath its own peculiar odour, but it must always be remembered that a stuporose or comatose patient with an alcoholic breath may be in this state due to some other cause than alcoholism. Paraldehyde lingers in the breath for a very long time after its administration. Certain foods, especially onions and garlic, give a readily noticeable odour to the breath. In uraemia the breath always has a fishy ammoniacal odour. In uncontrolled diabetics it smells of acetone, which imparts a sweet fruity odour. In severe liver disease the breath has a musty or mousy pungency. In bronchiectasis and with lung abscess, marked halitosis is often present.

THE TONGUE

White patches or patch
Whiteness of the tongue may be patchy or generalized, the commonest causes being furring (coated tongue), thrush and leukoplakia. A furred tongue nearly always causes a generalized whiteness, while in the other two conditions the involvement is nearly always patchy; but it may be generalized in the latter disorders, and furring may be patchy. Furring can be easily removed by wiping with a piece of gauze or scraping with a spatula, but thrush is more difficult to remove, and leukoplakia can never be removed by such methods.

*Sir Jonathan Hutchinson (1828–1913), a London surgeon who made many original contributions to several branches of medicine, wrote about the teeth in 1858.

It is no longer fashionable to pay attention to the tongue or even to bother to examine it as a routine in all patients, but it can give much useful information, helping in the diagnosis of many general diseases and assisting in the assessment of others. To many lay people the tongue is the mirror of the gastro-intestinal tract and a coated tongue is regarded as evidence of gastric disease or constipation. There is only a small element of truth in this viewpoint, because many patinets with organic gastro-intestinal disease – especially peptic ulceration – have a clean tongue and many with a furred tongue have no organic lesion. In the latter case the commonest cause of furring is mouth breathing, often due to nasal catarrh produced by excessive smoking. However, a furred tongue does occur in fevers, in toxic conditions such as uraemia and liver failure, and in acute abdominal conditions such as appendicitis and perforation (in fact, one should hesitate to diagnose an acute abdomen unless the tongue is furred).

Much more important than furring is the degree of dryness of the tongue, which is an indication of the state of hydration of the patient as a whole. Therefore in fevers, acute abdominal conditions and toxaemias, the furred tongue is also always a dry tongue. In uraemia the tongue, in addition to being dry and furred, is often brownish, and there are usually bleeding gums and an odour of urine in the breath. Moreover, the degree of dryness may be an important guide to the necessity for and the amount of fluid therapy required. In diabetic coma, however, although the tongue is dry it frequently remains clean – that is, without furring (the 'raw beef' tongue).

Thrush, due to *Candida albicans*, is much commoner in infants. In adults the fungus is normally saprophytic but becomes a pathogen when there is diminished resistance to infection as occurs with diabetes, steroid therapy (including the contraceptive pill), broad spectrum antibiotics (especially tetracycline), immuno-suppressive drugs and irradiation. The lesions often appear on the buccal mucosa and fauces as well as the tongue and often independently or simultaneously on the genitalia.

Leukoplakia is characterized by a painless, well-defined, white or yellowish-white patch or patches which cannot be wiped off. The commonest site is the tongue, but the lips, the buccal mucosa and the mucosa of the floor of the mouth may be affected. The condition is due either to chronic irritation by smoking, spirits, spices or stumps of teeth, or to tertiary syphilis. Its great importance is first that it may indicate the syphilitic aetiology of some other lesion, especially of the heart or the central nervous system, and secondly that it is precancerous. Syphilitic leukoplakia may be associated with a localized gumma or gummas of the tongue, forming an ulcer which has a punched-out edge and a base covered with a dirty yellowish (wash-leather) slough. Sometimes there is a gummatous infiltration of the floor of the mouth. It must be remembered, however, that in any patient with leukoplakia of the tongue, any swelling of the tongue may be malignant.

Atrophic glossitis

Normally the tongue is covered with small papillae giving to its surface a velvet appearance. The anterior two-thirds are covered with filiform papillae. Fungiform papillae are almost entirely localized to the tip and sides. The circumvallate papillae demarcate the posterior third from the anterior two-thirds of the tongue.

An atrophic (depapillating) glossitis is characterized by a smooth, red, glazed, clean and often painful tongue. The atrophy is always initially of the filiform and later of the fungiform papillae. The term should not be used unless the whole or the greater part of the tongue is affected. Atrophic glossitis is seen in the following conditions:

1. Dyshaemopoietic anaemias of any type (iron, B_{12} or folic acid deficiency).
2. Riboflavine and nicotinic acid deficiencies. In the former the tongue is frequently magenta-coloured, and there is often associated angular stomatitis (fissuring at the angles of the mouth) and cheilosis (thinning and cracking of the mucous membranes of the lips). Sometimes with riboflavine deficiency, because of enlargement of the fungiform papillae and loss of the filiform papillae, a pebbled appearance results. In nicotinic acid deficiency, a fiery red glossitis affects particularly the tip and sides of the tongue and is usually associated with marked ulceration. However, the distinction between riboflavine and nicotinic acid deficiency is often artificial because the two are usually associated.
3. With oral antibiotic therapy a complicating depapillating glossitis is frequent; although this is reputed to be due to interference with absorption of the vitamin B complex, it occurs too quickly for this to be a satisfactory explanation.

Geographical tongue

Geographical tongue is a condition characterized by coalescing areas of loss of papillae, the intervening portions of the tongue being either normal or coated. The condition may be associated with tongue fissuring. It is most often seen in the younger adult age groups. It is often painful and may be associated with dyspepsia, but has no other significance. It must not be confused with leukoplakia or atrophic glossitis, in which the atrophy of the papillae is always generalized.

Amyloid disease

Amyloid disease of the tongue is characterized by enlargement and induration, and there may be purplish nodules of the tongue and hypertrophy of the gums. The diagnosis may be proved histologically from a specimen removed by gingivectomy, which should always be done by an experienced dental surgeon. The presence of amyloid disease of the tongue should always arouse suspicion of the possibility of myelomatosis.

The tongue is described as being unduly large also in acromegaly, myxoedema, cretinism and mongolism, but such enlargement is impossible to assess accurately, is usually more apparent than real, and is certainly of no diagnostic importance.

Frenal ulceration

Frenal ulceration may help in the diagnosis of early whooping cough, although modern observers do not think that such ulceration is as important or as frequent as was previously taught.

Jaundice frequently first appears in the frenum, and this is usually the last place where it is seen when the jaundice is clearing.

Fissured tongue

A marked fissuring of the tongue ('scrotal tongue') is frequently seen in normal people and very occasionally with vitamin B complex deficiency, but more often in mental defectives, especially mongols. It is often stated that the tongue in mongolism is large but this rests on the false assumption that a constantly protruded tongue is necessarily large.

A very rare syndrome is the association of a congenitally fissured tongue with recurrent facial swelling (resembling angioneurotic oedema) and a lower motor neurone facial palsy.

Very painful ulcers, with undermined edges, of the lips and the tongue (mainly its tip) may be tuberculous due to infected sputum in patients with pulmonary tuberculosis.

Angiomas

A single angioma of the lips or tongue may indicate that some other lesion, especially a spinal or intracranial one, may be an angioma.

Multiple angiomas of the tongue, lips and buccal mucosa are often seen in hereditary telangiectasia (Osler–Rendu–Weber* syndrome), and this rare condition is the only one in which multiple angiomas of the mucous membranes occur, and involvement especially of the gastro-intestinal tract and uterus may cause severe bleeding.

Black hairy tongue

Dark brownish or black patches, especially on the posterior part of the tongue, are due to a fungus infection, and this may be associated with oral antibiotic therapy.

*The condition was described by H. J. L. M. Rendu (1844–1902, French physician) in 1896, by Sir William Osler (1814–1919, physician) in 1901 and by F. P. Parkes-Weber (1863–1962, London physician) in 1936.

Vesicles on the tongue are fairly common in cases of varicella with a widespread rash.

Neurological abnormalities of the tongue are discussed in Chapter 16.

Buccal mucosa

The significance of cyanosis and icterus of the buccal mucosa is described elsewhere, as is also that of leukoplakia and thrush.

Lichen planus often involves the mouth and is then nearly always associated with the typical skin lesions (flat, purplish, polygonal, waxy, shiny, striated and very itchy papules, especially on the front of the wrists and knees, the ankles, the genitalia, the medial aspect of the thighs and the lumbo-sacral region). When the lesions are confined to the mouth, they present diagnostic problems. On the buccal mucosa (especially opposite the molars) and on the tongue they show as ill-defined bluish-white linear, reticular (lace-like) or feathery areas which are very painful and persistent. Rarely there are whitish plaques which resemble leukoplakia, but the fact that they are painful is a distinguishing feature. Patches of lichen planus rarely ulcerate. The condition is of unknown aetiology and, when present in the mouth, often leads to cancerphobia.

Pigmentation, often confined to a small area, especially opposite the molars, is an important feature of Addison's disease. Because such brownish or bluish-black patches often occur on the hard palate, it is important when searching for them that any dentures be removed. Haemachromatosis is rarely associated with pigmentation of mucous membranes and when it is, it probably indicates gross iron deposition in the suprarenals, and it could be argued that then Addison's disease is present as a complication of the haemochromatosis.

Aphthous* ulceration is probably not a clinical entity. It is a very common condition characterized by crops of minute vesicles, which rupture and form shallow painful ulcers with a red rim and a whitish slough. They may occur anywhere within the mouth. The ulcers last for a few days and heal spontaneously without scarring. There may be a cyclical neutropenia with each bout of ulceration.

Ulceration of the mouth is common in acute leukaemia and also in agranulocytosis. In the latter condition, a distinctive feature is that the greyish-black ulcers are not surrounded by any redness (inflammatory reaction). Purpura from any cause may involve the buccal mucosa and the soft and hard palate, usually in petechial form and especially in acute leukaemia and septicaemias.

---

*Aphtha was a term used by Hippocratès to describe a condition resembling thrush, and has come to be used as a generic term for superficial ulcers in the mouth of unknown aetiology.

Behçet's* disease, which has a large number of synonyms, is a condition characterized by:
1. Recurrent superficial painful ulcers of the mouth, which last for only a few days and heal spontaneously;
2. Recurrent genital ulcers of the same type;
3. Recurrent eye infection, which is usually an angular conjunctivitis but may rarely be a recurrent iritis.

The condition is nearly always found in young women, and often there is a definite time relationship between any or all of the three components of the disease and menstruation.

Not all the three components are always present either at any one time or at any time in the same patient. Rare complications are arthralgia (actual swelling is very rare), phlebitis, and an encephalitis which usually involves the mid-brain and has a high mortality. If the skin is pricked with a sharp steel needle a painful red papule or vesicle develops and this has been described as a skin sensitivity test for this condition.

The Stevens—Johnson syndrome† is a condition characterized by:
1. Bullous eruptions of the skin and mucuous membranes, especially of the mouth;
2. Urethritis;
3. Severe conjunctivitis.

A widespread erythematous mascular rash may be present in addition to the bullous lesions. The condition is most frequent in children, but does occur in adults. It is usually of unknown aetiology, but may be a complication of sulpha drugs. It must be differentiated from pemphigus vulgaris, which can also cause bullous lesions of the skin and mouth.

In secondary syphilis there often develops on the fauces, on the tonsils, and rarely on the lips or tongue a greyish-white patch or patches which become confluent, with a red perimeter sharply differentiating the lesions from the surrounding tissues. These lesions are known as mucous patches. The patches may slough, leaving a serpiginous (snail-track) ulcer. Other mucous membranes apart from the mouth may be similarly affected. Nodular lesions of the hard palate occur with tertiary syphilis, lupus vulgaris and Wegener syndrome, and in any of these conditions destruction of part of the hard palate may occur. In leontiasis ossea bony nodules may be visible on the hard palate.

Koplik's‡ spots are very small superficial specks of a bluish-white hue, which usually become confluent, occurring on the buccal

*Hulusi Behçet, (1889—1948) a Turkish dermatologist, described the syndrome in four different papers written in either German or French between 1937 and 1940.
†Stevens and Johnson are American physicians.
‡Henry Koplik (1858—1927) a New York pediatrician.

mucosa, especially opposite the molars. They may be an important sign in the early diagnosis of morbilli because they precede the typical eruption by several days and disappear when the rash starts.

The abdomen

DIVISIONS OF THE ABDOMEN

There are several different ways of describing the divisions of the abdomen. It is essential to realize that these divisions are purely arbitrary in that they are for descriptive purposes only, and one way is not more correct than another. These different techniques are illustrated by diagrams (*Figure 3*). The author prefers scheme (*a*) because it avoids the term 'lumbar region', which is more often used when meaning the loin; the use of the word 'lumbar' to describe a part of the front of the abdomen may lead to confusion.

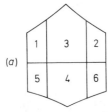

(*a*)

1. Right hypochondrium
2. Left hypochondrium
3. Epigastrium
4. Hypogastrium
5. Right iliac fossa
6. Left iliac fossa

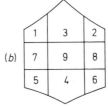

(*b*)

1–6 inclusive as (*a*)
7. Right lumbar region
8. Left lumbar region
9. Umbilical region

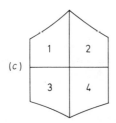

(*c*)

1. Right upper quadrant
2. Left upper quadrant
3. Right lower quadrant
4. Left lower quadrant

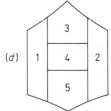

(*d*)

1. Right lateral
2. Left lateral
3. Epigastrium
4. Umbilical region
5. Hypogastrium

Figure 3. *Diagrams outlining the main areas of the abdomen. The curved lines at the top are the lower boundaries of the ribs; those at the bottom are the boundaries of the iliac crests*

INSPECTION

On inspection of the abdomen it is essential to look for skin lesions, scars, generalized or localized abdominal distension, the degree of abdominal movement with respiration, dilated veins, visible peristalsis, and abnormalities of the umbilicus.

Distension
Generalized distension may be due to fat, fluid, foetus or flatus (the last being associated with intestinal distension due to abnormality of motility or obstruction). Localized distension is seen in abnormal conditions of the belly wall such as hernias; with localized collections of fat; and with enlargement of any viscus.

Scaphoid abdomen
A scaphoid abdomen is characterized by a concave anterior abdominal wall and may occur in any patient with severe dehydration and/or marked weight loss.

Abdominal movement
The movements of the abdominal wall on deep inspiration and expiration become minimal or even absent when there is peritoneal irritation, and this is a very important diagnostic point. But if there is gross distension of the abdomen from any cause, its movements will be restricted, and this will also occur with conditions in which there is poor diaphragmatic movement, such as emphysema.

Venous obstruction
Large veins on the abdominal wall should always arouse strong suspicion of venous obstruction. This may be (1) of the inferior vena cava and/or iliac veins, and then the collateral veins are usually over the lower abdomen; (2) of the portal vein, and then they are usually on the lateral abdominal wall or, more rarely, radiating from the umbilicus; or (3) of the superior vena cava, and then the veins are over the upper abdomen as well as on the chest. However, the respective site of the engorged veins is sometimes not in the areas described above. It is often recommended that the direction of the blood flow in such veins be noted by pressing one of the largest veins with the index fingers of each hand, which are first held together and then gradually drawn apart along the line of the vein, the fingers then being lifted up each in turn and observation being made whether the vein which has been emptied then fills from above or from below.

Venous blood flow in the abdominal wall below the umbilicus is normally downward into the saphenous vein, while above the umbilicus it is upward into the veins of the thoracic wall. In portal distension, any dilated collateral veins will show a normal direction of blood flow, but inferior vena caval obstruction causes a reversal of the normal flow. Markedly dilated veins radiating from the

K

umbilicus are a very rare but pathognomonic sign of liver cirrhosis: it is called caput medusae from the resemblance to the character in Greek mythology whose head was adorned with snakes instead of hair. Occasionally with superior vena caval obstruction there are enlarged veins over the upper abdomen, and in these the blood flow will be downwards. In practice the direction of blood flow in collateral veins is rarely helpful as the findings are often equivocal.

Visible peristalsis

In thin people with poor musculature, and especially with divarication of the recti, visible peristalsis of the stomach or bowel is occasionally a normal finding. On the other hand, the recognition of such peristalsis may be diagnostic of intestinal or pyloric obstruction in a patient who is vomiting and/or has increasing constipation. Wavelike rounded elevations are seen, and these can often be accentuated by flicking or tapping the abdomen over the obstructed area. Unless there are antiperistaltic waves, the direction in pyloric obstruction is from left to right and in lesions of the transverse colon from right to left, while in small intestinal obstruction the elevations are seen mainly in the region of the umbilicus and form a ladder pattern of horizontal ridges extending across the abdomen (usually only in advanced cases). In large bowel obstruction they occur mainly laterally and form a horseshoe pattern from the right across the midline to the left. Visible peristalsis is more likely to be seen in subacute or chronic obstruction than in the acute forms, and should be regarded as a late and not an early sign.

The umbilicus

The umbilicus is normally recessed, that is, posterior to the plane of the anterior abdominal wall. If it is not (eversion), then an umbilical hernia or some cause of generalized abdominal distension should be sought.

The umbilicus should always be carefully examined for hernias; for infiltration with carcinoma (of which it is a very common site); for discharge due to infection or, less commonly, a sinus; and for any blue discoloration, which is a comparatively late sign of intraabdominal haemorrhage, especially due to ectopic or splenic rupture[9] or acute pancreatitis.

The groins

The groins should always be examined for enlarged lymph nodes and for herniae. A common cause of a tender groin swelling is a hernia and it must not be mistaken for a lymph node.

Hernial orifices should always be inspected as a routine. The region of the inguinal canals should always be palpated while the patient raises his head from the bed and coughs. An impulse will be detectable if a hernia is present. A hernia increases in size after standing and

usually decreases after lying down. If there is any suspicion of a
hernia, the patient must be examined while standing: an index
finger invaginates the scrotum, the finger is inserted into the external
inguinal ring or the canal itself, and an impulse is felt for at the neck
of the sac when the patient coughs.

A femoral hernia is situated more laterally than an inguinal one
and is always below Poupart's* ligament and below and lateral to the
pubic tubercle and the femoral artery is lateral to its neck. It enlarges
upwards to overlie the inguinal canal. It is much more difficult to
reduce than an inguinal hernia and an impulse on coughing is more
difficult to feel. It must not be mistaken for an enlarged lymph node.

The presence of a ventral hernia must always be sought for in
anyone who has had an abdominal operation. If a hernia is present,
whether it is reducible must be determined.

PALPATION

The art of palpation may appear to be crude and primitive compared
with radiology but, in fact, it often yields information of incompar-
able and immense diagnostic value.

During palpation of the abdomen, it is essential for both the
examiner and the patient to be as comfortable as possible in the
circumstances. The patient must be lying flat when the abdomen is
first palpated, preferably with no pillows. If possible the bed or couch
should be hard. It is very important in any doubtful case, or when a
definite swelling has been felt but its anatomy is uncertain, that the
patient be examined not only in the conventional position but also
lying on one side or the other and occasionally, when indicated,
either sitting or on his hands and knees. If the examiner is tall, and
especially if the bed or couch be low, he must sit or kneel by the
bedside.

Flexion of the patient's hips and knees often causes relaxation of
the abdominal muscles and aids palpation, but in other cases it is
easier with the lower limbs completely extended, so it may be useful to try both techniques. If, in spite of this, satisfactory relaxation
is not obtained, gradual pressure of the examiner's left palm on the
patient's sternum while palpating with the right hand may help. The
posture of the patient's upper limbs is very important. They should
always be held at his sides, adducted at the shoulders and extended
at the elbows. The patient should always be instructed to take deep
breaths through his wide open mouth.

Warm hands are essential for successful palpation. Rinsing the
hands in hot water is often the quickest way to warm them. The
abdomen must not be prodded, but the hand must be applied in a
gentle and delicate manner, and any pressure exerted must be gradual

*François Poupart (1616–1708), a French surgeon.

and not sudden or rough, otherwise lack of relaxation will not allow deeper and more detailed palpation. It is a good technique always to start by first palpating the whole of the abdomen with only a very light pressure and then to repeat this several times with firmer and deeper pressure on each occasion. It is important not to be casual and not to be satisfied with a perfunctory feeling of any swelling but all its details must be sought and noted.

The finger-tips are used when 'dipping', that is, feeling for a solid viscus in the presence of fluid, when intermittent pressure with the finger-tips in the region of the viscus will cause that organ to rebound against the finger-tips. This sensation can be imitated in some measure, but far from satisfactorily, by repeating a similar manoeuvre with a partially filled rubber hot-water bottle. When one is not adopting this particular procedure of dipping, the palmar aspect of the fingers and the palm of the hand itself and not the finger-tips should be used. The examiner's elbow and forearm should be on the same level as or even below the patient's anterior abdominal wall, as this will help to avoid the common error of having the wrist flexed making the examiner use his fingertips, which, as explained above, is a bad technique.

An especially valuable manoeuvre is the use of the ulnar border of the hand to attempt to cup and feel the outline of any swelling, instead of merely prodding its surface as is so often done. A very good practice is to feel the abdomen with such care that, without hesitation, an accurate diagram can be drawn of any swelling with special reference to its site, its size and whether its borders are well defined or not. Whenever an abdominal swelling is felt, it is an excellent plan for several observers each to draw such a diagram; the various representations different observers make are often surprising.

Palpation determines not only the presence of an enlarged viscus but also tenderness and guarding. The latter is a localized tenseness of the abdominal musculature, present even when the patient's attention is distracted and the rest of the abdominal musculature feels soft. Such localized guarding or rigidity, if accompanied by marked tenderness, indicates local peritoneal irritation and is generally felt over the site of the primary pathology. Generalized board-like ridigity with diffuse exquisite tenderness is found in any generalized acute peritonitis.

In cases of localized peritoneal irritation, deep pressure over the opposite side of the abdomen to that in which disease is suspected, followed by a quick release of the pressure, causes pain at the site of the disease. This is known as the rebound phenomenon. Especially in obese patients, it may provide valuable confirmatory evidence of localized peritoneal involvement, for example in acute appendicitis. This test should be done only at the end of abdominal palpation, because the pain induced may render further examination difficult.

In chronic peritonitis, especially tuberculous, tenderness is often not marked, and instead of a board-like rigidity there is a doughy feeling.

DIAGNOSTIC STAGES

As emphasized in relation to all systems discussed in this book, diagnosis is a matter of stages and it is essential to proceed by small steps, arguing from certainty to probability and leaving remote possibilities to the end of any discussion. In the case of the abdomen a stage 1 diagnosis should always be the anatomical one – that is, a statement as to which viscus or viscera, if any, is enlarged. In many cases, in fact in most cases, this is the only certain diagnosis which is possible. Discussion of the pathology gives at best only a probability and extremely rarely a certainty. It is, for example, quite incorrect to regard a patient as having a carcinoma of the caecum merely because a hard swelling is found in the right iliac fossa since, as shown on page 295, most caecal swellings – whatever their pathology, whether neoplastic or inflammatory – will feel the same. It is essential in clinical medicine to know the limitations of palpation, to have tactile insight, and to realize that palpation alone can never be a certain guide to histology. Inflammatory swellings may be as hard and irregular as any neoplasm, and a neoplastic swelling may be soft and tender. The emphasis, then, is on the fact that palpation can at best be merely a rough guide to pathology.

It is essential to note all the physical signs which may characterize any particular enlarged viscus. It is perfectly true that, for example, an enlarged spleen can frequently be correctly identified by the most casual palpation, and that there should be no necessity for considering a differential diagnosis of such a swelling. The reason why it is essential to know all the described signs is that occasionally the anatomy of an abdominal swelling is not obvious; for example, it may be very difficult to differentiate between a huge left kidney and a spleen. In such a case the correct diagnosis is made by balancing the evidence – that is, so many points in favour of one diagnosis and so many points in favour of the other – and unless the assessment is made on this basis, diagnosis becomes mere guesswork.

Moreover, a good diagnostician should always accurately name the enlarged viscus without resort to the 'penny in the slot' technique of successive multiple and haphazard radiological investigations. A very good way of assessing whether a man is a good clinician or not is to see how often, without any radiographs, he makes the correct anatomical diagnosis of abdominal swellings. Unless an anatomical diagnosis is correct, further discussion of a case is really impossible. For example, if a swelling is an enlarged kidney, then hydronephrosis, pyonephrosis and renal carcinoma will be the first probabilities to be considered, whereas these conditions would not be discussed if the swelling had been incorrectly diagnosed as an enlarged spleen.

ENLARGED LYMPH GLANDS
Palpation of the abdomen should always include feeling for enlarged lymph nodes in the groin. If the nodes are enlarged, their character should be noted. Whenever enlarged lymph nodes are found, the order of procedure should be first to feel for nodes elsewhere and for the spleen. If there is a generalized lymphadenopathy, especially with splenomegaly, the likely diagnosis is a reticulosis such as lymphadenoma or leukaemia, and a less likely diagnosis is that of inflammatory conditions such as glandular fever. On the other hand, if the enlarged glands are confined to one area, for example the groin, then the area of lymphatic drainage must be examined. In the case of the groin this includes the whole of the lower limbs, the abdomen, the genitalia and the pelvis.

The relative importance of percussion is discussed elsewhere.

AUSCULTATION
Auscultation very occasionally proves of value in the diagnosis of abdominal disease. Normal bowel sounds can be heard. The normal variations in the loudness, pitch and other qualities of these sounds cannot be described in words, and such knowledge cannot be acquired unless auscultation of the abdomen is done as a routine and not reserved for those cases in which it is likely to be of value.

Bowel sounds of an increased loudness and frequency but otherwise normal may be heard in any patient with diarrhoea, associated with increased peristalsis, from whatever cause. In acute peritonitis or other conditions in which there is paralysis of the bowel, bowel sounds will not be heard. In cases of intestinal obstruction, the sounds will be more marked than normal and are often described as being of a whistling or muffled bubbling character; moreover, they are continuous over a localized area.

The best place to auscultate is usually just below the umbilicus. The physician must engage in concentrated listening for at least 5 minutes before giving a definite opinion, and great care must be taken that the stethoscope is held perfectly still.

If an aneurysm of the abdominal aorta is suspected, very valuable confirmatory evidence is the hearing of a systolic bruit over the swelling. A systolic bruit, sometimes with a thrill, may be heard over a stenosed abdominal aorta or iliac artery. With stenosis of a renal artery, a systolic bruit is often heard over the central area of the abdomen, but it may be heard laterally or posteriorly. However any systolic bruit over the cardiac area may be conducted into the abdomen, and therefore a bruit heard over the abdomen is indicative of intra-abdominal aneurysm or arterial occlusion only if it is not heard also over the praecordium.

ENLARGED GALLBLADDER

An enlarged gallbladder is situated in the right hypochondrium unless it is huge, when it may extend into the right iliac fossa. It is felt as a smooth rounded swelling which is directed downward, inward and forward. It is very unusual to feel the whole of the gallbladder as a pyriform swelling, as often described; usually only the fundus is palpable, the rest of the organ being deep in the abdomen, and it is only the fact that it enlarges forward which enables it to be felt. It is not felt at the tip of the ninth rib along the outer border of the right rectus, as is frequently stated, that being the surface marking of the normal gallbladder, which is too deep in the abdomen to be felt. A grossly enlarged gallbladder may be movable from side to side. Contrary to what is frequently said, the gallbladder is often enlarged without the liver being palpable; when the liver edge and the gallbladder are both palpable, the two are not continuous but a sulcus can be felt between them. A distended gallbaldder is often more easily felt if the patient turns towards his left side.

An important law is that if a patient with obstructive jaundice also has a palpable gallbladder, then the cause is not gallstones but extrinsic pressure on the bile duct such as that produced by a carcinoma of the head of the pancreas or by enlarged nodes in the portal fissure. Cholelithiasis itself does not cause gallbladder enlargement because the associated cholecystitis (which is probably always present unless the stones are of a pure pigment type, as found in haemolytic anaemias) produces fibrosis and shrinkage of the gallbladder. There is only one exception to this law, and that is where there is a stone in the cystic duct or Hartmann's pouch (a normal sacculation of the neck of the gallbladder from which the cystic duct arises) which has produced a mucocele of the gallbladder and, in addition, another stone in the common bile duct has caused obstructive jaundice. Because stones are often multiple, this exception frequently occurs, but it is important to realize that it is the only exception to this fundamental law. A negative application of the law is that obstructive jaundice without a palpable gallbladder is unlikely to be due to extrinsic obstruction caused, for example, by a carcinoma of the pancreas.

When the gallbladder is enlarged due to extrinsic pressure, it is rarely tender. This contrasts with gallbladder enlargement due to cholecystitis or cholelithiasis producing a mucocele or empyeme of that viscus, which is then always tender.

ENLARGED SPLEEN

Enlargements of the spleen have the following characteristics:
  1. A swelling is present in the left hypochondrium, coming from

beneath the costal margin. This may extend into the left iliac fossa, but it is extremely rare for it to extend to the right of the midline.

2. The swelling has a well-defined medial border in which there may be a notch. (This is very important because it is pathognomonic of splenic enlargement; unfortunately it cannot always be felt, but it is most likely with chronic moderate or marked enlargements.)

3. It is impossible to get above the swelling.

4. The swelling moves on respiration and when moderately or markedly enlarged it can be felt to move medially as well as towards the iliac crest. This may be an important feature distinguishing splenomegaly from liver enlargement, especially when the latter is mainly or entirely of the left lobe.

5. It may be possible to get a finger between the swelling and the erector spinae muscle posteriorly, which is never possible with a renal swelling.

6. There is dullness over the swelling. This dullness is continuous with the normal splenic dullness which, if percussed along the axis of the tenth rib, does not normally extend further forward than the mid-axillary line. Percussion of the spleen is not recommended as a routine, but it may be of considerable help in a difficult case, for example in the differentiation from a large kidney.

There are various techniques for feeling for an enlarged spleen. The usual method is to push forward the palm of the left hand, which is placed immediately below the patient's left ribs posteriorly, while the right hand is placed anteriorly below the ribs and is pressed upwards towards the costal margin as the patient takes a deep breath. Alternatively, the left palm is placed over the lower left ribs anteriorly and the right hand below the costal margin anteriorly, and on deep respiration the left hand is pressed downwards and somewhat backwards while the right hand is pressed upwards towards the patient's axilla. With the latter technique, if the patient lies on his flexed left forearm, this may help to push the spleen forward and assist in its palpation. Sometimes the spleen can be felt much more easily if the patient half turns towards his right with flexed left hip and knee. The author uses all these techniques as a routine before giving an opinion that the spleen is not enlarged, and he advises the student to do likewise.

When feeling for an enlarged spleen, one should always start in the left iliac fossa and gradually feel towards the costal margin, because if a start is made from immediately below the costal margin, surprisingly enough a very large spleen can be missed. Also, it is important not to press too hard as otherwise one will miss a just palpable spleen.

Causes of splenomegaly

The causes of splenomegaly should be classified into groups, and the presence of additional findings must be taken into account when considering the probable diagnosis: for example, pallor or jaundice or plethora of mucous membranes, lymphadenopathy, skin pigmentation, arthritis of the hands, or any extra-abdominal manifestations of liver cirrhosis. Indeed, in most patients with splenomegaly, some clue outside the abdomen gives an inkling of the likely cause. It is never possible to find an enlarged spleen and be certain of the cause merely on palpation. The best that can be done is to discuss first probabilities and later possibilities, taking cognizance of any additional features which have been observed in the abdomen or elsewhere.

The common causes of splenomegaly are as follows:

1. Blood diseases such as chronic leukaemias, haemoglobinopathies, pernicious anaemia, myelosclerosis and polycythaemia vera. Primary thrombocytopenic purpura, acute leukaemia and iron deficiency anaemia are blood diseases in which it is unusual to find splenic enlargement.
2. Reticuloses, for example lymphadenoma, sarcoidosis and the lipoidoses such as Gaucher's* disease.
3. Infections, either acute or chronic. A large number of acute and chronic infections may be associated with splenomegaly, and for this reason the presence or absence of splenomegaly is of no help in the differential diagnosis of any obscure pyrexia.
4. Cirrhosis.
5. Amyloid disease. This should be discussed only if there is some known cause for it, because primary amyloid disease confined to the spleen does not occur.
6. Primary neoplasms of the spleen, which are very rare, and secondary deposits, which are even rarer, and when they do occur are nearly always from a pancreatic primary.

Whether the splenomegaly is moderately or grossly enlarged is of no diagnostic importance except for the fact that gross enlargement excludes an acute infection as the cause. Conditions such as chronic myeloid leukaemia may cause a huge spleen eventually, but at some stage of the illness the splenomegaly must have been only slight and later moderate before becoming gross.

JAUNDICE

Slight jaundice can easily be missed unless the patient is examined in a good natural light. Many cases are initially missed because of observation in artificial light.

*P. C. E. Gauchet (1854–1918), a French physician.

Jaundice may be obstructive, haemolytic or hepatogenous, and the physician's first task must always be to determine which of these types is present.

Cholestasis

It has become fashionable to replace the term 'obstructive jaundice' by the word 'cholestasis'. This is often defined as a failure of bile to reach the duodenum because of an extrahepatic or intrahepatic lesion anywhere along the bile pathway from the hepatocellular microsomes to the duodenum. However, the exact site of the obstruction cannot always be determined accurately even at autopsy, and in some patients no actual anatomical block can be found either macroscopically or microscopically. Most British experts reserve the term cholestasis for those cases where the obstruction is in the intrahepatic bile channels (the cholangioles), and I will follow this definition.

Because of interference with the entry of bile into the duodenum, any patient with chronic non-haemolytic jaundice from any cause is likely to develop steatorrhoea (interference with fat absorption), and this invariably leads to loss of weight which must not be interpreted as evidence of malignancy. Interference with the absorption of calcium and the fat-soluble vitamins (A, D and K) may also occur.

Obstructive jaundice may be due to prolonged extrahepatic bile obstruction, which secondarily causes cholestasis because of resultant infection of the cholangioles with their subsequent atresia (sclerosis). A similar process in the cholangioles may occur independently of any extrahepatic obstruction in patients with ulcerative colitis, but the mechanism of its production is obscure. Of course, jaundice complicating ulcerative colitis may be iatrogenic due to drug therapy or blood transfusions.

Primary biliary cirrhosis is a condition of middle-aged women and is characterized by painless, afebrile, persistent but often mild chronic cholestatic jaundice. It is doubtful whether it is a true cirrhosis. Its aetiology is unknown, although it is fashionable to classify it as an auto-immune disease. Congenital atresia of the intra- or extrahepatic bile ducts is a rare condition. A primary carcinoma may start in either hepatic duct, causing a cholestatic jaundice which may be intermittent and is difficult to diagnose without laparotomy.

Drugs producing jaundice

Today drugs have become a common cause of cholestatic jaundice, and an important offender is the phenothiazine group. The jaundice is nearly always of sudden onset, and although it may persist for a long time, the prognosis is good. The mechanism of the obstruction is not known, and the condition cannot be produced in animals. Only a small percentage of patients taking any drugs in this group actually develop jaundice. The jaundice is not dependent on dosage.

Other drugs which may also have this effect are the sulpha compounds, including tolbutamide and chlorpropamide, and erythromycin.

Other drugs are reputed to cause jaundice by precipitating a generalized hypersensitivity reaction which may be exhibited by fever, pain in joints, urticaria, lymphadenopathy and eosinophilia and is later followed by hepatocellular damage with jaundice and the development of a clinical picture resembling acute infective hepatitis. Drugs in this group are isoniazid and pyrazinamid and other hydrazine derivatives, phenindione, para-aminosalicylic acid, halothane, phenylbutazone and sometimes the sulpha compounds. Jaundice due to methyl testosterone, norethandrolone and oral contraceptives is also regarded as cholestatic, but occurs only after any of these compounds has been given in fairly large dosage for long periods.

Chloroform, carbon tetrachloride, gold, arsenic, tetracyclines, cytotoxic drugs, yellow phosphorus, cinchophen, trichlorethylene and some poisonous fungi such as muscarine amanita may cause jaundice, due to severe liver cell damage, which is often fatal. With this group of chemicals there is always also renal and bone marrow damage.

Some drugs produce jaundice which is haemolytic (*see below*).

Extrahepatic biliary obstruction
Extrahepatic bile duct obstruction may be due to (1) a lesion within the lumen, for example gallstones; (2) a lesion originating in the wall of the common bile duct, for example cancer; or (3) a lesion outside the duct and compressing it — for example, carcinoma of the head of the pancreas or enlarged nodes, from whatever cause, in the portal fissure.

Clinical differentiation between intra- and extrahepatic obstruction can be very difficult. Hepatomegaly is always present in chronic and nearly always in acute extrahepatic obstruction. Abdominal pain favours the latter condition.

Hepatogenous jaundice
Hepatogenous (hepatocellular) jaundice is due to primary disease of the liver cells themselves. It may be due to infections such as infective hepatitis, spirochaetosis ictero-haemorrhagica and yellow fever, and is an occasional feature of glandular fever, typhoid, brucellosis, and septicaemia from any cause. Chemicals which may cause hepato-cellular damage have been described above.

Haemolytic jaundice
The causes of haemolytic jaundice are obviously the same as those of haemolytic anaemia, the two terms being synonymous. They may be subdivided into the following types:
1. An intracorpuscular type due to the abnormalities of the red cells, the haemoglobinopathies.

2. An intravascular type due to abnormalities of the serum associated with (a) biological haemolysins, for example from incompatible blood transfusions; (b) chemical haemolysins, for example arsenuretted hydrogen, phenylhydrazine, lead, benzene derivatives and some snake bites; (c) bacterial and parasitic haemolysins, for example haemolytic streptococci, *Bacillus welchii*, malaria and blackwater fever; (d) unknown haemolysins, for example the paroxysmal haemoglobinurias (cold, exertion and nocturnal types) and some of the acquired idiopathic haemolytic anaemias which it is now fashionable to classify as auto-immune.

Patients with haemolytic jaundice do not have pruritis or brady-cardia, and their colour is lemon yellow rather than green.

A leading authority on liver disease, Professor Sherlock, has written:

'The place of biochemistry in the practical diagnosis of liver disease has been overemphasized. A careful clinical history and examination, together with simple urine testing and faecal inspection, will enable a correct diagnosis to be made in a jaundiced patient' (*Diseases of the Liver and Biliary System*, Oxford: Blackwell 1958).

THE LIVER

To feel for liver enlargement, always start low in the right iliac fossa and, with the right hand flat on the abdomen and its fingers parallel to the costal margin, press firmly while the patient breathes deeply, the pressure not being released until the end of inspiration. Palpation must be kept external to the rectus abdominis, or the muscle itself might be mistaken for the liver edge.

A liver swelling is characterized by the following:

1. A swelling in the right hypochondrium, which may be also in the epigastrium and even in the left hypochondrium. Sometimes the left lobe of the liver is much more enlarged than the right, and the swelling will then be mainly in the left hypochondrium, simulating a splenomegaly. If the liver is grossly enlarged, its lower border may extend into the iliac fossae.
2. A well-defined lower border which is roughly parallel with the costal margin.
3. Movement on respiration.
4. Impossibility of getting above the swelling.
5. Dullness over it which is continuous with normal liver dullness.

The upper border of the liver is about level with the upper border of the fifth rib in the right mid-clavicular line, with the eighth inter-space in the right mid-axillary line, and with the tenth interspace in the right scapular region. In the left mid-clavicular line, it is on a level with the sixth rib. The upper border must be defined by heavy and the lower border by light percussion, but attempts to define the upper border accurately are usually a waste of effort except when there is a strong suspicion that the liver has shrunken due to atrophy. Theoretically, the liver may be pushed down by a large right pleural effusion or pneumothorax or by an emphysematous lung, and determination of its upper border by percussion is reputed to help in arriving at such a diagnosis. Such demonstrable downward displacement is, however, very rarely possible. When it does occur, the upper border usually cannot be determined by percussion because of the practical impossibility of distinguishing between liver and fluid dullness and, in the case of emphysema, because the area of liver dullness is itself grossly diminished.

In theory, the upper border of the liver will be raised in any case of hepatomegaly, but in fact this is rarely if ever demonstrable. Indeed, attempts at accurate definition of the liver borders are usually neither necessary nor helpful.

Percussion is a valuable method, and in fact is the only way, of demonstrating liver atrophy. Gross diminution of liver dullness in the area, and its replacement by tympany or hyper-resonance, can be a valuable confirmatory sign of emphysema, pneumothorax or pneumoperitoneum (due to perforation of a hollow viscus).

Many clinicians claim to be able to feel the liver edge just below the right costal margin in most healthy non-obese people. The author personally doubts this ability, and if the consistency of a normal liver is remembered, this sceptism appears justified.

Riedel's* lobe

This is a fairly common normal finding, especially in women. It is a tongue-like projection from the inferior surface of the right lobe. It may be felt in the right hypochondrium and very rarely also in the right iliac fossa. It is a normal anatomical variation which has no clinical significance and must not be mistaken for a hepatoma, hepatic cyst, or single secondary, or even large liver nodule or a renal swelling. In my experience the error is more often the other way round and wrongly diagnosing any of the conditions just mentioned as a Riedel's lobe.

Nodular liver

Having felt the hepatic enlargement, it is then extremely important to determine whether any nodules are present and, if so, the characteristics of these nodules. A nodular liver is nearly always due to metastases, and if a depression (umbilication) is felt in the centre of any of the nodules, then this diagnosis is certain. In cirrhosis, nodules other than post-necrotic ones (*see below*) are exceptional. Secondary nodules are frequently tender and cirrhotic nodules rarely so, but this

*B. M. C. L. Riedel (1846–1916), Jena surgeon.

is not a reliable sign. Moreover, the size of a nodule is no guide to its pathology. Rare causes of hepatic nodules are gummas due to tertiary syphilis or schistosomiasis.

Cirrhosis of the liver

In any classification of cirrhosis it is best to avoid eponyms, also aetiological classifications and those based solely on histology. The simplest classification is into biliary and portal cirrhosis. Some experts insist on adding a third type, designated post-necrotic, which is secondary to viral hepatitis or chemical poisoning, but undoubtedly both these conditions may be followed by either typical portal or typical biliary cirrhosis. Post-necrotic cirrhosis is characteristically multilobular in contrast with the monolobular portal type.

Cirrhosis is not synonymous with a merely fibrous tissue reaction within the liver. A true cirrhosis implies that the primary lesion was hepatocellular and the fibrosis is secondary to this.

Biliary cirrhosis

Biliary cirrhosis is caused by any condition which produces prolonged obstruction to biliary flow, whether primarily extrahepatic or primarily intrahepatic (cholestasis).

When biliary cirrhosis is due to chronic extrahepatic obstruction, the patient usually gives a history suggestive of gallbladder disease and fever due to an ascending cholangiitis. When the biliary obstruction is partial or valvular, the fever is likely to be high and intermittent and associated with rigors. The gallbladder may be palpable and tender, and the liver is always enlarged and tender but is never nodular.

When the biliary obstruction is cholestatic, the liver is often not palpable, and if it is, it is not tender. The gallbladder in these cases is not palpable, and cholangiitis is not a feature. Primary biliary cirrhosis is described previously.

In biliary cirrhosis, jaundice is always an early sign and may be very marked, producing an almost grass green discoloration of the skin. Splenomegaly is an early and constant manifestation. Ascites is not present except very rarely as a terminal event. Because of the associated hypercholesterolaemia secondary to the prolonged jaundice, xanthomas of the skin and subcutaneous tissues are common.

Portal cirrhosis

Portal cirrhosis is the end result of liver damage caused by a large variety of deleterious agents — chemical, infective, nutritional and circulatory (cardiac cirrhosis). In England, in about half the cases the aetiology is obscure.

The consensus of opinion is that malnutrition by itself rarely gives rise to cirrhosis. However, in certain areas of the world, especially in Africa, children may suffer from kwashiorkor where malnutrition is prevalent. The affected children are irritable yet apathetic, grossly oedematous and depigmented. The depigmentation of the skin produces an appearance like that of flaking paint, and the hair becomes reddish. Kwashiorkor is due to a diet very low in protein although the total calorie intake may be adequate.

Haemochromatosis produces a portal type of cirrhosis, but in contrast with most cases of portal cirrhosis, ascites and collateral veins are unusual. Hepato-lenticular degeneration is a combination of a portal type of cirrhosis with extrapyramidal lesions due to a genetically determined abnormality of copper metabolism.Schistosomiasis is reputed to cause a portal cirrhosis, but most authorities dissent from this view because although the disease produces marked hepatic fibrosis, there is little or no generalized liver cell destruction.

In portal cirrhosis, jaundice is a late sign and is rarely very marked. At an early stage of the disease, the liver may be enlarged and is usually hard and sometimes irregular, but is rarely nodular. In the later stages, the liver shrinks considerably and ceases to be palpable. With portal cirrhosis the spleen may be enlarged, but not so frequently or so markedly as with biliary cirrhosis.

Signs of portal cirrhosis
1. The presence of an enlarged or atrophic liver.
2. The presence of portal hypertension, as shown by ascites, collateral veins and splenomegaly. The ascites is probably not caused entirely by portal hypertension; lowered plasma osmotic pressure due to hypoproteinaemia, secondary to defective albumin synthesis, is also a factor.
3. The presence of telangiectases ('spider naevi' or 'arterial spider'). These are dilated capillaries which are nearly always small (about 5 millimetres). They occur on the face, chest and upper limbs, especially on the dorsum of the hands, but are extremely rare below the level of the thorax. They are not pathognomonic because they occur in a few normal people, rarely in rheumatoid arthritis, and sometimes in late pregnancy, disappearing after delivery.
4. The presence of a persistent redness of the palms.
5. Leuconychia — the presence of whiteness of the nails.
6. Occasionally sexual changes are shown by loss of pubic hair, testicular atrophy and gynaecomastia. These endocrine changes are very common in the cirrhosis associated with alcoholism and also in haemochromatosis, and are reputed to be due to failure of the liver to destroy oestrogens.
7. Dupuytren's contracture is commoner, especially in alcoholic cirrhosis, than can be explained by mere coincidence.
8. Purpura is common in severe liver disease.

9. Patients with portal cirrhosis are very liable to relapsing pancreatitis, chronic pyelonephritis and pulmonary infections.
10. A low grade fever is very common even in the absence of complicating infection.
11. Parotitis is fairly common.
12. Between 5 and 10 per cent of patients with portal cirrhosis develop a serous pleural effusion at some stage of their illness.

Liver failure

The manifestations of liver failure are mainly encephalopathic — headache and delirium, epilepsy and focal brain signs. The delirium has no special features (*see* Chapter 16) distinguishing it from any other type of delirium. The encephalopathic signs fluctuate markedly, and considerable spontaneous improvement and even apparent recovery are common.

The flapping tremor of liver failure is described in Chapter 16.

Hepatic failure may be precipitated by gastro-intestinal haemorrhage, an alcoholic bout, morphine, barbiturates, chlorothiazide derivatives, and surgery of even a minor variety such as paracentesis or liver puncture.

THE COLON

Although the colon is situated in all described divisions of the abdomen, it is unusual to feel a distended colon or a mass in the colon except in the right or left iliac fossa.

The upper part of the sigmoid (pelvic) colon may be palpable in normal people as a sausage-shaped movable swelling anteriorly situated immediately posterior to the anterior abdominal wall. The actual size and consistency of such a swelling depends mainly on the tone of the abdominal and bowel musculature and the amount of its faecal content. In very constipated patients, hard scybalae (never a single mass) may be palpable; these can be indented and altered in shape by firm pressure, and this is their most important diagnostic feature.

The normal transverse colon is not palpable except rarely in very thin people, in whom it may be felt as a movable tube across the upper abdomen. The ascending colon and the caecum, if they contain a great deal of fluid material and faeces, may be palpable in a normal person a few hours after a main meal.

The hepatic and splenic flexures are not normally felt because they are deep in the abdomen. Pathology at these sites is unfortunately very common, especially carcinoma, but because of the deep position of the flexures and the fact that such carcinomas are usually of the scirrhous type, it is extremely unusual to be able to feel a malignant mass at these sites unless it is very large. This will be palpable below the left or right costal margin, and can easily be confused with either an enlarged liver or spleen or a huge kidney unless the characteristics of the swelling are carefully sought for.

The usual colonic swelling is felt, as stated above, in the right or left iliac fossa (and for this purpose caecal swellings are also included). Such a swelling may have fairly well defined lateral borders, but its upper and lower borders are always ill defined, as may also be the lateral borders. The colonic swelling never moves on respiration; it is only slightly mobile from side to side, and never up and down. It may give the impression that one can roll it under one's hand and the attempt to do so often produces gurgling, a very important sign that the swelling is colonic. Whatever its pathology, a colonic swelling is always a comparatively although not completely fixed swelling, and therefore fixity of a colonic or caecal swelling is no evidence of malignancy. The colonic swelling cannot be pushed forward from the loin. A swelling of the sigmoid colon is much more likely to be faeces than a neoplasm.

The percussion note over the swelling will depend upon its nature. If the distended colon is due to constipation, to some abnormality of motility or to intestinal obstruction, it will be tympanitic. On the other hand, if an inflammatory or neoplastic mass is felt in the colon, then percussion over this area will give a dull note.

Distension of a large part of the colon occurs with a low intestinal obstruction from any cause, with a toxic dilatation of the colon such as may occur in ulcerative colitis, and in Hirschsprung's* disease. Hirschsprung's disease is an inherited condition in which there is an absence of the ganglion cells of the mesenteric plexus. It always affects the distal colon but the involvement may be very extensive. It is commoner in males and although symptoms and signs may start in childhood they may be delayed until adult life. The main symptom is constipation. It may cause an extremely distended tympanitic abdomen in which it may be possible to feel large faecal masses which can be indented on pressure. Rectal examination will show a normal and not distended rectum. X-ray will show not only the distended colon but also a well-defined narrow segment distally.

Some diseases of the caecum, ileum or appendix produce a fixed sausage-shaped swelling in the right iliac fossa. The commonest pathologies in this region giving rise to a palpable mass are malignancy, tuberculosis, regional ileitis, actinomycosis, appendix abscess, intussusception and, rarely, amoebiasis. Again it must be emphasized that any of these swellings may be hard and nodular and that all are fixed and immobile.

The presence of sinuses over the swelling should arouse suspicion of actinomycosis. Search should then be made for the 'sulphur granules' in the depths of the sinus, which are yellowish bodies, the size of a large pin-head and consisting of a conglomeration of mycelial

*Harald Hirschsprung (1831–1916), a Danish physician, wrote his paper in 1887.

filaments. A very useful point, which should always lead to the thought that any sinus in the abdomen, neck or chest is secondary to an actinomycotic lesion, is the fact that such sinuses have a purplish granulation tissue. Rarely tuberculosis and, still more rarely, regional ileitis may give rise to sinuses.

The differential diagnosis between these conditions can seldom be made with certainty at the bedside. The barium meal in all of them will show a filling defect in the area, and therefore the radiograph also is not diagnostic. In the case of regional ileitis, because it involves a fairly extensive part of the ileum and caecum, the radiographs often show an extensive filling defect, the affected part of the ileum being converted into a very narrow channel (the 'string sign'). However, this radiographic appearance is not always seen in this disease and may rarely be seen in the other pathologies mentioned above. Even on laparotomy it is not always possible to distinguish between these conditions, and therefore it will be apparent how unlikely one is to be able to make a certain pathological diagnosis on palpation alone.

THE STOMACH

A distended stomach often causes distension of the upper part of the abdomen and is seen rather than felt, because its borders are rarely definable even if the gastric enlargement is gross. A splash may be felt and heard if the firm pressure of the examiner's hand be suddenly released or the area be percussed with the ends of all the fingers of one hand simultaneously. The decision whether or not a splash is present must be made after a single performance of either manoeuvre, because repetition is certain to cause abdominal muscle guarding which will interfere with the test. Gastric splashing is significant if it is present more than four hours after the last full meal or two hours after only fluids.

A tumour in the pyloric region is often readily palpable, even when small, as a hard, fixed, usually irregular mass in the epigastrium in the midline or immediately to the right of it. In infants with congenital pyloric stenosis, a knotty lump is often palpable in the upper half of the abdomen near the outer border of the right rectus muscle, especially if the examiner is fortunate enough to feel the abdomen while active pyloric contractions are present.

Tumours arising from the cardia, the lesser curvature or the posterior wall of the body of the stomach are very unlikely to be palpable unless they are very large. Occasionally tumours of the body or the greater curvature are palpable, and palpation may be facilitated by examining the patient while he is turned towards his right side.

Tumours arising from the anterior wall of the greater curvature are often palpable, while those from the body or the cardia are rarely so because they are deep beneath the left costal margin. How-ever, a large hypertrophic carcinoma may be felt as a hard mass with an irregular lower border coming from below the left rib margin and extending into the left hypochondrium and epigastrium. Its upper border will not be palpable and it is very unlikely to move on respiration. Turning the patient on his left side may help one to feel the mass. Rarely in linitis plastica ('leather bottle stomach') the out-line of the greater part of the stomach can be felt.

THE PANCREAS

Because the pancreas is situated deep in the abdomen, a swelling arising from any part of it is rarely palpable unless it is huge, as cysts may be but neoplasms very rarely are.

A pancreatic swelling is situated in the epigastrium with its long axis across the abdomen. It is fixed, not moving on respiration, and its borders may be rounded but are usually ill defined. There is dull-ness over the swelling and resonance between it and the normal liver and spleen dullness. It often exhibits pulsation transmitted from the abdominal aorta. If due to a large cyst, it may be ballotable and a fluid thrill may be demonstrable.

RETROPERITONEAL MASSES

The kidneys, suprarenals and pancreas are all retroperitoneal structures, but apart from swellings in these sites, swellings may arise from nodes or from connective tissue (especially between the muscles). Such primary tumours may be benign, such as fibroma or lipoma, but are more often malignant. Masses arising from the lymph nodes may be primary lymphosarcoma but are usually secondary to any intra-abdominal malignancy. They may, however, be part of a reticulosis such as lymphadenoma or, less likely, of an inflammatory lesion, for example, tuberculosis.

A retroperitoneal mass is usually situated in the region of the umbilicus. It is always firm, irregular and fixed, with at least one of its borders, usually the upper, well defined. It may have the features of a mass arising out of the pelvis. A retroperitoneal mass may cause displacement of the stomach, bowel or ureter as shown radiologically.

PELVIC SWELLINGS

A swelling arising in the pelvis in a male may be of the bladder or colon or may be a mass of retroperitoneal nodes. In the female, to the above list must be added swellings arising from the internal genitalia. In the latter connection, it is important to note that a large ovarian swell-ing is often a midline one.

The features of swelling, other than those of the colon, arising out of the pelvis are their site in the hypogastrium or the right or left iliac fossa, the fact that they have a well-defined upper border, and the fact that it is impossible to get below the swelling, which is felt to recede into the pelvis.

The bladder swelling is always a midline swelling with a smooth rounded upper margin, and firm pressure over it produces an urgent desire to micturate. Proof is obtained by emptying the bladder, which causes the swelling to disappear. When there is a diverticulum of the bladder, the swelling is asymmetrical and not the more usual hemispherical shape. Diverticulum of the bladder is fairly frequent in patients with neurological disease complicated by retention of urine, for example tabes dorsalis. Prostatic enlargement interfering with urinary outflow causes hypertrophy of the detrusor with subsequent bladder trabeculation and later diverticula.

Before giving a final opinion on the anatomical nature of any pelvic swelling, it is always advisable to ask the patient to empty his bladder and then to palpate the abdomen again.

ANEURYSMS OF THE ABDOMINAL AORTA

These are usually found in elderly people and cause a swelling which may be difficult to diagnose anatomically. Such a swelling may be felt anywhere in the abdomen, but is usually in the upper half. It may appear to come from below the costal margin. It does not move on respiration and is not mobile, and usually some part of it is well defined, smooth and regular. The main clue, however, is often provided by the fact that it just does not fit in with the signs of any other viscus, so that whenever an unusual swelling is felt, especially in an elderly person, an abdominal aneurysm must be considered. The proof would be the demonstration of an expansile sensation — that is, pulsation in all directions, felt by gripping the swelling either between the palms of the hands or, if the examiner's hand is large, between the thumb and fingers. Where there is still doubt as to whether the swelling shows an expansile or merely transmitted pulsation, examining the abdomen with the patient on his hands and knees may be decisive because transmitted pulsation cannot be readily felt in this position and expansile pulsation can.

The hearing of a loud bruit over the swelling, in the absence of such a loud bruit over the heart, is very strong supporting evidence. A straight radiograph of the abdomen will show a soft tissue mass, and this may exhibit linear calcification along part of its border. The lateral view of the spine may show a smooth erosion of the vertebral bodies, leaving the intervertebral discs unaffected and producing a scallop effect.

Aneurysms of the abdominal aorta, unlike those of the thoracic aorta, are rarely syphilitic, usually being atherosclerotic. They are often found on routine examination in a patient complaining of vague abdominal pain. They may, however, give rise to symptoms and signs due either (1) to pressure on any vessels, nerves, viscera or bones or (2) to leakage or rupture into the peritoneal cavity, into retroperitoneal tissues, into any viscus or, more rarely, into a large vein.

ASCITES

Ascites is the presence of free fluid in the peritoneal cavity. Such fluid may be either a transudate or an exudate and may be serous, purulent or chylous. The fundamental signs of ascites are as follows:
1. A generalized distension of the abdomen.
2. A stony dullness in the flanks, which shifts.
3. A fluid thrill.
4. Where there is hepatomegaly, splenomegaly or other enlarged viscus, it can be felt only by dipping and does not appear to be immediately beneath the palm of the examiner's hand.
5. Eversion of the umbilicus.

It is necessary to describe these signs in more detail and especially the wording used. Most textbooks emphasize distension in the flanks, and this is done to stress the differentiation from swellings arising out of the pelvis, where the distension is only central. On the other hand, 'generalized distension' is a better description, because with ascites there is not only distension in the flanks but central distension as well. Marked distension in the flanks only, without any distension centrally, is found where there is marked colonic distension, for example, in severe constipation, in Hirschsprung's disease, and in gross bilateral renal enlargement due to polycystic renal disease or bilateral hydronephrosis.

With regard to sign (2) above, the usual wording is 'shifting dullness'. However, the phrase 'stony dullness which shifts' is preferable because it is desired to emphasize that unless it is possible to demonstrate marked dullness in the flanks, no attempt should be made to exhibit a shifting dullness, a sign which is frequently wrongly interpreted to fit in with a preconceived notion of the diagnosis. Therefore, in a patient with a distended abdomen the procedure should be first to note whether the distension is generalized; if it is, to percuss the flanks, and if these exhibit a marked impairment of percussion note, then and only then to attempt to demonstrate a shifting dullness.

Regarding sign (3), a fluid thrill is never present unless the amount of fluid is large, that is, it is under tension, and even then the thrill is often difficult to elicit. A large cyst, for example, an ovarian cyst, may also give a fluid thrill. A help in differentiating a very large ovarian cyst from ascites is to place a ruler, or something of a similar shape, across the abdomen at the level of the superior iliac spines. With a cyst pulsation of the aorta will be visible and palpable transmitted from the abdominal aorta, but not with ascites. A less reliable guide is that with ascites the umbilicus is often everted and its slit is transverse but with a large ovarian cyst the umbilicus may be drawn upwards and its slit become vertical. A common mistake is to diagnose ascites when it is not present merely because it is thought that it should be there, for example, in a patient who has cardiac failure with marked oedema of the lower limbs, or in a patient with suspected cirrhosis of the liver. It is impossible to diagnose ascites unless at least two pints of fluid are present, but it is surgeons in particular who attempt to impress by demonstrating on percussion the presence of even less than one ounce of peritoneal fluid.

THE KIDNEYS

Renal swelling
A renal swelling has the following characteristics:
1. It is felt in the loin and has a well-defined rounded lower border.
2. It can be felt bimanually; that is, with one hand in the loin and the other hand anteriorly, the swelling can be lightly pressed between the two hands and, moreover, can be pushed from one hand to the other. The latter manoeuvre is usually referred to as 'ballotting'. However, some clinicians prefer to reserve this term for feeling a viscus which is surrounded by fluid. It is important that the front hand be pressed towards the hand in the loin immediately at the end of inspiration.
3. It may be possible to get above it and, if this is so, this immediately rules out splenic or hepatic enlargement.
4. It moves on respiration. It is surprising that several textbooks say that it does not. However, any competent radiologist knows that an opacity in the kidney, for example a calculus, can on a radiograph be shown to alter its position on deep inspiration and deep expiration. The only exceptions to this rule are a perinephric abscess and occasionally a renal carcinoma.
5. It is impossible to insert a finger or fingers between the swelling and the erector spinae muscle because the upper part of the kidney is situated immediately anterior to this muscle. This sign is a difficult one to demonstrate, but on rare occasions it may help to distinguish between the enlarged kidney and splenic swelling.
6. There is a band of resonance over the kidney anteriorly.

With regard to percussion of a kidney, a correct sense of values must be observed. Percussion is rarely necessary or informative, but can be an extremely useful sign in differentiating between a very big kidney and a liver or spleen. It is only when the kidney is very large that this sign will be demonstrable, but it is the very big kidney and not the slightly enlarged one that is more likely to be mistaken for some other viscus. It is often stated that the lower pole of the right kidney is frequently palpable in normal people. It occasionally is in thin patients, almost without exception female, but in others such a finding should never be dismissed lightly as being of no significance. Even in thin females, the additional presence of urinary symptoms or pain of renal distribution demands further investigation.

Polycystic kidneys
If enlargement of both kidneys is found, the probability is that polycystic disease of the kidneys is present, the less probable cause being a bilateral hydronephrosis.

The usual first symptom of polycystic disease of the kidneys is recurrent painless haematuria. Other symptoms are those referable either to uraemia or to an associated hypertension or recurrent pyelitis. It is unusual for symptoms to appear before the age of forty years, although the condition is a congenital abnormality. The proof of the diagnosis will be established by pyelography, which will demonstrate long, thin, attenuated calyces ('spider calyces'). Because the lesion causes poor renal function, retrograde pyelograms usually give better pictures than intravenous ones due to better concentration of the dye. The nephrotic syndrome, amyloid disease and leukaemia also give rise to bilateral renal enlargement, but such enlargements are rarely palpable.

Clinical manifestations of uraemia
Uraemia is a word which has been in use for over 100 years to indicate the manifestations of renal failure from any cause. Many of the symptoms and signs, for example purpura and anaemia, have no accepted explanation. Other signs, especially the encephalopathic ones, may in fact be due to the accompanying hypertension. Of recent years there has been an emphasis on the fact that uraemia is associated not only with the retention of products which should be excreted but with excessive excretion of other substance which should be retained, with resultant deficiency defects.

Uraemia and renal involvement are not synonymous, but many physicians, who should know better, when discussing the symptoms of uraemia list such things as nocturia, which in itself can never be an indication of actual renal failure.

There is no single clinical picture, but the symptoms and signs can be usefully classified under system heads as follows:

Encephalopathic. This includes headache; epilepsy; focal signs in the brain and cranial nerves, including the optic nerve, which are often transient; and delirium (*see* Chapter 16), which may be associated either with gradually increasing drowsiness passing into stupor and coma or with an acute mania.

Respiratory. There is a marked liability to infection. Whether there is a (histologically) distinctive pneumonia is controversial. Acute pulmonary oedema, usually secondary to left ventricular failure, is common. Dyspnoea may be continuous, paroxysmal, Cheyne–Stokes, or rarely of Kussmaul type (*see* Chapter 14).

Gastro-intestinal. The tongue is always very furred, brown and dry. This is often associated with an ulcerative stomatitis and marked halitosis. Thirst, anorexia, nausea, vomiting, hiccup, and severe diarrhoea are all common symptoms. Melaena or haematemesis may occur terminally.

Skin. This may show a flaky white deposit, especially on the face, called urea frost. Purpura and pallor of the skin and mucous membranes are very common. An extensive blotchy macular erythematous eruption is occasionally seen. Pruritus may be a troublesome symptom.

Other manifestations. A low-grade fever independent of any obvious infection is very common, as is also pericarditis, which very rarely develops into an effusion.

The rectum and anus

The adage that if you do not put your finger in it you will put your foot in it is hoary but still true. Rectal examination is an essential component of every complete abdominal examination. It must be explained to the patient exactly what you are going to do, and he must be warned that the procedure will probably be unpleasant but usually not painful. The commonest cause of marked pain on rectal examination is an anal fissure which may be very difficult to see. The patient turns on his left side with his buttocks at the edge of the bed and his spine, neck and lower limbs fully flexed. The anus is inspected for skin lesions, especially for signs of excoriation due to scratching, fissures and external haemorrhoids (dilated veins). A lubricated gloved finger is next gently inserted into the anal canal and then into the rectum. If there is marked anal spasm with resultant difficulty in inserting the finger, the cause must be sought. It is often due to nervousness or to some psychogenic abnormality, but the presence of fissures, fistulas, thrombosed haemorrhoids, eczematous lesions of the anal margin or prostatitis should be looked for.

The walls of the anal canal and rectum should feel smooth and soft. In the male the prostate is felt anteriorly, and its medial groove should be easily discernible. The normal prostate has a rubbery feel and is slightly movable. A non-malignant prostatic enlargement feels boggy and soft. An enlarged, irregular and fixed prostate is almost certainly malignant. What constitutes prostatic enlargement or abnormal hardness is learnt only by long experience. A great problem concerning an enlarged prostate is that the degree of obstruction to the expulsion of urine which it causes, and therefore its effect on the bladder and kidneys, is not always proportional to its actual size. Furthermore, the apparent degree of enlargement as felt *per rectum* is often not in agreement with the assessment on cystoscopy. Above the prostate the seminal vesicles are often normally just palpable on either side.

In the female the cervix is felt as a mobile firm knob through the anterior rectal wall. Any other swellings felt in either sex must be pathological. To help in feeling such swellings, the patient should take deep breaths while the physician's left palm is pressed above the pubis down towards the examining finger in the rectum. After palpation of the whole circumference of the rectum and as high as possible, the patient must then be asked to bear down, because by this manoeuvre a mass otherwise out of reach of the finger may be pushed down and become palpable.

If faeces are felt in the rectum, their hardness should be assessed. A rectum full of faeces or one which is ballooned but empty is more likely to be associated with a functional constipation than with an organic obstruction, in which the usual finding is an empty but normal-sized rectum. A large rectum may be due to unsuspected homosexual practices.

A carcinoma of the rectum is usually palpable unless it is beyond the examining finger. Internal haemorrhoids are never palpable unless they are thrombosed. They may be seen, especially when prolapsed, when the patient strains down. After its withdrawal the gloved finger must always be inspected for blood and pus and any faeces on it must be inspected carefully.

The male genitalia

THE PENIS

The size of the flaccid penis varies very much and should never be considered as abnormally small unless it is markedly so. The penis is small in patients with infantilism from whatever cause. The commonest congenital abnormality of the penis is hypospadias, which is characterized by an abnormal opening of the urethra.

Pseudo-hermaphroditism is a congenital condition due to hyperplasia of the foetal suprarenal cortex with resultant overproduction of adrenal androgens, causing some modification in the development of the external genitalia. The genital abnormality is visible at birth and it may be impossible to say definitely whether the infant is male or female. For example, in severe cases the genitalia may be interpreted as representing either a bifid scrotum with hypospadias or fused labia with a large clitoris. Usually the gonads are ovaries and the chromosome pattern is female, so that the person is really female although the external genitalia may more resemble the male pattern.

Oedema of the penis and scrotum may be found in congestive cardiac failure and in renal disease associated with marked oedema. It is an unusual finding in inferior vena caval obstruction. Lymphatic oedema of the penis is nearly always accompanied by oedema of the scrotum and usually also by inguinal lymph node enlargement. The most marked examples are seen in filariasis, but the condition may rarely occur with malignant bilateral metastases in the inguinal lymph nodes.

A chancre, due to primary syphilis of the penis, usually involves the glans or prepuce. It starts as a reddish papule, which enlarges and ulcerates with a marked, almost cartilaginous induration of the surrounding tissues. A chancre is always painless and usually single, but multiple lesions may occur.

Chancroid is due to Ducrey's* bacillus, which causes vesicles on the penis. It is common in tropical and subtropical countries. These become pustular and later form punched-out small superficial ulcers, nearly always located around the corona. The ulcers increase in size and are associated with oedema of the prepuce and often with phimosis. The inguinal lymph nodes become markedly enlarged and often suppurate (buboes). Involvement of the male and female genitalia is part of both the Behçet and the Stevens—Johnson syndromes.

Epithelioma of the penis usually affects the glans but occasionally the prepuce, and has the characteristics of an epithelioma elsewhere. The penis is fairly often affected in many common skin diseases, especially scabies, herpes simplex, herpes zoster, multiple papillomas and eczematous lesions. Herpes simplex of the male and female genitalia has become a common condition which nowadays is often sexually transmitted. It causes vesicles and often small superficial ulcers with enlargement of the inguinal lymph nodes and the condition often after healing spontaneously recurs in the same site repeatedly. White patches on the genitalia, especially the penis may be due to leukoplakia, psoriasis or lichen planus. Candia infection may affect the penis and genitalia and may be sexually transmitted. It causes a balanitis (an inflammation of the epithelial tissues of the glans) and also often of the prepuce. The glans become bright red and very tender, and white lesions such as occur on the tongue are very unusual.

Urethritis will not be readily seen unless it is acute or the patient has complained about it. The commonest causes are gonorrhoea and so-called non-specific urethritis:

*Augosto Ducrey (1860—1940), an Italian dermatologist.

THE SCROTUM

Oedema and some development abnormalities have been described previously. The two commonest abnormal swellings in the scrotum are hydrocele and inguinal hernia. A hydrocele is a collection of fluid in the tunica vaginalis which envelops the testes. It feels cystic, and the swelling is well defined and smooth and exhibits translucency when a strong light is shone behind it, but has no impulse on coughing. The swelling is usually lax allowing the testes to be felt within it. Acute hydrocele may be a complication of an acute orchitis or epididymitis. Chronic hydrocele is a condition common in middle-aged and elderly men, and its cause is usually obscure.

Normal testes vary in size, but the two should be roughly equal in size and feel firm, with a rubbery but not hard consistency. The testes are usually asymmetrical, the left being lower than the right. Except when diseased and in tabes dorsalis, they are normally exquisitely tender when squeezed. Very small testes are a feature of infantilism, but are not an essential finding in Klinefelter's* syndrome.

The epididymis is behind and slightly above the testis and has an irregular, poorly defined outline. It feels softer than the testis, and attached to it is the spermatic cord. This contains the vas deferens, which feels like a piece of whipcord. Enalrgement of the pampiniform plexus (venous) of the spermatic cord causes a varicocele, which is palpable above and behind the testis and may be visible. It is usually left-sided and may be painful, but is otherwise of no importance.

Cryptorchidism (ectopic testis) is an incomplete descent of either or both testes through the inguinal canal. It may be found in an otherwise normal boy, but if it persists it may be a manifestation of infantilism, the undescended testis often being smaller than normal.

Acute orchitis, which may be associated with epididymitis, is a common complication of urethritis, but is also seen as an important complication of mumps and occasionally of brucellosis. It may follow prostectomy. Tuberculosis produces an irregular enlargement of the testis and the epididymis, which often becomes adherent to the scrotum posteriorly and may form a sinus. It is not a very painful condition. A gumma of the testis produces a smooth, very hard (billiard ball) swelling which may become adherent to the anterior part of the scrotum and may form a sinus. Cancer of the testis has the features of a malignant swelling elsewhere, but is often slowly growing and may be either ignored by the patient or wrongly ascribed to some remembered injury. It is painless and the epididymis and cord are rarely affected. Often the first manifestation seen by the physician is the presence of intrathoracic or intra-abdominal secondaries.

*H. F. Klinefelter (1912–   ), an American physician.

16 The Nervous System

In any case of neurological disease, an attempt should be made to answer three questions in the following order:
1. *The anatomical site of the lesion.* This is usually determined by the physical signs and, in the great majority of cases, is the only diagnosis that can be made with certainty clinically. Moreover, nearly always this should be the first stage diagnosis. The exact site of the lesion is very important, because most neurological diseases have a predilection for only one or a few sites.
2. *The general pathology of the lesion.* The history, with special reference to the mode of onset and the subsequent progress, usually constitutes the main guide. If the condition came on with dramatic suddenness reaching its maximum in about twenty-four hours but occasionally in about forty-eight hours and rarely longer – and especially if subsequently it improved, even though not completely – the likely pathology is vascular. Acute inflammatory lesions may come on fairly suddenly but rarely reach their maximum severity within twenty-four hours, usually taking several days to do so. If the condition came on very gradually and has slowly become worse, then the likely pathology is either neoplastic or degenerative. However, sometimes a chronic inflammatory lesion follows this pattern, and a patient with a rapidly growing neoplasm may have a sudden severe exacerbation of symptoms due to a spontaneous haemorrhage within it. It must be remembered that disseminated sclerosis is not the only disease which may show spontaneous remissions. For example, peripheral neuritis may exhibit remissions, whether spontaneous or due either to therapy or to removal of the offending toxic agent causing the condition. Any inflammatory lesion, particularly one amenable to therapy such as neurosyphilis, may have such a history, as may also some diseases of unknown aetiology such as myasthenia gravis.
3. *The special pathology.* Signs observed outside the nervous system often give the main clue to the aetiology of a cerebral or spinal lesion. For example, the finding of a cardiac arrhythmia, evidence of infective endocarditis or hypertension, or

signs of generalized vascular disease should arouse immediate suspicion that any neurological lesion is probably secondary to this. Or else the patient may have a congenital anomaly such as a skeletal deformity of skull or spine, indicating that any neurological lesion is likely also to be congenital. If a patient shows evidence of malignant disease anywhere, the probability is that any neurological signs are due to metastases or to carcinomatous encephalopathy or neuropathy.

Scheme for examination

Examination of the nervous system must be methodical and thorough, and this can be achieved only by always following a set pattern, thus guaranteeing a reasonable speed without omitting anything important. The table below gives such a scheme.

EXAMINATION OF THE NERVOUS SYSTEM

General	Assessment of intelligence, including memory. Observation of speech. Examination of the skull. Test for nuchal rigidity.
Cranial nerves	Detailed examination of the cranial nerves in correct order. While examining the ocular nerves, the pupillary details are carefully scrutinized and nystagmus is looked for.
Limbs and trunk	Involuntary movements.
Motor	Weakness of any muscle group (always examine in some fixed order – for example, from peripheral to proximal groups). Wasting – if present, its distribution. Muscle tone.
Reflexes	Tendon. Superficial. Plantar.
Co-ordination	With eyes open and closed.
Sensory	Touch. Pain (pin-prick). Position. Vibration. Deep pain. Thermal.
Gait	Including Rombergism.
Spine	Essential to examine if any evidence of root or cord lesion.

Intelligence

Intelligence is a concept which is incapable of precise definition. It consists in a variety of types of mental ability which include verbal and mathematical reasoning, conceptualization and interpretation and logical deduction from facts. There are many unsolved problems with regard to intelligence the discussion of which is outside the scope of this elementary account. Is intelligence synonymous with an ability to learn from experience and teaching? What are the proportional roles of hereditary and environmental factors in its development? Perhaps it depends mainly on the choice of parents, teachers and friends. Is intelligence a fixed quotient that remains unaltered by experience? Intelligence may signify primarily an ability to learn but the learning processes are not understood. Does intelligence include an ability not only to learn more but quicker than other people? In spite of frequent snide remarks such as, 'That is only a feat of memory', there is no doubt that memory and its development (and with proper training such development is possible) are an important and integral part of intelligence.

Intelligence is such a complex phenomenon that it is extremely doubtful that it can be measured in a truly scientific way, although a rough assessment may be possible. The ordinary physician is very reluctant to use any standard intelligence tests and their value to them is very limited. Perhaps such tests merely test an ability to do those tests. However useful they may sometimes be they cannot define an individual's ability or measure those human virtues such as curiosity, imagination and emotional predisposition which are all very important factors contributing to a person's character, and many components of intelligence are not measurable. If intelligence includes the capacity for mental development then it follows that a completely illiterate person may be highly intelligent, but no tests have ever been devised to demonstrate this. Intelligence tests cannot assess the global ability to think rationally and to deal effectively at all times with the changing environment and unusual situations. Moreover an intelligent person is capable of behaving unintelligently and indeed often does so.

The intelligence quotient is defined as the ratio of the mental age as assessed by the special tests and the chronological age.

Mental state

It is impossible in a book of this size to give anything but a few clues to a consideration of the mental state. A rough guide to the person's mental state should have been obtained by noting the manner he gave his history, his mode of answering questions, his attention and alertness and his general behaviour during the interview. A patient's mental state is a complex summation of intellect, memory, behaviour patterns and emotions. Any alteration of mental state may be the first indication not only of brain damage but also of disease of other parts of the body acting indirectly on the brain, such as severe renal, hepatic or pulmonary disease.

A normal person has the ability to reflect with some degree of objectivity on his inner feelings and experiences, and is capable of appreciating that his thoughts and feelings and the sensations he is experiencing truly belong to him. This awareness and its acceptance is often called insight. A psychotic does not recognize that his thoughts, sensations and emotions and his auditory and visual impressions belong to him and may be abnormal. He lacks insight and is unlikely himself to seek medical advice without great persuasion.

When assessing mental state it is important to attempt to evaluate the person's mood by observing him during the interview and by asking direct questions, noting if he appears to be depressed, agitated, anxious or euphoric. Remember that there are other things apart from mental disturbance which can cause a patient either not to answer questions satisfactorily or to give a poor account of his symptoms – for example, deafness, aphasia or an incomplete understanding of English. The earliest manifestations of any mental disease will be first noticeable only to close friends and acquaintances. Indeed, except in gross cases, before suggesting that any person is mentally abnormal the physician must find out from close relatives, friends and acquaintances whether or not his behaviour has become abnormal in any way or whether he has always been the same, and whether it really matters either to others or to himself.

MEMORY

'Great is the force of memory, excessive great, O my God, a large and infinite roominess. Who can plummet the bottom of it? . . . Great is this power of memory, a thing, O my God, to be amazed at, a very profound and infinite multiplicity, and this thing is the mind, and this thing am I.' St Augustine over 1,600 years ago in his tenth book of *Confessions.*

Memory can be defined as the capacity or faculty of relearning and recovering impressions or of recalling or recognizing previous experiences. Memory is related both to learning and intelligence and without it we cannot learn and intelligence depends upon a capacity to learn. The exact nature of that capacity is difficult to define. Memory is a complex depending on attention, retention, recall and recognition and those are its components. The patient who is stuperose, comatose, delirious or depressed, or markedly occupied with some extraneous activity, will have memory defect because of lack of attention. The hysteric's memory suffers because of lack of recall. But nobody has the ability to remember everything which they have ever seen or heard and we all possess the subconscious power of forgetting. There is no sharp borderline between normal forgetfulness and the earliest manifestations of a pathological defect of memory. Whatever the mode of its manifestation pathological loss of memory, as with any other mental defect, always indicates a lesion of the cerebral cortex, but more accurate localization is impossible.

Testing of the memory is often more informative to the neurologist than any formal intelligence test. The commonest initial disturbance in any psychosis is a failing memory, and this may for a long time be the only manifestation. Therefore, when rapidly assessing the patient's mental state one should always ask some questions relative to memory defect and make a distinction between defects for recent and remote events (anterograde and retrograde amnesia respectively). Retrograde amnesia is defined as the period before an accident or illness the details of which the patient cannot fully recall. With head injuries a general rule is that the longer the period of retrograde amnesia the more severe the lesion. Anterograde amnesia is an impaired ability to acquire and store new information. The patient may also be asked to give the dates of important national events or to name distinguished personages. A test for recent memory is an ability to recall three unrelated nouns such as chair, ship and ball, or fictitous names and addresses, five minutes after they have been repeated to the patient with a request to remember them. An inability to count in reverse from twenty, to spell simple words such as 'chair' or 'table' backwards, or to recite the days of the week or the months of the year in reverse after first demonstrating that he can do these things in the normal order may indicate early mental dysfunction.

Terminology

It is essential to know the definitions of commonly used terms in psychiatry.

An *hallucination* is a sensory impression (visual, auditory, olfactory, and so on) without sensory stimulus.

An *illusion* is an incorrect interpretation of a sensory impression – for example, failure in correct recognition of an object. Disorientation in time and/or space is an example of an illusion.

A *delusion* is an erroneous idea impervious to reason.

A *phobia* is an irrational fear, for example, of closed spaces (claustrophobia) or open spaces (agoraphobia) and when such a person is unable to escape from or avoid the situation causing the phobia he develops acute anxiety and distress.

Stupor is an absence or gross diminution of all voluntary movements and of speech without loss of consciousness. It is possible to get the patient to respond to external stimuli, which, however, may need to be marked, even vigorous and possibly painful. When so roused the patient is capable of answering only the simplest of questions and his co-operation is minimal.

Coma is a condition in which the patient is unconscious and incapable of responding to any external stimulus, however strong. There is no clearcut borderline between stupor and coma and the patient may pass from one state to the other. Whatever its cause, coma is likely to be associated with dilated fixed pupils, absence of tendon reflexes, and bilateral extensor plantar responses.

When attempting to discover the cause of coma whenever possible a history should be obtained from relatives, friends and witnesses to the onset of the coma. The patient's personal belongings may indicate that he is a diabetic, or epileptic, or on drugs, or attending a hospital for any reason.

The commonest causes of coma are injuries (especially of the head), epilepsy, renal, liver or respiratory failure, hyper- or hypoglycaemia, chemical poisonings (including alcohol and a large number of drugs), septicaemias and gross lesions of adrenal, pituitary or thyroid.

The depth of the coma should be evaluated and the skin noted for marked pallor, cyanosis, jaundice, bruisings or the cherry red colour of carbon monoxide poisoning, as any of these may be a very important clue. Emaciation may be a valuable diagnostic finding. The whole body must be carefully examined for evidence of injury. The tongue may show scars of previous tongue biting in an epileptic. In the nervous system the most important points are nuchal rigidity, fundi, and the eyes. A unilateral dilated fixed pupil suggests pressure on the third nerve by a haemorrhage, spontaneous or traumatic, in the temporal lobe area. Bilateral very small pupils suggest a pontine lesion. Fixed lateral deviation of the eyes suggests a lesion of the opposite cerebral hemisphere. When the depth of coma is marked both pupils are likely to be dilated and unresponsive to light but this has no localizing value. Evidence of limb paralysis can be judged by raising each limb in turn and letting it fall, a paralysed limb falling limply and heavily instead of with a gentle returning to its initial position. The tendon reflexes are helpful only if they are grossly asymmetrical.

Delirium. Delirium is an acute mental confusion of short duration, lasting for only a few hours or a few days, during which there is disordered perception and abnormal motor activity. The disordered perception takes the form of visual or auditory hallucinations and/or illusions, especially disorientation in time and space. In some cases of delirium the hallucinations or illusions dominate the picture, whereas in others the abnormal motor activities are more obvious.

L

It is especially in acute alcoholism and in delirium associated with fevers that hallucinations are likely to be the marked feature.

The motor excitement concerns movement of the limbs, which may vary from the mildest form — for example, repeated picking at the bedclothes — to extreme varieties in which the patient throws himself about, struggling and fighting. It is shown, in addition, by uncontrolled speech, which may be of a mild form in which the patient keeps on muttering to himself, or an extreme maniacal form with screaming.

Delirium is associated with stupor of variable degree, so that the patient is incapable of sustained thought. Delirious patients invariably have impaired concentration, and so if they recover they will have impaired memory of the events which occurred during the period of their delirium. If the delirium persists, the patient becomes increasingly lethargic and later stuporose, from which state it is not possible to arouse him except for brief moments. Stupor may be followed by coma.

The common causes of delirium are as follows:

1. It may be associated with infections, especially typhoid fever, septicaemias, pneumonia pre-eminently of the upper lobe (particularly in the very young and in very old or debilitated patients), facial erysipelas, and malaria of the so-called cerebral type. But delirium may, on occasions, occur in any severe infection.

2. It may be toxic due to known chemical poisons such as alcohol, the belladonna group of alkaloids, benzedrine, cannabis indica ('hashish'), mescaline, lead and organic arsenic and steroids. It has also been described as an occasional complication of a large variety of chemical compounds, and may even rarely be caused by hypnotics such as barbiturates, bromides and morphine. Delirium commonly occurs as a toxic manifestation of the unknown poisons of uraemia, hepatic failure and toxaemias of pregnancy.

3. It may be a manifestation of any organic disease of the brain or meninges — for example, meningitis, severe head injury, neoplasm, general paralysis of the insane, and occasionally cerebral vascular lesions.

4. It may result from metabolic disturbances, myxoedema, Addison's disease, hypoglycaemia, hypokalaemia, acute porphyria, thiamine deficiency and cerebral anoxia, especially with carbon dioxide retention due to severe cardiac or lung disease or paralysis of the respiratory muscles. S. S. Korsakoff (1853–1900) wrote in Russian in 1887 describing a syndrome which may be seen in alcoholics and consisting of disorientation in time and space, loss of memory of recent events, confabulation (recounting false memories and activities) and peripheral neuritis. Cognition, intelligence and consciousness all remain normal.

Speech

While obtaining the history, one should have assessed whether or not the patient had any speech defect, but even if no obvious defect was found, special attention should be devoted to eliciting such an abnormality before further neurological examination is undertaken. It is important that when examining a patient with a view to eliciting and diagnosing any speech disturbance one does not rely on questions, such as his name or age or 'How are you?', which can be answered in monosyllables or automatically even by an almost speechless patient. It is therefore imperative to ask only those questions which will demand from the patient a formulation of ideas. An opening remark such as 'Tell me all about yourself' is likely to be effective.

It is impossible to give an entirely satisfactory definition of speech in a short sentence. However, as a basis for discussion it may be defined as the construction of propositions, auditory and visual, in order to communicate ideas. Not only speaking itself, but also the comprehension of the spoken and written word is implied. Speech is essentially an intellectual process. Important considerations of speech such as its relationship to gesture, mime and music, and how it developed in the course of evolution, are problems beyond the scope of this book. The expression of emotions and the language of gesture are innate but speech is learned.

No scientific evidence has ever supplanted the view that speech is the prerogative of man and is a divine gift. Certainly no animal can write. Birds and animals communicate with one another by sounds and by other means but only human beings can utter and understand sounds which they have never heard before. The great British neurologist J. Hughlings Jackson (1835–1911) emphasized that speech is simply the expression of a capacity to make propositions and I agree with the American linguistic expert Noam Chomsky that the sovereignty and mystery of language makes man uniquely 'the language animal'. It is indeed an awesome but indisputable fact that sounds other than human speech, however produced or reproduced (for example, electronically), can always be differentiated from speech and, moreover, that speech can always be recognized as such even when it is in some exotic language and recorded by some mechanical instrument. To regard the brain merely as a complex computer is to accept a mechanistic view of the mind and to ignore completely the fact that we have been granted free will. A person speaks because he has the desire to do so and because he wants to communicate with others or talk aloud to himself.

Furthermore, much of our thinking is done in words and, as a consequence, loss of verbal memory will cause impairment of speech. Speech implying as it does an exchange of ideas, it follows that any intellectual disturbance will result in a paucity or absence of ideas and thus in an impairment of speech. Speech is not synonymous with memory, but the two cannot be completely dissociated, and speech must be regarded as a component of intelligence.

In regard to the way in which a child learns to talk, special emphasis must be given to the importance of hearing, for if an infant is born deaf or develops deafness in infancy or early childhood he is likely to remain speechless and may be considered mentally defective unless special educational techniques are used.

If a patient cannot talk properly he must have one of four possible lesions: dementia, dysphasia, dysarthria or dysphonia. It must be emphasized that these are four different things, each giving rise to a different and distinctive type of speech defect, and that the diagnosis of one of them constitutes the first stage diagnosis in any patient with an abnormality of speech. Moreover, the diagnosis of each condition gives an important clue to the probable, or sometimes certain, localization of the lesion. More than one type of speech abnormality may occur in the same patient, but it is more usual for the patient to have only a single variety, and when dysphasia and dysarthria do occasionally occur together, as for example following an internal carotid artery occlusion, the dysphasia is the more important diagnostically because of its more certain localizing value.

APHASIA

'Aphasia' and 'epilepsy' are perhaps the only commonly used words in neurology which defy a simple and short definition acceptable to everybody, although any competent neurologist has no doubt of what he means by either of these terms. The other great difficulty concerning aphasia is its classification, and in this book discussion is purposely on a very elementary basis so that some first principles can be understood and used to build upon later if desired.

Aphasia may be defined as a loss of those means, vocal and written, by which we normally exchange ideas. A normal person does not speak unless he wants to, but an aphasic patient cannot speak even if he does want to. Aphasia is the inability to understand or use properly the spoken and written symbols of speech. It is a disturbance of the comprehension, elaboration and expression of speech concepts and may be either motor or sensory. A combined motor and sensory aphasia is fairly common. Motor aphasia not only affects speech but also seriously disrupts thinking and intelligence. Incomplete forms of aphasia are more common than complete loss and are sometimes referred to as dysphasias.

Motor types (expressive)

Motor aphasia is when the patient appears to understand all ideas, written or spoken, put to him but is unable himself to express any ideas because of inability to formulate recognizable word patterns, although he has no weakness of any of the muscles that produce the sounds of speech. The condition can be diagnosed because by gesture and facial expression the patient clearly indicates that he knows what he wants to say, but cannot express himself because he has lost the power of spontaneous speech: he has forgotten how to speak, although he can understand spoken words and therefore obey commands. Motor aphasia may be described as an apraxia (*see* page 412) of speech. The patient can often still use monosyllabic words such as 'yes' and 'no' and, especially under emotional stress, expletives, curses and the like. He may even speak fluently when under great emotion. A patient with aphasia is speechless but not wordless. As speech gradually recovers, his vocabulary becomes increasingly extensive and his speech disturbance more difficult to appreciate as a dysphasia.

The cause of motor aphasia is always a lesion in the dominant cortex which in right-handed persons is the left Broca's area, which is the posterior part of the inferior frontal convulation immediately anterior to that part of the motor cortex which controls the muscles of speech. Any pathology whatsoever affecting this area will cause motor aphasia, but the commonest is a cerebral vascular lesion involving the middle cerebral artery or its inferior frontal branch. As mentioned above, aphasia does not always indicate organic disease, as it may be a transitory phenomenon in a normal person – for example, in an oral examination.

Sensory types (receptive or comprehensive)
Sensory aphasia may be auditory or visual. Auditory aphasia is an inability to comprehend the significance of the spoken word in a patient who is neither demented nor deaf. When such a patient is commanded, for example, to close his eyes, he does not respond to the request, but if the clinician does the action himself, the patient may imitate him. Frequently the loss of comprehension is not complete and may involve, for example, only proper nouns. The condition may affect not only the patient's recognition of what he hears but also the range of his own vocabulary and his grammar and syntax (correct arrangement of words), and, moreover, he may not appear to be aware of his mistakes and in a severe case his speech becomes mere gibberish. With more extensive lesions he may not be able to read what he himself has written, and this may interfere with his writing. It is now appreciated that a form of dyslexia is common in which the child although he has normal vision and intelligence (often being good at mathematics) has great difficulty in learning how to read and spell. The condition is regarded as a development lack of normal dominance of the appropriate cerebral hemisphere.

Dyslexia is an inability to read in the absence of visual defect, although the patient may be able to name individual letters. This may be regarded as a form of visual aphasia.

Visual aphasia is an inability to comprehend the significance of written symbols in a patient who is neither demented nor blind. Such a patient will be unable to obey a written command. He will be unable to name objects, but may succeed in doing so if he is allowed, when appropriate, to feel, taste or smell them. He can speak normally and may be able to write and read but cannot understand either. He can copy without understanding what he is copying and cannot transfer the printed words in books into his own cursive handwriting. The term 'nominal aphasia' is sometimes used for such difficulty in naming an object or some specific quality of an object, such as colour, although the person can form and verbalize even complex sentences. Visual aphasia may be described as a visual agnosia (*see* page 410), and auditory aphasia as an auditory agnosia.

Auditory aphasia is due to involvement of the superior temporal gyrus or of association fibres from Broca's area to that gyrus. A combination of dyslexia and agraphia points to a lesion of the angular gyrus which is immediately posterior to the visual cortex. Visual aphasia is due to a lesion of the visual (occipital) cortex or of association fibres from Broca's area to the occipital cortex.

The reason why such a simple classification is a far from complete answer to the study of aphasia is that a large number of cases cannot be subdivided into these simple divisions. Pure auditory or pure visual aphasia is very rare. A patient with a gross sensory aphasia and a consequent lack of comprehension of vocal and written speech will also be unable to express himself properly, especially as regards the names of things he talks about, so that he misplaces words and uses wrong words and may even become incomprehensible. Such a patient also often keeps repeating the same word or phrase (perseveration). However, perseveration of speech is not considered to be a manifestation of aphasia, but rather to be due to an associated intellectual disturbance caused by cortical damage. Similarly, a patient with motor aphasia usually also has some defect of speech comprehension that is, some degree of associated sensory aphasia. In other words, in many patients aphasia is mixed, being both sensory and motor.

Moreover, severe damage to these cortical areas is often associated with intellectual impairment, and failure of attention, with consequent variable replies, makes the speech defect difficult to analyse. Furthermore, speech is an intellectual process and it may be deemed illogical to localize any part of the intellect, including its components of speech, to any cortical area. The motor and sensory speech areas, sometimes called 'centres', are connected by subcortical commissural tracts, and it may be lesions of these circuits rather than of localized centres which cause the speech defect.

Tests for aphasia
Tests for aphasia are useless in any patient who is an ament, a dement, stuporose or delirious. It must always be known whether or not

the patient has a gross defect of hearing or vision, and he must be able to understand the language, spoken or written. Whether he is right- or left-handed is a matter of great importance.

Elementary tests for aphasia may be summarized as an assessment of the patient's ability:

1. To express himself — for example, so as to give a coherent account of his symptoms.
2. To obey both vocal and written commands.
3. To name common objects or parts of his own body or clothing and pick out from a group of objects any named individually by the physician, for example, asking him to point in sequence to a window, a pillow and then a radiator. He may also be asked to do some more complex act with objects placed in front of him such as putting a coin into a glass and a piece of card underneath that glass.
4. To read aloud with obvious understanding.
5. To write spontaneously and to dictation, and to read and understand what has been written. Do not ask him to write something which he has done very often such as his name and address because he is likely to be able to do this although he cannot do anything else satisfactory.

DYSARTHRIA

Dysarthria is a failure of proper articulation and is a disorder of articulation. It affects essentially those consonants which are produced by properly co-ordinated action of the lips, tongue and palate. The term refers to any type of lesion of any of these structures, not necessarily a neurological one. The labial consonants are B, M, P and W; the lingual consonants are D, L, R and T; the labio-dentals are F, S, Th and V; and the palatal consonants are N and the final K and NG. So, for example, any disease of the lips, whatever its nature, will interfere with the pronunciation of the labials and produce dysarthria without interfering with the production of other consonants.

Commonly used phrases which the patient is asked to repeat to elicit dysarthria are: 'The humming of innumerable bees' (tests labials); 'Around the rocks the ragged rascal ran' (tests linguals); and 'The Leith police dismisses us' (tests labio-dentals). However, the use of only one stock phrase may not be enough to elicit dysarthria. The following phrases test a variety of types of consonants: 'Engaging in rabid biblical criticism'; 'A roving dark hippopotamus roaring in Constantinople'; 'The true Methodist Episcopal Church'; 'Irretrievable voluntary contributions to national hospitals'.

Having decided that the patient's difficulty is essentially one of articulation, the examiner must first carefully examine the lips, the tongue and the palate.

Bulbar palsy dysarthria
In true bulbar or pseudo-bulbar palsies, which are labio-glosso-palato-pharyngeal palsies due to bilateral involvement of these structures, there will be great difficulty with all consonants and the speech will be nasal and lacking in modulation. Donald Duck of Disney cartoon fame is a good example of bulbar palsy speech, which may be imitated by pressing one's throat immediately below the jaw between one's index finger and thumb and attempting to talk while such pressure is applied. Hearing such a type of speech arouses suspicion of a bulbar palsy; to confirm this, look for a bilateral paralysis of the tongue and weakness of the soft palate and lips.

Palatal palsy dysarthria
With a paralysis of the soft palate the speech becomes nasal so that 'b' sounds like 'm' and 'd' like 'n'. This dysarthria may be accentuated by getting the patient to flex his head on to his chest.

Cerebellar dysarthria
This is characterized by speech which is slow, jerky and monotonous, with undue separation of the syllables, slurring of some syllables and undue accentuation of others. This is often referred to as staccato or scanning speech (from a supposed resemblance to the scanning of Greek verse). Sometimes, however, in a cerebellar dysarthria it is better described as sounding as if the patient were talking with his mouth full. In either case such speech suggests a lesion of the cerebellum. In such a dysarthria no obvious lesion of the lips, tongue or palate will be seen as the mechanism producing it is a defect of co-ordination of these structures, but confirmatory evidence of a cerebellar lesion, such as nystagmus, should be sought for, the speech defect never being the sole manifestation.

Dysarthria due to general paralysis of the insane
In general paralysis of the insane the patient's speech is described as 'lalling' — that is, like baby talk — because it is slow and monotonous, with elision and omission of syllables and even of words and with an almost complete inability to pronounce linguals. Moreover, the patient frequently makes mistakes which he makes no attempt to correct. This latter feature and the elision suggest that, in addition to the dysarthria, the mental impairment plays an important part in the production of the speech defect.

Extrapyramidal dysarthria
In Parkinsonism and other extrapyramidal lesions the speech is slow, monotonous and low-pitched, and may be feeble (due to an element of dysphonia) so that he cannot talk loudly or shout. It may rarely, like the gait, acquire a 'festinant' character, going more and more quickly the more the patient talks, so that final syllables and the words at the ends of sentences are articulated hastily and thus indistinctly.

Facial palsy

It is frequently not realized that a patient with a facial palsy of any type often complains of an inability to talk properly which, of course is due to a weakness of his lips. Stammering and stuttering should be regarded as dysarthrias of psychological aetiology.

DYSPHONIA

Dysphonia is hoarseness, the speech also lacking volume. The disorder is one of vocalization. It is always due to a lesion of the vocal cords, the patient being able to express his ideas and to articulate properly. The vocal cord lesion may be of any pathology: it may be inflammatory, neoplastic or traumatic, or it may be neurological, function or organic (discussed on page 368).

The skull

It is always advisable that examination of the central nervous system should include palpation, percussion and auscultation of the skull, and such examination is essential when clinical signs indicate a cerebral lesion because the skull examination may give an important clue to the cause of a neurological finding. Inspection and palpation of the skull have been discussed previously.

Percussion, although useful only in the very occasional case, should be done as a routine because only in this way will deviations from the normal be appreciated. With a fractured skull or an internal hydrocephalus a 'cracked pot' note may be elicited, and this will be easier to appreciate if the dilatation of the lateral ventricle is unilateral. It is not, however, a very useful sign.

Auscultation is rarely revealing, but should always be done as a routine (especially over the temporal region, mastoid and orbit) because the finding of a bruit in an adult indicates an aneurysm or an angioma. On account of wide conduction, it may be heard even though the lesion is deep. Its site of maximum intensity is not of localizing value. Rarely with Paget's disease involving the skull a bruit can be heard. In infants a bruit over the skull is unlikely to have any significance. A bell and not a diaphragm must be used, and only light pressure exerted with the stethoscope because heavy pressure may itself produce an abnormal sound. If a bruit is heard, the effect on it of ipsilateral carotid compression should be observed. In any patient with focal brain signs, auscultation must be practised over both carotids. If a bruit is heard, especially a unilateral one, which is not conducted from the base of the heart, this is very suggestive of a carotid artery occlusion but is not proof. During auscultation over the carotids the patient's head should be extended and his breath held.

Nuchal rigidity

Nuchal rigidity should always be sought. It occurs not only in meningitis but also with neoplasms in the posterior fossa and intracranial haemorrhage or any other cause of meningeal irritation, and with arthritis of the cervical spine, and destructive lesions of the cervical vertebrae. In nuchal rigidity there is a persistent spasm of the muscles of the back of the neck, which feel hard and firm, and attempted flexion of the neck is difficult and extremely painful.

The triad of severe headache, photophobia and nuchal rigidity is called meningismus and indicates either meningitis or meningeal irritation. In the presence of either of these conditions, there is often marked pain on stretching the brachial or lumbar plexus nerve roots. This can be demonstrated in the lower limbs by fully flexing the hips and knees and then attempting to extend the knee, which causes marked pain and resistance. Often attempted flexion of the neck causes an involuntary flexion at the hip and knees. If one lower extremity is passively fully flexed, an involuntary flexion of the opposite side occurs. These limb signs may be present with lesions of the upper cervical nerve roots but in those cases nuchal rigidity is unlikely.

The first cranial nerve

The first cranial nerve is the olfactory nerve and is entirely sensory. The nerve endings arise from ciliated receptors in the mucous membrane of the upper part of the nasal cavity, and the nerve fibres pass from there through the cribriform plate of the ethmoid to end in the olfactory bulb. They are then relayed via the olfactory tract to the mammillary bodies of the hypothalamus and to the uncinate and hippocampal gyri of both temporal lobes.

Smell is usually tested for by simply asking the patient whether he can smell things satisfactorily. If interference with such function is suspected, then more detailed testing is done by using various scents, testing each nostril separately. A practical difficulty is that many people, especially men, are confident that they can recognize a scent although they cannot name it. For this purpose pungent and irritating odours such as ammonia, acetic acid, formaldehyde, menthol or camphor must not be used as they stimulate the endings of the first division of the fifth and not the olfactory nerve.

Loss of smell is rarely of importance in neurology because the majority of people with such loss (anosmia) are suffering not from a neurological but from a nasal lesion. Because olfactory nerve fibres go to both sides of the brain, it follows that anosmia of neurological significance must be due to a lesion of the olfactory nerve or bulb (for example, fracture of the anterior fossa, meningioma of the olfactory groove or sphenoidal ridge, or basal meningitis) and not of the brain unless the lesion is extensive and bilateral, which is most unusual.

The second cranial nerve

The fibres of the second cranial nerve – the optic – originate in the ganglion cells of the retina. In the optic nerve the fibres from the upper part of the retina lie in the upper half and those from the lower part of the retina in its lower half. The optic nerve itself has no

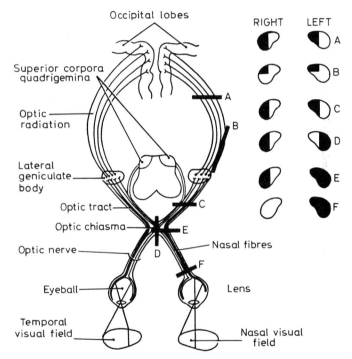

Figure 4. *Schematic diagram of the optic nerves and tracts. The visual field defects are shown shaded at various (lettered) sites*

receptor organ and this explains the normal 'blind spot' in the temporal field of vision. The macular fibres (papillo-macular bundle) are at first in the outer part of the nerve, but at the chiasma they are central. The nerves are surrounded by layers of arachnoid pia and dura, and their subdural and subarachnoid spaces are continuous with those around the brain. Each optic nerve exits from the orbit with the ophthalmic artery via the optic foramen, where each optic nerve is close to the internal carotid artery. At the base of the brain the two nerves join to form the optic chiasma, which is situated near the sella turcica. In the chiasma the fibres from the nasal half of the retina (from the temporal visual field) cross to the other side; those of the temporal half of the retina (from the nasal visual field) stay on the same side (*Figure 4*).

From the optic chiasma the pathway is known as the optic tract. This terminates on each side mainly in the lateral geniculate body (which is situated immediately lateral to the pulvinar of the thalamus). The fibres concerned not with visual appreciation but with the light reflex terminate in the superior corpora quadrigemina. From the lateral geniculate bodies the next relay, called the visual radiation, passes through the posterior limb of the internal capsule. The fibres from the upper retinal quadrants pass more or less directly to the medial aspect of the occipital pole, but the lower quadrant fibres have a long pathway in the parietal and temporal lobes, sweeping around the descending horn of the lateral ventricle before reaching the occipital cortex. The upper retinal quadrants are represented in the cuneate and the lower in the lingular gyri, respectively above and below the calcarine fissure, and the macula in the most posterior part of the occipital pole; but from the fact that central vision is often preserved in a patient with radiation defects, it is inferred that the macula has bilateral cortical representation.

The pathway for the light reflex is along the optic nerve to the optic chiasma and via the optic tract to the superior corpus quadrigeminum on the same side. From there connections are made with both third nerve nuclei. The efferent path for the reflex is along both third nerves to both ciliary ganglia, and so to the sphincter pupillae via the short ciliary nerves.

The pathway for the accommodation-convergence reflex starts in an area, not precisely known, in the cortex. Initiation of the reflex depends upon the co-operation of the patient and his willingness to look at a near object. From the cortex the pathway is to both third nerve nuclei in the mid-brain and along both third nerves to the ciliary ganglia, the ciliary nerves and the sphincter pupillae. The reflex produces contraction of the pupils, convergence of the eyeballs and drooping of the upper lids.

Clinical evaluation of the optic nerves involves examination of (1) visual acuity, (2) visual fields, and (3) the fundus oculi.

VISUAL ACUITY

Impairment of visual acuity is usually due to an error of refraction or some other ocular lesion and not to a neurological defect. Moreover, it is possible to have a lesion of the optic nerve — for example, papilloedema or optic atrophy — with retention of a fair degree of visual acuity.

Visual acuity is assessed with test cards placed 6 metres away. Each eye is rested separately while the other eye is covered with an opaque glass or a card rather than a hand which may allow light between the fingers. The result is expressed as a fraction with 6 as the numerator. If, for example, the patient can read at 6 metres only those letters which a normal person can read at 60 metres, then the visual acuity is expressed as 6/60.

VISUAL FIELDS

Examination of the visual fields must never be neglected. They are the portions of space in which an object can be seen while the gaze is fixed in a given direction, usually straight in front. Absence of visual symptoms does not exclude even a gross field defect; indeed, it is common for patients with lesions of the optic radiation to be unaware of their disability, so that it behoves the physician always to test visual fields as a routine. The macula represents the centre of the visual field and therefore the temporal and nasal fields are differentiated not by a vertical line through the disc but through the macula.

They are tested by rough confrontation techniques. For example, a patient is asked to keep looking straight ahead at the observer's nose, and a careful watch is kept that he observes this rule. The patient's eyes are then covered one at a time by the observer's hand, or preferably by a card, and a small source of light (for example, from an ophthalmoscope) or a coloured object of about 5 mm diameter such as an old-fashioned hat-pin is held 2—3 feet away from the patient and is slowly brought forward at a uniform rate from behind the patient who, still looking at the observer's nose, informs him as soon as he can see the moving object. The test is best performed with the patient's back to any window or room light. The temporal and then the nasal halves of the visual field of each eye are tested separately, and also the central part of the fields (moving the object in the vicinity of the examiner's nose). Another method is for the examiner to hold up the index finger of each of his hands keeping them about 18 cm apart and roughly midway between himself and the patient whilst he looks at the patient's eye and asking the patient to concentrate on the examiner's nose.

Visual field testing done in a slipshod fashion is worse than useless, but if it is performed with care, even a small defect can be located. If there is any doubt whether the patient has a visual field defect, then recourse must be had to the use of a mechanical perimeter for more accurate assessment, and this usually means referring the patient to an ophthalmologist experienced in such methods.

Hemianopia and hemianopsia

Hemianopia is the loss or diminution of vision over half the visual fields. A similar term, applied to the retina, is hemianopsia. A temporal hemianopia is the same as a nasal hemianopsia because the rays of light entering the lens cross to the opposite side. A homonymous hemianopia is one affecting the temporal half of one field and the nasal half of the other. A heteronymous hemianopia is either bitemporal or binasal. Quadrantic defects involve half of both superior or inferior quadrants and may be homonymous (temporal on one side and nasal on the other) or binasal or bitemporal.

It is important to know the type of field defect which is likely to occur as a result of lesions in various parts of the visual pathway. A lesion of the optic nerve causes a disturbance of vision of that eye only, and this initially takes the form of a central scotoma which may later progress to complete unilateral blindness. A scotoma is an area of depressed vision within the visual field (increase of the blind spot). A central scotoma is a feature of optic nerve or macula lesions. Scotomas of peculiar shapes are nearly always due to ocular lesions other than those of the optic nerve. A lesion of the optic chiasma, if centrally situated, will give rise to bitemporal hemianopia (often asymmetrical), whereas lesions affecting only the periphery of the chiasma on either side will give rise to a unilateral nasal hemianopia. In the early stages of chiasmal compression there may be either a superior or inferior homonymous quadrantic defect. The commonest causes of pressure on the chiasma are pituitary and suprasellar tumours and a dilated third ventricle.

The commonest cause of a binasal hemianopia is a bilateral incomplete secondary optic atrophy. To produce this condition otherwise it would be necessary to have two lesions, one at each end of the chiasma. A lesion of the centre of the chiasma spreading to one side will produce ipsilateral total blindness and contralateral temporal hemianopia.

Any lesions between the optic chiasma and the mid-brain if it involves the optic tract — will give rise to a homonymous hemianopia, but this is often incomplete (less than half) and incongruous (grossly asymmetrical in the two eyes). Homonymous hemianopia may be due to a lesion of the optic tract between the chiasma and the lateral geniculate body but a far commoner cause is a lesion between the latter structure and the occipital cortex, and in such cases the defect may be quadrantic and not hemianopic.

Temporal lobe lesions usually produce a homonymous hemianopia but, because the optic radiation expands into a sizeable area, sometimes only the lower retinal fibres are involved as they sweep around the descending horn of the lateral ventricle, and then a superior quadrantic defect results. The latter is less commonly due to involvement of the lingual gyrus, and an inferior quadrantic defect to a lesion of the cuneate gyrus of the occipital lobe. With homonymous hemianopia due to a temporal lobe lesion, there is no macular sparing. Lesions of the parietal lobe are likely to cause a crossed inferior quadrantic defect, or less probably a homonymous hemianopia without macular sparing. With lesions localized to the area of the calcarine fissure there will always be macular sparing. By macular sparing is meant that often on careful visual field screening of a patient with an homonymous hemianopia a small central area extending for about five degrees into the blind area can be mapped. The explanation for this is controversial. An extensive unilateral lesion of the visual cortex, for example due to a posterior cerebral artery occlusion, will give rise to a homonymous hemianopia which does not include the macular region. Lesions of either the middle or the posterior cerebral artery sometimes do not cause visual field defects because of the rich arterial anastomoses in their areas of supply. A medial lesion, for example neoplasm or injury, involving both cuneate or both lingual gyri of both occipital lobes, may result in a horizontal hemianopia with blindness above or below the horizontal meridian. Superiorly placed lesions cause inferior homonymous quadrantic defects and inferiorly placed lesions cause superior quadrantic defects. Very localized lesions of the cortex will cause central defects if posteriorly placed and peripheral defects if anteriorly placed.

If in a patient with a homonymous hemianopia the lesion is between the chiasma and the mid-brain, there will be interference with the light reflex. This will not be so if the lesion is between the mid-brain and the occipital lobe. Such interference will be demonstrable only if a narrow beam of light is focused solely on the affected half of the retina: this is an extremely difficult thing to do, and therefore this guide to localization is rarely of practical value.

OPHTHALMOSCOPY

Ophthalmoscopy is a technique which to many is very much a hit-and-miss affair. Practice should be obtained on all patients regardless of whether they are likely to have any lesion of the fundus, for it is only by such frequent experience that a clinician really gets to know how to use his ophthalmoscope properly and to appreciate the enormous variations of normal fundi. If the examiner has studied coloured pictures of the various common abnormalities of the fundi, he will recognize them instantly when he sees them in a patient if he has developed a satisfactory degree of skill which enables him to see almost any fundus under almost any conditions. Again it must be emphasized that such an ability can be achieved only by practice, looking at every patient's fundus regardless of the nature of his illness. Incorrect diagnosis is usually due not to wrong interpretation of what is seen but to poor visualization of the fundus. All aspects and details of the fundus differ in normal people and this represents a difficulty for the inexperienced who are likely to interpret such normal variations as significant abnormalities. Moreover, from the normal fundus the ophthalmoscope light is reflected, as from watered silk, and this may disturb the beginner by obscuring the finer details of the fundus. Oedema of the retina which is often accentuated by papilloedema (*see later*) alters the light reflex especially in the central area of the fundus so that it appears as if it is produced by a polished but dented metal surface rather than watered silk and thereby the fundus loses its normal granular and striated appearance.

The physician must appreciate that it is extremely unlikely that he himself will see the fundus with such clarity as is depicted in any good colour atlas of the fundus oculi, and that he will not recognize the lesions he sees with his ophthalmoscope unless he has mastered the use of that instrument. It is preferable to hold the ophthalmoscope in the right hand, to stand on the patient's right side, and to use one's own right eye to look at the patient's right eye and one's left for observation of the left eye so as to get the instrument as close to the patient's eye as is necessary. The instrument must be held very close to the physician's eye and initially at most about three inches from the patient's eye, bringing it nearer if necessary. If possible the patient should be seated. It is often advisable to keep the patient's head steady with the observer's free hand, and it occasionally helps to keep the patient's upper lid elevated by gentle upward pressure with the index finger of the hand steadying the head. The physician himself should attempt to keep both eyes wide open and not to accommodate for near vision but to focus as though looking at some distant object.

The ophthalmoscope should be used to visualize all the ocular structures and not only the fundus. As emphasized previously the first stage diagnosis must always be an anatomical one, not only noting lesions such as haemorrhages or abnormal opacities but also accurately localizing them to the particular part of the eye affected, and this must always be done before the actual pathology of the lesion is considered. Correct diagnoses can be achieved only by a sure ability to make the correct anatomical diagnosis.

If the patient or the observer is hypermetropic a suitable plus lens, and if myopic a minus lens, must be used in the ophthalmoscope. The plus lenses, marked in red on the dial, are convex and the minus lenses are concave. The dial number represents the focal length expressed in diopters, one diopter corresponding to a focal length of one metre, two diopters to half a metre, and so on.

The correct way to use an ophthalmoscope is to start with at least a plus eight lens (sometimes a much stronger lens will be found to be even better) and report on the pupil, the cornea and the iris. Its head should be pressed firmly against your brow or nose and kept in that position and about a foot away from the patient. A uniform red glow (the red reflex) is seen which is due to the light being reflected back. The presence of a red reflex indicates (1) that the media in front of the retina are transparent, (2) the retina is adposed to the choroid. The three main causes of absence of a red reflex are lens opacities, vitreous haemorrhage, and retinal detachment. The physician should approach gradually nearer and nearer to the patient until his own forehead almost touches the patient whilst at the same time as he is moving nearer the patient he gradually reduces the strength of the lenses while examining the structures of the eye from the front backwards, including the lens and vitreous. Finally he should bring the vessels and optic disc into sharp focus by further rotating the lenses but never by himself attempting to accommodate for near vision. However, many physicians are content with visualizing only the fundus.

The fundus oculi
To examine the fundus, first focus sharply one of the four principal retinal arteries, preferably the superior nasal, and follow this towards the centre of the fundus until the disc is seen. The disc is the ophthalmoscopic view of the optic nerve and is round or oval (the long axis in the vertical) depending on the presence of any error of refraction. Details of the disc as regards colour, contour, cup and cribrosa are noted. Normal elevations or depressions of the disc or of any part of the fundus can be brought into sharp focus by the introduction of a plus lens for elevations and a minus lens for depressions.

The hallmark of the tyro is that he keeps bobbing his own head about in his attempts to visualize the whole of the retina. The correct way is first to scrutinize the disc, noting its colour, cup and cribrosa and the four main arteries and veins emerging all around the vicinity of the disc. One then observes the more peripheral parts by asking the patient, with his head stationary, to look directly upwards and then upwards and inwards, then directly inwards, then downwards and inwards, then directly downwards, and finally upwards and outwards. Only by such a technique, even if one is using a wide angle lens ophthalmoscope, will it be possible to visualize the whole of the retina.

Colour of disc
The colour of the disc is normally whitish (a shade paler on the temporal side), but in disease it may be whiter or pinker than normal. In optic atrophy of any type the whiteness (pallor) of the disc is enhanced and in papilloedema the disc becomes pinker than normal. It is important to realize that where the lesion is unilateral, diagnosis becomes easier by comparison with the other disc. Thus, if there is a difference in the degree of whiteness of the two discs, then one of them must be abnormal. On the other hand, if the lesion is bilateral, and especially if it is symmetrical, there is no such means of comparison and the only guide is experience. Therefore, when the change is marked it is usually easy to make such an assessment, but the early degrees of such change must always be very difficult to appreciate even by the expert. The mistake is too often made of

diagnosing pallor of the disc, for example, in disseminated sclerosis, just because the examiner knows it frequently occurs. Moreover, one must remember that the temporal side of the disc is normally paler than the nasal but the normal limits of difference cannot be readily defined and for this reason it is better not to use the term temporal pallor. Whenever in doubt one should regard the disc as normal, especially if the patient has never had any visual disturbance, or consider sending the patient to an expert ophthalmologist.

It is also important to realize that there are other criteria (*see later*) which help in the diagnosis of optic atrophy. Moreover, to state that a patient has pallor of the disc is not a diagnosis at all, because if there really is pallor there must be optic atrophy since these are synonymous, and optic atrophy should be the firm diagnosis. Furthermore, optic atrophy may not affect all the nerve fibres of the optic nerve head, which consists of bundles of many fibres. In disseminated sclerosis it often happens that only the fibres comprising the temporal half of the disc are affected, but it is important to realize that this is optic atrophy, admittedly of only part of the nerve but nonetheless optic atrophy. Too often clinicians refer to the occurrence of optic pallor in disseminated sclerosis as though it were something different from optic atrophy. It must be borne in mind that with a high myope the disc always looks paler and larger than normal.

Contour of disc
Normally the disc margin is well defined, but in papilloedema or secondary optic atrophy the margins become blurred. Assessment of such blurring depends upon experience gained by much practice and upon paying due regard to the fact that the commonest cause of inability to focus the disc margins properly is a refractive error and not a lesion of the optic nerve (in other words, the examiner is not using his ophthalmoscope properly) and that the nasal margin is always more difficult to focus than the temporal. Unless the examiner has had considerable experience, he should beware of diagnosing any swelling of the nerve head merely on the grounds that there is an apparent slight blurring of the nasal side of the disc. This Procrustean crime is often committed with hypertensive patients.

Cup and lamina cribrosa
The physiological cup and the lamina cribrosa are both normal appearances and should always be seen if the ophthalmoscope is used properly. The cup, a funnel-shaped depression which is normally paler than the rest of the disc, may not be clearly definable even in normal people. The cup's shape, comparative size and actual position within the disc vary enormously, but these details are not important except in glaucoma. The cribrosa is situated in the centre of the cup and has a sieve-like pattern produced by the piercing of

the sclerotic by the optic nerve fibres of the retina. The lamina cribrosa cannot always be identified even in normal people. The changes in the lamina cribrosa are always comparable with those in the cup; both are very well marked and concave in a primary optic atrophy, and both become increasingly obliterated in palpilloedema and in optic atrophy which has followed papilloedema. It will thus be realized from the above description that the optic nerve head is not a flat surface but a concave surface which, if correctly focused, will be seen to have a distinctive pattern — what artists call 'modelling'.

Fundus circulation
The arteries do not normally run a straight course but a sinuous one. The vessels branch dichotomously. The centre of their blood column is normally lighter than the periphery (the central axial light reflex) and occupies about a third of the width of the column of blood. Whereas with the arteries pathology causes narrowing, for example in atherosclerosis or following optic atrophy, with vein pathology such as caused by raised intracranial tension, leukaemia, polycythemia and obstruction of the central vein, the veins become considerably distended. The normal relationship between the calibre of veins and that of arteries is 3 : 2. Any deviation from this proportion will obviously be difficult for the inexperienced to diagnose except when marked. The central retinal artery and vein are situated very close to each other and emerge from the centre of the cup. Each has four main branches supplying the four retinal quadrants. The arteries are a lighter red and narrower than the veins. The macula is two to three disc diameters away from and a little below the disc itself. It is best seen by asking the patient to look directly at the ophthalmoscope light. Sometimes it helps by elevating the ophthalmoscope head, if this is possible, and so narrowing the light beam or by using a green filter. The macula is normally a darker red than the surrounding retina. The fovea is a small round even darker and brighter area with a brilliant light reflex and can be identified in the centre of the macula. The macula area is very important because any lesion there however small such as a haemorrhage or exudate will cause marked visual impairment. In Tay—Sach's* disease and related conditions a cherry red spot develops in the macula and this is surrounded by a usually well defined whitish-grey halo. Later in the disease the whole retina becomes pale and optic atrophy develops. Occlusion of the central artery of the retina may also cause a cherry red spot, but without the surrounding halo.

*Warren Tay (1843—1927), a British ophthalmologist, described the condition in 1881 and Sachs, an American neurologist, in 1887.

Haemorrhages in the retina are seen as reddish patches which may be of any shape or size. Old haemorrhages become darker and darker and may even become blackish.

Subhyaloid haemorrhage

A subhyaloid haemorrhage is a bleeding into the tissue space between the internal lining membrane of the retina and the hyaloid membrane of the vitreous. It causes a dark red area in front of the disc (that is why it is disconcertingly persistently visible to the patient) which, provided that the patient is not lying down, has a fluid level with a well-defined upper limit and convex lower border. By far the commonest cause of a subhyaloid haemorrhage is a ruptured aneurysm at the base of the brain.

Exudates are white patches which may also be of any size or shape. Having noticed these, one's immediate task must be to localize them and determine whether they are in the retina or in the choroid. This distinction is made by noting the relationship of blood vessels to the patches because, in the case of choroiditis, the blood vessels run over (that is, are superficial) to the exudates, whereas in retinitis the blood vessels are interrupted by the exudates.

Because of the close proximity of the choroid and retina and the fact that the outer layers of the retina are supplied by choroidal vessels, it is not surprising that any inflammatory lesions of the former are likely ultimately to affect the retina and lead to choroidoretinitis. Even then, however, it is very important and usually easy to determine which is the dominant lesion, because the causes of retinitis are different from those of choroiditis (which are usually inflammatory), and diagnosing a choroido-retinitis merely shirks the issue. Primary lesions of the retina are rarely inflammatory and therefore are very unlikely to spread to the choroid.

Myopic crescents

A myopic crescent may be found in a patient with a high degree of myopia and is a well-defined (if focused properly) white crescentic patch immediately contiguous to one or other side of the disc, nearly always on the temporal side but it may be of any size, occasionally surrounding even more than half the disc circumference. It is not always proportional to the degree of myopia. Sometimes a similar crescent can be seen on the inferior disc margin in hypermetropia and/or astigmatism. Crescents have to be distinguished from opaque (medullated) nerve fibres, which are a unilateral or bilateral congenital abnormality of no significance. In the latter condition the white patch, abutting on the disc, has a brushlike irregular free margin. Opaque nerve fibres usually have a silky finely striated appearance. There is never a clear normal area between the disc and the medullated (opaque) nerve fibres. This contrasts with an area of choroiditis near the disc which is very rarely at the disc margin itself. Opaque nerve fibres may be so large and so white as to be mistaken for the disc itself and optic atrophy wrongly diagnosed.

Pigment

The tyro is often distinguished by the readiness with which he boasts that he can see pigment in the fundus not appreciating that pigment, which is almost entirely in the choroid, is a normal finding. Its amount varies from virtual complete absence in an albino, so that the whole retina appears white with a profusion of normal choroidal vessels, to the extreme chocolate-brown pigmentation, often with a greenish tinge, seen in Negroes. In blondes, other than albinos, the fundus has an orange-red tinge and in brunettes dark pigmentation is present of various sizes and shapes in patches between the orange-streaked network of choroidal vessels giving a tessellated appearance (the tigroid fundus) which has no significance.

In any chronic lesion of the retina or choroid, pigmentation occurs around the areas and that pigmentation is of no diagnostic value other than indicating chronicity. It is the lesion which the pigment surrounds that is far more important than the pigmentation itself, which is but a secondary phenomenon.

Retinitis pigmentosa

Retinitis pigmentosa is the only condition in which retinal pigmentation is itself important. This is a rare genetically determined disease in which blackish pigmentation of spidery shapes occurs in the periphery of the retina. Later the lesions may be complicated by an optic atrophy.

Papilloedema

Papilloedema is swelling of the nerve head as seen on ophthalmoscopy. It is found in raised intracranial tension, in retinitis, due to hypertension (including when secondary to renal disease), diabetes and blood diseases (including polycythaemia vera). With occlusion of the central retinal vein the papilloedema is always unilateral and marked with gross venous dilatation and the fundus becomes splashed with haemorrhages which may be large or small and are often flame shaped radiating in all directions from the disc. Occasionally only one of the four main tributaries is affected (most often the superior temporal) as a result of which the haemorrhages are confined to a quadrant of the retina. It is an extremely rare finding in either superior vena caval obstruction or with chronic cor pulmonale. The author sees no good reason for the introduction of special words such as 'papillitis', 'optic neuritis' and 'choked disc' to differentiate swelling of the nerve head due to different causes because the appearance of the disc is the same whatever the cause. The appearance of the fundus in papilloedema is that the colour of the disc becomes redder, approximating to that of the rest of the retina, its contour becomes blurred and the cup and cribrosa are filled in.

In raised intracranial tension the veins are distended and if the degree of papilloedema is marked, then and only then will there be haemorrhages radiating from the disc. When papilloedema is associated with any retinitis other than retinitis pigmentosa the haemorrhages are scattered throughout the fundus and not maximum around the disc. This is in contrast with retinitis, for example due to hypertension, where the haemorrhages are an early sign present when the papilloedema is absent or of only minor degree.

The earliest manifestation of papilloedema is engorgement of the veins. Obviously, unless this is marked, a great deal of experience is required to recognize it, and papilloedema should never be definitely diagnosed unless the examiner is certain that it is present, because the implications of such a diagnosis are so important. Papilloedema is a rare finding in retrobulbar neuritis. The viewpoint that fluorescein angiography is necessary for the diagnosis of early papilloedema is absurd. To measure the amount of papilloedema, the fundus must be examined with both of the observer's eyes wide open and completely unaccommodated as if looking at a far distant object. This is not easy and requires diligent practice. The lenses are then rotated until a vessel near the centre of the disc is sharply focused with the highest possible plus lens. The same vessel is followed and again carefully refocused at its emergence from the disc margin. The difference in diopters between the two focusings gives a measure of the papilloedema, three diopters being equivalent to one millimetre of swelling.

Papilloedema is always associated with enlargement of the blind spot, with a consequent diminution of visual fields and gradual loss of visual acruity, but a fair acuity may remain until the papilloedema becomes marked.

Retrobulbar neuritis
Retrobulbar neuritis is a lesion of the optic nerve between the eyeball and the optic chiasma. The physical signs to which it gives rise are as follows:

1. A visual field defect, which is usually but not necessarily a central or paracentral scotoma especially with colours and with enlargement of the blind spot. It always seriously interferes with vision.
2. A large pupil, which is circular and reacts sluggishly to direct light but briskly to consensual light (light shone into the other eye) and to accommodation. These pupillary changes will be much more obvious with a unilateral lesion.
3. If the lesion extends to the nerve head, which it very rarely does, then papilloedema will result.

The common causes of retrobulbar neuritis are:
1. Disseminated sclerosis. In this disease the condition is usually unilateral and, in fact, disseminated sclerosis is by far the commonest cause of unilateral retrobulbar neuritis.
2. Neurosyphilis.
3. Chemical poisons, particularly lead, alcohol (especially methanol), organic arsenic (especially the pentavalent tryparsamide), quinine and tobacco, thallium used as a depilatory and carbon disulphide used in rubber manufacture. A large number of other chemical compounds may, on rare occasions, cause this lesion. When due to chemical causes a retrobulbar heuritis is sometimes called a toxic amblyopia.

Rarer causes are diabetes, spread of infection from local sinuses, B_1 or B_{12} vitamin deficiency and neuromyelitis optica (in which a bilateral retrobulbar neuritis is associated with a transverse myelitis). The natural history of a retrobulbar neuritis is that it either gets completely better or progresses to an optic atrophy.

Optic atrophy
The classification of optic atrophy is obfuscated by the fact that there are rival schemes, and many clinicians are unaware that the terminology they use is not used by everybody else. The simplest classification is into primary and secondary optic atrophy, the primary condition being one which has not been preceded by papilloedema, and the atrophy being termed secondary when it has followed papilloedema. In primary optic atrophy the disc is wholly or partly paler than normal; its contour, cup and cribrosa are all well defined, and the circulation shows a narrowing (attenuation) of the arteries. The pallor is due to grossly diminished vascularity and involves the whole or half of the disc extending uniformly from the centre to the periphery and is never confined to a crescentic shaped rim. In secondary optic atrophy the colour of the disc is paler than normal; its contour, cup and cribrosa are ill defined, and there is attenuation of the arteries. Moreover, while primary optica atrophy may involve only some of the nerve fibres, secondary atrophy always affects the whole nerve.

It will be seen from the above that the diagnosis of an optic atrophy and of its type depends on other criteria than pallor. Moreover, as explained above pallor may be difficult to assess and must often be merely an impression based on experience. An important point to note is that it is impossible to have an optic atrophy with normal visual fields carefully measured on a proper screen.

The commonest causes of primary optic atrophy are the same as those of a retrobulbar neuritis, but other causes are injury to the nerve and pressure by tumours in the. region of the optic nerve or chiasma, for example pituitary tumours. Primary optic atrophy may also be associated with the hereditary and familial cerebellar ataxias;

it may rarely occur as a hereditary sex-linked clinical entity, present without any other neurological abnormality. It may follow severe haemorrhage, especially from the gastrointestinal tract, and also occlusion of the central retinal artery. The last-named condition is unilateral and of sudden onset, producing gross diminution of visual acuity (unless the patient is lucky enough to have a cilioretinal artery) due to optic atrophy which is accompanied by pallor of the whole of the fundus with diminution of the calibre of the vessels. If the occlusion is only of a branch of the main artery the retinal changes are confined to a quadrant and optic atrophy will not be present. If the occlusion persists, marked perimacular oedema may result; the macula itself is then seen as a cherry red spot, but without the white halo which surrounds the area in cases of Tay Sach's disease. A choroiditis or retinitis pigmentosa may be followed by an optic atrophy which the author would designate primary optic atrophy because it has not been preceded by papilloedema and is indistinguishable from any other optic atrophy.

The term consecutive optic atrophy is a controversial one and is better avoided. Some use it as an equivalent or alternative term for what has been described above as a secondary atrophy, but others use the term to indicate an atrophy complicating a choroiditis or rarely a retinitis.

Glaucoma
In glaucoma the disc becomes very pale and the cup well marked and large extending at least in part to the rim of the disc so that there appears to be only a narrow lip of disc surrounding the cup. The cribrosa is at first well marked but later may be obscured by neuroglial proliferation. The vessels appear crowded together over the disc and pushed to one side and if a vessel near the centre of the disc is followed it seems to disappear in the region of the lip and then to reappear at the disc margin. Glaucoma is due to an elevation of intraocular pressure produced by any of a possible variety of mechanisms. Primary glaucoma is nearly always bilateral but secondary glaucoma is often unilateral and due to pre-existing eye disease.

Choroiditis
Choroiditis is diagnosed by the presence of exudates of various shades of white, grey and yellow, with arteries superficial to them. There may or may not be an optic atrophy. If the lesions are chronic, the exudates will be surrounded by blackish pigment. The choroid is part of the uveal tract, which also consists of the iris and the ciliary body. The common causes of choroiditis are inflammatory lesions such as syphilis, tuberculosis (not associated with any active tuberculous lesions elsewhere except in miliary tuberculosi in which the finding of an acute choroiditis may be important diagnostically), sarcoidosis and toxoplasmosis, but injury is also a fairly common

cause, and idiopathic cases are seen. The choroid may be the site of a primary melanoma malignum.

Retinitis

A frequent and stupid quibble is the replacement of the word 'retinitis', which is presumed to mean an inflammation of the retina, by the word 'retinopathy', while the same authors, with no regard for consistency, talk about retinitis pigmentosa.

Retinitis is characterized by the presence in the retina of haemorrhages and whitish patches (exudates) and sometimes papilloedema, which is not an essential feature. The retinal vessels are interrupted by the exudates and not superficial to them as in a choroiditis. The haemorrhages and exudates may be of any size or shape.

Papilloedema when present usually indicates a bad prognosis, but may be reversible with drug therapy. It is never marked. The student should beware of automatically diagnosing it, for example in a patient with hypertensive retinitis, merely because it is known that it occurs, and should remember that the earliest degrees of papilloedema are extremely difficult to recognize. The papilloedema of raised intracranial tension is usually readily differentiated because in this condition haemorrhages do not occur unless the papilloedema is marked, whereas in retinitis the haemorrhages are the earliest sign and the papilloedema is late and always comparatively slight. With raised intracranial tension the haemorrhages are always maximum near and around the disc, appearing to radiate from it like the spokes of a wheel. The common causes of retinitis are hypertension, nephritis (albuminuric retinitis), diabetes and blood diseases, especially leukaemia and severe anaemia. The distinction between these is often impossible on ophthalmoscopy. Retinal haemorrhages due to anaemia are always small and flame or spindle shaped, lying close to the vessels except when due to massive acute bleeding. In acute leukaemia marked distension of the veins occurs and the haemorrhages may exhibit whitish centres. Sickle cell anaemia causes vitreous and retinal haemorrhage with micro-aneurysms. Polycythaemia vera causes a purplish hue to the whole retina with gross vein distension. There may be papilloedema and/or retinal vein thrombosis. The retinal changes of nephritis are probably secondary to any associated hypertension. However, the classical description of albuminuric retinitis is the presence of large flame-shaped haemorrhages and 'cotton-wool' exudates which are maximal at the macula, producing the so-called star or fan. Cotton-wool exudates are variously described as being due to localized collections of oedema, to small retinal infarcts, or organized haemorrhages or bulbous swellings on the terminal nerve fibres (cytoid bodies). Although previously cytoid bodies were thought to be peculiar to renal retinitis, they may also occur in malignant hypertension, in diabetic retinitis, in severe anaemia, and rarely in systemic lupus erythematosus. With hypertensive retinitis part or the whole of the retina may be oedematous causing pallor and shinyness of any part of it but especially the macular area.

Diabetic retinitis is characterized by the fact that the haemorrhages and exudates are usually small and round (presumably because they are in the deeper layers of the retina), and they may have a yellowish waxy appearance. The exudates are frequently described as 'hard', meaning well defined. A mild degree of papilloedema may be present.

In diabetic retinitis, sometimes, but it is important to realize not always, small aneurysms may be seen, and to the inexpert these will look exactly like small haemorrhages adjacent to the vessel wall. They are round or ovoid and arise on the capillaries, which are normally too small to be visible on ophthalmoscopy. These micro-aneurysms are sometimes regarded as the earliest sign of a diabetic retinitis but, although suggestive, are not pathognomonic, occurring also in malignant hypertension, macroglobinaemia and sickle cell anaemia, Unfortunately, many clinicians diagnose micro-aneurysms if the patient is a known diabetic and has a retinitis, but such an uncritical approach is very bad. Indeed, fluorescein studies, producing an *intra vitam* staining of the retina, have shown that most of the 'dot' lesions are in fact small exudates or haemorrhages and not aneurysms, and fluorescein staining may be essential if the academic distinction is to be made for certain. Moreover, many diabetics have hypertension with or without atherosclerosis, and any retinitis which they have may well be due to atherosclerosis or diabetes, or combinations of these, and not to the diabetes *per se*.

In diabetic retinitis, retinal oedema is conspicuously absent. Diabetic retinitis is always bilateral but often asymmetrical. Retinitis is a rare complication of young diabetics however severe their disease.

Retinitis proliferans is a term used by some to indicate proliferation of new arterioles or veins, which are usually seen crossing in front of the other retinal vessels and emerging as small tufts near the disc and later forming arcades alongside the main vessels. The commonest cause of this is long-standing diabetes, but it may also occur in malignant hypertension and rarely in sickle cell anaemia. Other experts use the term only when this appearance is associated with a marked fibrous tissue reaction, seen as fronds or bands or sheets of whitish or yellowish tissue on the surface of the retina. It is this inclusive picture which is seen only in diabetes. Retinitis proliferans may be complicated by retinal detachment.

It is very important to realize that hypertensive retinitis and atherosclerotic retinitis are two different things, although they are often seen in the same patient. Atherosclerotic retinitis is characterized by narrowing and undue tortuosity of the vessels, a silver wire appearance of the arteries because of an increase of the centre axial light reflex of the artery and a nipping (apparent partial constriction) of the veins where they are crossed by an artery.

It is very questionable whether ordinary doctors can measure arteriolar narrowing, or the effects produced by the intersection of arteries and veins, especially as diameters vary between individuals and different parts of the same retina. Many doctors pontificate on such matters, spuriously grading the vascular changes and deluding themselves that they were being impressive.

Angioid streaks are a feature of pseudo-xanthoma elasticum and consist of brownish-black, sometimes with white borders, fine or broad tapering bands surrounding and radiating from the disc. They are due to rupture of Bruch's choroidal elastic membrane.

The third cranial nerve

ANATOMY

A useful technique when describing the anatomy of the various cranial nerves is to label the different parts of the pathway, because each part gives rise to distinctive clinical signs.

Part 1 of the course of the third nerve may be considered to be the nucleus. Each third nerve nucleus is situated in the mid-brain at the level of the superior quadrigemina and is in the anterior part of the grey matter surrounding the aqueduct of Sylvius. The two nuclei are close together and each consists not of a single nucleus but of a conglomeration of nuclei, each supplying a different muscle. In addition there is one which is concerned with the light reflex and another concerned with accommodation-convergence. The two third nerves are connected by commissural fibres via the posterior longitudinal bundle, which is situated immediately anterior to the aqueduct of Sylvius.

Part 2 of the nerve is its pathway through the mid-brain (*see Figure 5*). Both third nerves course forward through the substance of the mid-brain, where they are in close proximity to the red nucleus, the substantia nigra, and the pyramidal and cortico-cerebellar fibres of the crura. Part 3 of the nerve is its course in the posterior fossa, which is in the interpenduncular space at the base of the brain as it emerges internal to the crura cerebri (cerebral peduncles). In this space there is also the circle of Willis* (*see Figure 6*) and the hypothalamus, and each third nerve passes between the posterior cerebral and the superior cerebellar vessels. Part 4 of its course, which is in the middle fossa, is in the cavernous sinus, which it leaves by piercing the dura in the region of the posterior clinoid process. In the sinus are also the fourth, the ophthalmic division of the fifth, and the sixth nerves. In part 5 of its course the nerve exits from the skull, together with the above nerves, via the superior orbital fissure. Within the orbit it gives

*Thomas Willis (1621–75), an English anatomist and physician.

off its terminal branches to supply all the external ocular muscles (except the superior oblique and the external rectus) and, in addition, the levator palpebrae superioris and the sphincter pupillae.

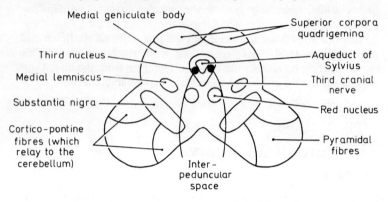

Figure 5. *The mid-brain showing the pathway of the third cranial nerve*

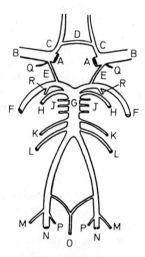

A—Internal carotid
B—Middle cerebral
C—Anterior cerebral
D—Anterior communicating
E—Posterior communicating
F—Posterior cerebral
G—Basilar
H—Superior cerebellar
J—Pontine
K—Internal auditory
L Anterior inferior cerebellar
M—Posterior inferior cerebellar
N—Verebral
O—Anterior spinal
P—Posterior spinal
Q—Anterior choroid
R—Posterior choroid

Figure 6. *Schematic diagram showing the arteries at the base of the brain*

The fourth cranial nerve

ANATOMY

The fourth nerves arise from paired nuclei situated in the mid-brain in the grey matter of the aqueduct of Sylvius, immediately anterior and inferior to the third nuclei. Both fourth nerves run backwards and inwards and decussate in the posterior medullary velum, and then wind around the cerebral peduncles. Thereafter they follow the course of the third nerves into the cavernous sinus and through the superior orbital fissure into the orbit to supply the superior oblique. The latter, acting alone, depresses the globe (maximum on adduction). The same muscle also intorts the globe and abducts it.

The sixth cranial nerve

ANATOMY

Part 1 of the course of the sixth nerve is within the pons (*see Figure 7*), the nucleus being situated dorsally and immediately dorsal to the nucleus of the seventh nerve, the fibres of which wind around the nucleus of the sixth. The sixth nerve, together with the seventh, then courses directly forward through the substance of the pons where, anteriorly, both are in close association with the pyramidal fibres.

Part 2 of its course is in the cerebello-pontine angle. Both the sixth and the seventh nerve emerge from the inferior border of the pons, and although at first the two are close together, with the seventh nerve laterally placed, they diverge, the sixth nerve never becoming much more lateral and the seventh nerve remaining nearer the midline until just before its exit from the skull. Soon after the sixth nerves leaves

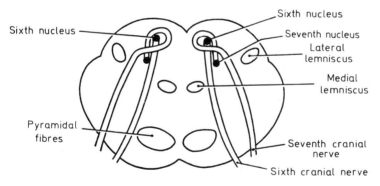

Figure 7. *The pons showing the pathways of the sixth and seventh cranial nerves*

the pons it comes into close relationship with the circle of Willis, passing between the anterior inferior cerebellar and the internal auditory vessels. In the most lateral part of its course in the cerebello-pontine angle, it pierces the dura overlying the basilar portion of the occipital bone. Beneath the dura, it lies on the petrous portion of the temporal bone, where it is near the fifth nerve.

The nerve's main direction is then forward and inward and it enters upon part 3 of its course. This is in the cavernous sinus, where its relationships have been described in the section on the third nerve.

In part 4 of its course, the nerve exists through the superior orbital fissure to enter the orbit and supply the external rectus muscle.

Testing the third, fourth and sixth cranial nerves

These nerves are examined collectively by looking for squint, testing ocular movements, asking about diplopia, examining the pupils and looking for ptosis. It is convenient to search for nystagmus at this stage of the examination.

Important points when examining ocular movements are as follows:

1. It is far easier to assess these movements if the patient is sitting up.
2. The observer's finger or a thin object, such as a pencil, which the patient is asked to follow should be held at eye level, or even a little above, so that the eyes are fully open and therefore can be properly observed.
3. The moving object must be at least 20 inches away (not 10 inches, as often advised, because the patient may be hypermetropic and unable to focus properly at this distance).
4. The patient's head should be kept fixed by the examiner's other hand, otherwise even a slight movement of his head will prevent him from carrying out full lateral eye movements. This is exceptionally important when looking for nystagmus, which is frequently brought out only on extreme conjugate deviation.
5. He must always be asked whether he has or has had diplopia.

THE PUPILS

Most people find great difficulty in assessing pupuils, and this is often because their observations have been perfunctory. Attention must be paid to size, equality or inequality, shape, regularity or irregularity, briskness of reaction to light (directly and consensually), and reaction to accommodation.

Whether the pupils are large or small is merely a clinical impression, as actual measurement is not usually done. The term 'pin-point' should be used only when they are extremely small, literally the size of a pin-point, which occurs only in pontine haemorrhage and in opium poisoning. The size of the pupils is normally controlled by the opposing forces of the sympathetic, supplying the dilator pupillae, and the parasympathetic component of the third nerve, supplying the constrictor pupillae.

Reaction to light can be properly assessed only if a strong light is used; the patient must look into the distance and must not be allowed to look towards the light used, which must be brought obliquely and not directly to the eye, otherwise the examiner is testing light and accommodation at the same time and this is a frequent cause of incorrect assessment. After about three minutes the light should be rapidly transferred to the opposite pupil and this moving of the light should be repeated several times and both pupils carefully scrutinized each time. The reaction to light must be tested not only directly but also consensually — that is, noting the pupillary reaction in one eye on shining the light in the opposite eye.

Reaction to accommodation involves the co-operation of the patient and should be observed most carefully. If the patient is blind, it is still possible to test accommodation by asking him to look in the direction of his own nose, which the examiner should touch with his finger. The dilatation of the pupils on bringing one's finger further and further away from the patient is often easier to assess than the contraction on near vision, because in the latter the upper eyelids are lowered and therefore, unless held open, will interfere with proper observation of the pupils. By far the commonest cause of a pupil which appears to react normally to light but poorly to accommodation is faulty technique and is only very rarely due to a lesion in the upper part of the midbrain.

It cannot be over-emphasized that the normal range of pupillary response to both light and accommodation can be learnt only by experience, and that complete failure to react to either or both is unusual, the far commoner finding being a comparative sluggishness or lack of maintenance of the contraction. For careful observation of pupils, the use of a hand lens is strongly recommended, or looking at them with the ophthalmoscope switched to a plus 20 lens. If pupils are very small, they cannot contract much more to either light or accommodation and may be wrongly regarded as non-reacting unless a slit lamp is used.

Irregular pupils

The commonest cause of an irregular pupil is iritis. Another important cause is neurosyphilis, especially tabes dorsalis and dementia paralytica. Any iritis, even in the absence of neurological signs, may be syphilitic but then keratitis is usually present. Neurosyphilitic pupils are discussed below, and iritis in Chapter 8.

Mydriasis

Mydriasis is the presence of an abnormally large pupil.

1. It may be caused by a third nerve lesion, in which case the pupil will be large, regular, circular, and reacting not at all or sluggishly to direct and consensual light and to accommodation.

The fixity of the pupil is designated internal ophthalmoplegia, and occurs only in a third nerve lesion or in iritis complicated by synechiae. The confirmatory evidence that the mydriasis is due to a third nerve palsy is the presence of an external ophthalmoplegia and ptosis. If the only manifestation of a third nerve lesion is an internal ophthalmoplegia, then the lesion must be confined to its parasympathetic portion and is most often due to drugs such as atropine and its derivatives.

2. It may be due to sympathetic stimulation, in which case the pupil will be large, circular, regular, and reacting normally to light and to accommodation. The confirmatory evidence may be overaction of the levator palpebrae superioris and perhaps excessive facial sweating. Apart from emotion, the commonest cause of cervical sympathetic stimulation is drugs such as adrenaline and its relatives and cocaine.

3. Lesions of the optic nerve may be associated with mydriasis, and then the pupil will be large, regular, circular, and reacting sluggishly or not at all to direct light or if it does react normally initially the reaction is not sustained but the pupil reacts briskly to consensual light and to accommodation. The confirmatory evidence is either an optic atrophy or a retrobulbar neuritis. The pupillary changes will be modified if there is an associated or coincidental iritis.

4. With lesions of any part of the eye which interfere with vision, the pupil is often dilated in order to allow as much light as possible to enter the eye to compensate for the disability.

5. In iritis, the pupil may be large but will then be irregular and non-reactive to either light or accommodation. The mydriasis may be explicable as in paragraph 4, but is often due to atropine therapy, which is the standard treatment.

6. In any patient who is deeply comatose from whatever cause, the pupils are usually dilated and not reacting to light.

7. The myotonic pupil (Adie—Holmes* syndrome) is usually large and always circular and regular, and the condition is often unilateral. On testing the light reflex by conventional methods, the myotonic pupil appears to react poorly and sluggishly. However, if a strong and persistent stimulus is used it can be shown that the pupil contracts excessively to a very small size, and when the stimulus is removed it returns to its former size only very slowly, hence the term myotonic. Alternatively, if the patient is kept in the dark the affected pupil becomes very large, and when the patient is brought into the light it will be several minutes before the pupil contracts to its normal size. The pupillary reaction to accommodation is likewise

*W. J. Adie (1886–1935) and Sir Gordon Holmes (1876–   ), British neurologists who jointly described the syndrome in 1931.

excessive. A myotonic pupil is often associated with sluggishness of some of the tendon reflexes, so the condition has a superficial resemblance to tabes dorsalis. Both the pathology and the aetiology of the condition are obscure.
8. In markedly myopic people the pupils are often large.

Meiosis

Meiosis is an abnormally small pupil, and may be due to parasympathetic stimulation or to cervical sympathetic paralysis. The only common cause of parasympathetic stimulation is drugs, especially pilocarpine and physostigmine. The manifestations and causes of cervical sympathetic paralysis are discussed later. In pontine haemorrhage and also in opium poisoning the pupils are very small, being contracted to the size of a pin-point. The pupils in neurosyphilis are often but not necessarily small.

Argyll Robertson pupils

In neurosyphilis the pupils, as originally described in four cases by Argyll Robertson of Edinburgh in 1869, are small, irregular and unequal, not reacting to light but reacting briskly to accommodation, and there is patchy atrophy of the iris and depigmentation. A stupid quibble relating to the eponymous term is that it should not be used unless all the above features are present. This represents the crime of diagnostic greed at its worst.

The pupils often are not small and may react a little to light, or may react fairly briskly but without the contraction being maintained – that is, subsequently dilating even though the light stimulus is still present. Such findings have the same significance as no response to light. The basis of assessment of a sluggish light reaction is by comparison with the reaction to accommodation, which is always normal in the neurosyphilitic pupil. However, if the pupils are very small it will be difficult to demonstrate reaction to accommodation because the pupils are incapable of contracting much more than their permanent meiotic state.

Altered shape, the pupils not being circular, is just as significant as irregularity. The commonest cause of an irregular pupil is iritis (which itself may be syphilitic), but then the reaction to accommodation will also be affected and iris adhesions (synechiae) may be seen.

The diagnosis of general paralysis of the insane (G.P.I.) or tabes dorsalis in a patient with completely normal pupils is very likely to be wrong, but in other forms of neurosyphilis it is very common to find normal pupils. The exact site of the lesion causing the pupillary changes in neurosyphilis is extremely controversial, and many experts do not place the lesion in the mid-brain as is frequently done.

M

PARALYSIS OF CONJUGATE DEVIATION

There is no such thing as a supranuclear lesion of any one of these cranial nerves. The nearest equivalent — and this is at best only a very rough approximation — is paralysis or spasm of conjugate deviation.

With a paralysis of lateral gaze, the patient cannot move his eyes completely to either the right or the left: this is a combined movement involving the external rectus muscle of one eye and the internal rectus muscle of the other, and as these muscles are supplied by different nerves, such a paralysis cannot be regarded as a supranuclear lesion of either the third or the sixth nerve. It is a paralysis of movement rather than of individual muscles. Moreover, it can be shown on accommodation-convergence that the internal rectus muscle is not actually paralysed but does not act together with the opposite external rectus. With paralysis of conjugate deviation, the eyes remain parallel and therefore there is neither squint nor diplopia. Paralyses of conjugate deviation are rare, and their exact location is controversial. Paralysis of lateral gaze in either direction suggests a lesion of the upper part of the pons which is often neoplastic, or extensive unilateral subcortical damage, usually of the frontal lobe and commonly due to a vascular lesion. A paralysis of vertical gaze suggests a lesion in the region of the superior corpora quadrigemina.

SPASMS OF CONJUGATE DEVIATION

Spasms of conjugate deviation are much commoner than paralyses and are seen in the following circumstances:
1. At the commencement of an epileptiform attack.
2. At the onset of a cerebrovascular lesion, when the head and eyes turn temporarily away from the lesion (that is, towards the paralysed limbs) and later to the other side. Such spasm is not always present.
3. In encephalitis lethargica, when they are known as oculogyric crises.
4. Rarely as an hysterical phenomenon.

The exact site of the lesion causing the spasm is unknown but is probably in the frontal cortex.

SIGNS OF OCULAR NERVE LESIONS

The cardinal manifestations of a lesion of one or more external ocular muscles are (1) strabismus (squint), which is a deviation of the eye from the optical axis; (2) defective ocular movement; and (3) double vision (diplopia).

Strabismus

A strabismus is usually obvious, but minor degrees can be more readily recognized by asking the patient to concentrate his gaze on some object held about a foot away and then covering each eye in turn and carefully observing the uncovered eye. If this moves to fix upon the object, it indicates a strabismus. The most important classification of strabismus is into paralytic and concomitant types. In lesions of the third, fourth or sixth nerve, the resultant strabismus will be paralytic. However, a concomitant strabismus due to a relative increase in tone of one ocular muscle compared with its synergic muscle (muscle imbalance) is a far commoner type. This condition is usually first seen in infancy or childhood and frequently follows one of the exanthems. It is incorrect to refer to it as a congenital squint, as if often done, because all newborn infants have a squint and do not develop the power of fixation for several months.

In concomitant strabismus, ocular movements are full (which can best be shown by testing each eye separately, covering first one and then the other) and, because of suppression of the image from the squinting eye, there is no diplopia. The affected eye usually has a high degree of refractive error. It follows that, in a patient with a squint, it is impossible to state whether it is paralytic or concomitant unless one knows (1) whether he has diplopia, and (2) whether his ocular movements are full.

Diplopia
Diplopia is the most important sign of any type of ocular palsy because it may be the only manifestation. Except in rare conditions – for example, dislocation of the lens – it always indicates an ocular palsy. It is therefore imperative that when testing ocular movements the examiner asks the patient whether he has or has had diplopia, because, even if his ocular movements appear to be full, if he has diplopia he must have or have had a paralysis of the third, fourth or sixth nerves, or weakness of the muscles themselves due to myasthenia gravis, even if his ocular movements appear full.

The fundamental rules of diplopia are as follows:
1. It is seen when the object is moved in the direction of action of the paralysed muscle. The physician must first determine the position of gaze with both eyes open which produces the diplopia with the maximum separation of the images. Each eye is then covered in turn as this will determine which eye produces the more peripheral and usually less distinct image, and this comes from the defective eye. For example, if the maximum separation of the images is seen when looking to the right this would indicate a right lateral rectus or left medial rectus palsy but if the more peripheral image comes from the right eye the right lateral rectus must be the affected muscle.
2. As the object is moved further in this direction, there is increasing separation of images. This sign is more valuable in recent than in chronic ophthalmoplegias.

From the above rules and by noticing any defect of ocular movement, it is frequently possible to diagnose correctly the affected
muscle. However, this simple technique does not always suffice for
the following reasons:

1. The patient may have a diplopia — for example, on looking
   to his right — with full ocular movements, and in that case
   the examiner would not even know which was the affected
   eye, because such diplopia could be due to a lesion of either
   the right external rectus or the left internal rectus. This
   problem is often encountered in disseminated sclerosis and in
   myasthenia gravis.
2. The patient may have more than one muscle affected, and the
   muscles may be supplied by different cranial nerves.
3. Because, apart from the external and internal recti, the muscles
   have a compound action, the superior rectus elevates the eye
   (maximal in abduction) and also intorts and adducts; the
   inferior rectus depresses the eye (maximally in abduction) and
   also intorts and adducts; the superior oblique depresses the eye
   (maximal in adduction) and also intorts and abducts and the
   inferior oblique raises the eye (maximal on adduction) and also
   extorts and abducts. Stated differently and perhaps more
   simply, the superior rectus elevates when the eye is turned
   outwards; the inferior rectus depresses when the eye is turned
   outwards; the superior oblique depresses when the eye turns
   inwards; and the inferior oblique elevates the eye when it turns
   inwards. The resultant false image, if any of these muscles is
   affected, is not truly vertical or horizontal but tilted. Tilting
   is especially likely with either superior or inferior oblique
   involvement. There are simple rules about tilting, but such
   detailed knowledge is quite unnecessary except for the
   specialist. A brief account is as follows. If the images are
   vertical and parallel then the muscles affected must be either
   the medial or lateral rectus. If the images are horizontal or
   tilted the superior or inferior recti or either of the obliques
   must be affected.

The technique to be followed in attempting to identify the
muscle or muscles affected in a case where the simple rules are
unhelpful is to place glasses of different colours in front of each
eye so that the examiner can immediately determine which image
is coming from which eye. A small light is then slowly moved through
a complete circle, the patient being asked to say throughout the whole
range of movement whether or not he has diplopia and, if so, to
describe the exact position and colour of the images. A diagram is
thus obtained which can be interpreted by anybody conversant with
this type of work. However, as stated above, no purpose is to be
gained by the non-specialist memorizing any such examples.

Chameleon eye movements are rolling and rotatory independent movements of the two eyes and are reputed to be pathognomonic of tuberculous meningitis.

THIRD CRANIAL NERVE

Localization

A complete paralysis of the third nerve produces the following signs:

1. An external ophthalmoplegia affecting some or all of the external ocular muscles (except the external rectus and superior oblique) with resultant diplopia, squint and defective ocular movement.
2. A large circular and regular pupil, which does not react to light directly or consensually and does not react to accommodation (a fixed pupil — an internal ophthalmoplegia).
3. Ptosis, which is a drooping of the eyelid and the inability to elevate it completely. When ptosis is due to a third nerve palsy, unlike when due to other causes, it is frequently complete.

Third nerve palsies are more often partial than complete and the examiner must be prepared to diagnose a third nerve lesion with only a few signs, but ptosis is never the sole evidence of such a lesion. As a general rule, the nearer the lesion is to the nucleus the more likely it is to be partial.

The next task must be to attempt to locate the lesion more accurately. If it is at site 1, the nucleus, it is frequently partial and usually bilateral as anatomical considerations indicate. The commonest nuclear lesions are a plaque of disseminated sclerosis, neoplasms, inflammatory lesions such as encephalitis lethargica, small haemorrhages, and aplasia (lack of development).

If the lesion is at site 2, within the substance of the mid-brain, then it is likely to be associated with involvement of any of those structures near which it passes. The commonest association is that of an ipsilateral third nerve lesion with a contralateral upper motor neurone hemiplegia (Weber's* syndrome) due to a lesion of the crus. This is an example of a crossed or alternate paralysis, which means an ipsilateral lower motor neurone lesion of a cranial nerve and a contralateral upper motor neurone hemiplegia. The importance of any crossed paralysis is that it localizes the lesion to the brain stem (mid-brain, pons or medulla) — in Weber's syndrome, to the mid-brain. The commonest cause of this condition is thrombosis of a branch of the posterior cerebral artery.

Much rarer syndromes involving the third nerve in the mid-brain can be worked out from *Figure 5*. There may be an ipsilateral third nerve palsy with involuntary movement of the contralateral upper

---

*Sir Herman Weber (1823–1918), a London physician.

limb, usually a coarse compound tremor but perhaps choreiform or athetoid. This is due to involvement of the red nucleus and/or the substantia nigra, both of which are extrapyramidal structures. Or the patient may have an ipsilateral third nerve palsy plus ataxia, with the eyes open of the ipsilateral limbs, due to involvement of the nearby corticocerebellar fibres of the crus. Both the syndromes described above are extremely rare.

If the patient has an isolated unilateral third nerve lesion, the probable cause is a lesion in part 3 of the course of the nerve in the interpeduncular space, the commonest causes being aneurysms, neurosyphilis, tuberculous meningitis and a fractured base of the skull. It must be appreciated that a patient with a unilateral third nerve lesion may also have an ipsilateral fourth nerve lesion which will be difficult to recognize. An important feature of part 3 of the course is its relationship to the circle of Willis, and this explains why the third nerve is so commonly affected by aneurysms, a common site of which is the junction of the posterior cerebral artery with the posterior communicating artery. A partial or complete third nerve palsy may then be due to direct pressure by the aneurysm, to leakage from it, or to actual rupture.

Whatever may be the reason, the third nerve is frequently involved in raised intracranial tension and, moreover, such involvement by itself has no localizing value. An explanation has been given that this involvement occurs because with raised intracranial tension there is distension of the whole of the intracranial venous system, including enlargement of the posterior cerebral and superior cerebellar veins between which the third nerve passes, with a consequent nipping of this nerve between the distended veins. This appears to be a rather far-fetched explanation, but so is the more usual one that the involvement occurs because the nerve has a long and tortuous course and so is likely to be compressed by any displacement of the brain stem, a feature which is not peculiar to the third nerve.

In part 4 of the course of the nerve, its involvement is likely to be associated with that of any or all of its neighbours — the fourth, the ophthalmic division of the fifth, and the sixth nerve. The common lesions of the cavernous sinus are aneurysms and thrombosis. Cavernous sinus lesions may also be associated with exophthalmos (undue prominence of the eye), which is then likely to be bilateral although asymmetrical. When the lesions are caused by sinus thrombosis, chemosis (oedema and redness of the bulbar conjunctiva) and sometimes papilloedema are also present.

Because part 5 of its course is within the orbit, which is also entered by the fourth, the ophthalmic division of the fifth and the sixth nerve, any of these may be affected together with the third nerve. In this case the distinction from a lesion at site 4 may be difficult, but a unilateral exophthalmos strongly favours the localization of the lesion to the orbit. The common lesions of the orbit are fractures and retro-orbital swellings such as primary and secondary neoplasms, reticuloses and aneurysms.

Any ocular palsy may be due to a lesion of the muscles themselves, as seen in myasthenia gravis and exophthalmic ophthalmoplegia.

Ptosis

Ptosis is a drooping of the upper eyelid associated with an inability to elevate it completely. A ptosis can be easily missed unless the patient is sitting up and his head is held by the observer. Any ptosis may be partial or complete, unilateral or bilateral, and asssociated or not associated with overaction of the frontalis. The causes of ptosis are as follows:

1. It may be due to a third nerve lesion, when it is likely to be unilateral and associated with overaction of the frontalis. It is often complete. Supporting evidence may be an external and an internal ophthalmoplegia.
2. It may be due to a sympathetic paralysis, in which case it is always partial, is very rarely bilateral, and is usually unassociated with any frontalis overaction. Meiosis and lack of sweating on that side of the face will be supporting evidence.
3. It may be due to a muscle lesion such as myasthenia gravis, facio-scapulo-humeral myopathy, or dystrophia myotonica. It will then always be bilateral, usually be partial, and be unassociated with any frontalis overaction because that muscle is also affected.
4. An hysterical ptosis is always complete and associated with spasm of the orbicularis oculi, but there is no overaction of the frontalis. It is likely to be unilateral.
5. Congenital ptosis is common. It may be unilateral or bilateral, and is always partial and associated with frontalis overaction. It is present since birth and is unassociated with any other positive findings in the nervous system.
6. Tabes dorsalis and dementia paralytica usually cause a bilateral ptosis, which is always partial and accompanied by overaction of the frontalis. This important cause is mentioned separately because the site producing it is controversial.

FOURTH CRANIAL NERVE

Clinical Aspects

Paralysis of the fourth nerve does not produce an obvious squint, but when the patient looks outwards and downwards a wheel movement of the globe may be noticed, especially if a conjunctival vessel is carefully observed (this is a difficult sign to be sure of). Diplopia is usually found in every position of the eyeball except when looking directly upwards.

An isolated fourth nerve lesion is very unusual and is likely to be due to a lesion at the base of the brain in the interpeduncular space, most commonly a fracture of the base. Sometimes at this site the third nerve is also involved. If, in addition, the ophthalmic fifth or the sixth nerve is affected, then the lesions will be further forward in the cavernous sinus or orbit.

SIXTH CRANIAL NERVE

Clinical Aspects

The sole manifestation of sixth nerve involvement is a paralysis of the external rectus. Any lesion in part 1 of the nerve pathway is likely to be associated with a crossed paralysis, with ipsilateral lower motor neurone lesions of the seventh nerve together with a sixth nerve palsy and a contralateral upper motor neurone hemiplegia. Frequently this crossed paralysis is only partial, the sixth nerve palsy being absent, and in that case the lesion may be in the upper part of the pons and will then be associated with a paralysis of conjugate deviation. Any lesion of the pons may give rise to such a crossed paralysis, either partial or complete. However, in the case of haemorrhage into the pons the resultant lesion will be very extensive, causing upper motor neurone paralysis of all four limbs with rapidly increasing depth of coma. Paralysis of the facial or ocular muscles and the limbs in such a patient will be extremely difficult if not impossible to recognize. Suspicion that the lesion is pontine will be created by the presence of pin-point pupils and hyperpyrexia in a patient with a rapidly increasing depth of coma.

The description of part 2 of the course of the sixth nerve explains why it may be involved with aneurysms of the circle of Willis, and may provide a possible explanation (*see* section on third nerve above) why occasionally the nerve is affected by raised intracranial tension without this being a localizing sign. The nerve may be involved in any of the common lesions of the cerebello-pontine angle, which are: (1) neoplasms, for example acoustic neuroma; (2) basal meningitis, especially tuberculous or syphilitic; (3) fractured base; (4) aneurysms.

The fact that the sixth nerve crosses the petrous temporal bone explains why, as a complication of otitis media, an ipsilateral sixth nerve palsy may occur and very occasionally there may be pain in the distribution of any part of the sensory fifth. This is because the infection has spread and caused an osteomyelitis of the apex of the petrous bone, and meningitis or cerebral abscess is then likely unless the condition is urgently treated. Parts 3 and 4 of the nerve, and the results and causes of such involvement, have been discussed in relation to the third nerve.

The fifth cranial nerve

ANATOMY

This is a mixed nerve with motor and sensory divisions. Both the sensory and the motor nuclei are situated in the mid-pons, but the former extends downwards through the medulla as far as the third cervical segment of the cord. This extension explains why sensory disturbance of the face may occur with lesions of either the medulla or the upper cervical cord. The two roots exit from the lateral border of the pons and in the cerebello-pontine angle pass almost directly outwards, the motor root being beneath the sensory one. Both branches in the outermost part of their course lie on the petrous portion of the temporal bone in the middle cranial fossa, and here the sensory division has on it an enlargement called the Gasserian* ganglion, the motor division being immediately beneath this. From the sensory division emerge three branches – the ophthalmic, the maxillary and the mandibular.

The ophthalmic division of the sensory fifth nerve runs near the lateral wall of the cavernous sinus together with the third, fourth and sixth nerves; it is joined by fibres from the cervical sympathetic, and then enters the orbit via the superior orbital fissure. It supplies sensation to the conjunctiva, the cornea, the upper eyelid, part of the nasal mucosa, the bridge of the nose, the forehead, and the scalp as far back as the vertex. There is much overlap in the distribution of the supply from each of the three sensory branches of the fifth and with the supply from the second, third and fourth cervical roots. The sympathetic fibres which travel alongside those of the ophthalmic division of the fifth supply the dilator pupillae and the levator palpebrae superioris (also supplied by the third nerve) and control the sweat mechanism of the face and possibly lacrymation.

The maxillary sensory division exits from the skull via the foramen rotundum. It passes across the pterygo-palatine fossa and along the infra-orbital canal to emerge from the infra-orbital foramen on the anterior aspect of the maxilla, 1½ inches below the lower rim of the orbit. From there its terminal twigs branch out and supply sensation to the cheek, the lateral aspect of the nose, the upper teeth and jaw, and the mucous membranes of part of the nasal cavity, uvula, hard palate and nasopharynx.

The mandibular sensory division, together with the motor root, leaves the skull via the foramen ovale and supplies sensation to the lower teeth and gums and to the mucous membranes of the floor of the mouth and the buccal surface of the cheeks. The motor division supplies the pterygoid, temporalis and masseter muscles as well as small muscles, for example, the anterior belly of the digastric and the mylohyoid, which cannot be tested clinically.

*Johann Laurenz Gasser (1723–63), Professor of Anatomy in Vienna, 1757– 65.

EXAMINATION

The sensory fifth nerve is tested clinically by examination of the corneal reflexes and sensations of the appropriate area of the face. The motor fifth is tested by asking the patient to clench his teeth, when the muscles can be seen and felt. Patients who for any reason have lost a good deal of weight will develop a thin face with hollowing of the cheeks but this is due to loss of fat and not muscle-wasting and must not be mistaken for a neurological lesion. The simplest way of testing the pterygoids is to ask the patient to open his mouth against slight resistance: if the jaw persistently involuntarily deviates to one side, then provided he has not got a dislocated jaw, he must have a weakness of the pterygoid muscles. The deviation is always to the paralysed side. Because of their position, wasting of the pterygoids cannot be seen but the weakness is shown by deviation of the jaw. On the other hand, although wasting of the temporalis and masseters can be seen above and below the zygoma respectively (this is easier to appreciate if the lesion is unilateral), the power of these muscles is difficult to assess, especially if the lesion is unilateral. It is important, therefore, to test both groups of muscles.

Bilateral lower motor neurone lesions of the fifth nerve muscles are commonly seen with the muscle diseases and occasionally with motor neurone disease and in all these conditions there is also likely to be bilateral wasting of the facial muscles supplied by the seventh nerve. Unilateral lesions of the motor fifth nerve are rare and must be of lower motor neurone type because these muscles are bilaterally innervated. A bilateral upper motor neurone lesion of the fifth nerves is due to a lesion above their nuclei and an important piece of evidence is the presence of a jaw jerk or actual jaw clonus which can therefore be of great importance when localizing the cause of an upper motor neurone quadriplegia. The jaw jerk is elicited by asking the patient to half open his mouth and allowing the jaw to sag and the examiner puts a finger horizontally below the lower lip, which he then percusses with a tendon hammer. The response is normally difficult to appreciate but if there is a bilateral upper motor fifth lesion it results in a very brisk response which might even amount to a true clonus.

Loss of the corneal reflex is often the first manifestation of fifth nerve involvement. This reflex is tested rather than the conjunctival because the latter may be lost in hysteria, whereas loss of the corneal reflex is always organic. Before doing the corneal reflex the patient must be told what you are going to do so as to avoid any flinching which would make the interpretation of the result difficult. It is a reflex of which the afferent arc is the ophthalmic division of the fifth nerve and the efferent arc is the facial nerve branch supplying the orbicularis oculi. Theoretically, therefore, a lower motor neurone lesion of the seventh nerve will also cause a loss of the corneal reflex. In this case, however, because the cornea is still sensitive, stimulating it will cause closure of the opposite eye and withdrawal of the head away from the stimulus.

TRIGEMINAL NEURALGIA

Trigeminal neuralgia (tic douloureux) is a condition of unknown aetiology without demonstrable pathology. When considering this diagnosis the following points are important:
1. The condition is unusual before late middle age.
2. It is rarely bilateral.
3. The pain is always paroxysmal and never continuous; it is localized to the distribution of one (least commonly the first) or more divisions of the nerve, and never radiates to areas not supplied by the fifth nerve.
4. The pain is either spontaneous or evoked by any stimulus applied to the affected zone, and there are often complete spontaneous remissions lasting weeks or even months.
5. On clinical examination there are no motor, sensory or reflex changes of the fifth nerve, and no positive signs in the nervous system apart from the trigger zones of hyperaesthesiae which, when stimulated, produce the pain.

The Gasserian ganglion may be involved by herpes zoster, causing vesicles over the affected segment or segments (always unilateral), together with pain and loss of sensation in the area. If the ophthalmic division is affected, then the cornea may be seriously involved, either because of the development of vesicles which become infected, or because of a neurokeratitis secondary to anaesthesia of the cornea. Oedema of the upper lid, conjunctivitis especially of the lid margins, scleritis, episcleritis and iritis are all fairly common complications.

The seventh cranial nerve

ANATOMY

Part 1 of the course of this nerve in the pons (*see Figure 7*) and part 2 of its course in the cerebello-pontine angle have already been described in the section on the sixth nerve.

Part 3 of its course is in the facial canal. The nerve exits from the skull through the internal auditory meatus, together with the eighth nerve, the pars intermedia and the auditory artery, and enters the facial canal. In the canal the nerve has on it an enlargement known as the geniculate ganglion, which is joined by the pars intermedia and also by the great and small superficial petrosal nerves. The small superficial petrosal has connections via the otic ganglion with the fifth and ninth nerves, and the great superficial petrosal with the maxillary fifth via the spheno-palatine ganglion, and both petrosals have central connections with the nucleus solitarius via the pars intermedia. These petrosal nerves carry parasympathetic fibres to the salivary and lacrimal glands. Within the canal, the seventh nerve gives off the nerve to the stapedius and the chorda tympani (perhaps more correctly stated, the chorda tympani joins the facial nerve), and the nerve then exists from the stylomastoid foramen.

Part 4 is the peripheral distribution. The nerve, winding around the angle of the jaw, enters the substance of the parotid gland, where it divides into its terminal branches which supply all the facial muscles except the levator palpebrae superioris.

TASTE

The pathway for taste is complex and much of it is controversial, but some practical elementary considerations should be understood.

Substances placed in the mouth probably initiate complex chemical reactions. The various chemical products thus created stimulate the receptor end-organs, the taste buds, which are situated in the papillae at the tip, sides and back of the tongue. From the anterior two-thirds of the tongue, taste sensation is transmitted along the lingual nerve (a branch of the fifth nerve), then via the chorda tympani nerve to the facial nerve, and thus to the geniculate ganglion and thereby, via the pars intermedia, to the nucleus solitarius in the medulla. From there the pathway is to both sides of the cerebral cortex (probably temporal), appreciation of nuances of taste being an intellectual pastime. Taste sensation from the posterior third of the tongue is usually described as travelling along the glosso-pharyngeal nerve directly to the nucleus solitarius (which lies lateral to the dorsal nucleus of the tenth nerve) and then to the temporal cortex. Another view holds that the pathway is via the glosso-pharyngeal nerve, through the petrosal plexuses, to the otic and spheno-palatine ganglia, via the petrosal nerves to the geniculate ganglion, and thence via the pars intermedia to the nucleus solitarius.

Testing taste is not a routine procedure, but in a patient with a lower motor neurone facial palsy it may help to localize the lesion, because if it is lost over the anterior two-thirds of the tongue on the same side, then the lesion must be in the facial canal. There are four fundamental tastes — sweet, sour, bitter and salt — and the technique involves the successive application to the part of the tongue to be tested of powders or solutions which represent examples of the above fundamental tastes, such as sugar, lemon, quinine and common salt. The tongue is firmly held during the whole procedure, and by some prearranged sign the patient intimates what he believes to be the nature of each substance applied to his tongue. The mouth must be rinsed between each test. He must not be allowed to talk because this would necessitate letting go of his tongue and the dispersal of the substance over a larger area than that to be tested. Testing taste sensation over the posterior third of the tongue is a waste of time.

CLINICAL ASPECTS

A methodical technique is needed for testing the facial muscles, which comprise a group of muscles. Merely asking the patient to smile or show his teeth, as is so frequently done, is therefore a grossly inadequate performance. Perhaps the best way is to test the muscles from above downwards. The frontalis wrinkles the forehead. The orbicularis oculi closes the eyelids tightly, so that the upper lid cannot be raised by the examiner. The nasal muscles wrinkle the nose and dilate and narrow the nostrils. The buccinator blows out the cheeks. The orbicularis oris is demonstrated on whistling, the levator anguli oris and risorius by smiling and showing the teeth, and the platysma by drawing down the lower lip and the angles of the mouth while wrinkling the skin of the neck. Mouth closure is tested by the patient tightly apposing his lips and attempting to prevent the examiner from pulling the upper lip upwards and the lower lip downwards.

In any facial palsy, whether upper or lower motor neurone, the patient may have only two or three muscles affected. It is far better to consider the actual muscles than to refer to upper and lower halves of the face and regard an upper motor neurone lesion as one that spares the frontalis and/or the orbicularis oculi muscles, which have identities of their own and which have been tested separately. Moreover, it is important that if either of these muscles is affected, and not necessarily both, then the lesion must be of a lower motor neurone type.

The error of diagnosing a non-existent facial palsy is far commoner than that of missing one. This could in large measure be obviated by hesitating to diagnose a facial palsy merely on a slight degree of facial asymmetry, because the majority of normal people have a minor degree of such asymmetry at rest — for example, the naso-labial groove being more prominent on one side than on the other. Moreover, although it is true that the earliest manifestations of an upper motor neurone type of facial palsy may be observed only on spontaneous emotional movement, such a diagnosis requires a great deal of experience and is likely to be wrong when made by the inexpert. Remember that a patient with any facial palsy may have dysarthria and dysphagia due to paralysis of the lips.

An upper motor neurone facial palsy is, in the great majority of cases, part of an upper motor neurone hemiplegia. It may, however, occur by itself. The lesion is then in the opposite frontal cortex and, if the facial paralysis is right-sided, is likely to be associated with a motor aphasia because the face and the motor speech areas are contiguous. This area is fairly frequently involved as the result of a cerebral thrombosis affecting the inferior frontal branch of the middle cerebral artery.

If the facial palsy is of lower motor neurone type, the next task is to localize the lesion, which may be anywhere from the facial muscles to the nucleus. If it is due to muscle disease such as myasthenia gravis, facio-scapulo-humeral myopathy or dystrophia myotonica, it is always bilateral and usually symmetrical and, in addition to weakness of the muscles supplied by the facial nerve, the levatores palpebrae superioris are usually involved, causing a bilateral ptosis (without compensatory overaction of the frontalis), and there is often bilateral involvement of the fifth nerve muscles. Bilateral facial nerve involvement is rare and, when present, is generally due to a peripheral neuritis, for example, acute infective polyneuritis. If the lesion is in part 4 of the course of the nerve, the result will be a lower motor neurone facial palsy without neurological accompaniments. The cause of this lesion is most often a Bell's palsy, but it may be due to pathology of the parotid gland or to an injury, for example a mastoid operation. If the lesion is in the facial canal, there will be a lower motor neurone facial palsy with loss of taste in the anterior two-thirds of that side of the tongue. In addition there may be hyperacusis from involvement of the stapedius, but this is extremely rare. When the geniculate ganglion itself is affected, usually by the herpes zoster virus, a syndrome results which is characterized by a lower motor neurone facial palsy, plus loss of taste of the anterior two-thirds of the same side of the tongue, plus the occurrence of herpes vesicles in the region of the external auditory meatus. Such vesicles are extremely painful, and the pain may precede the onset of the facial palsy. Occasionally pain also occurs in the region of the ipsilateral fauces, and vesicles may then be found in that area.

Bell's palsy is a lower motor neurone facial palsy of unknown aetiology, although often considered to be due to a virus infection. The site of the lesion is probably in the region of the stylomastoid foramen, but if taste is involved, this must mean that the involvement has spread up the canal. It is wrong to describe other lower motor neurone facial lesions — for example, those due to a parotid tumour — as Bell's palsy. Lower motor neurone facial palsies due to lesions in part 2 and part 1 of the course of the nerve are considered with such nerve lesions.

The eighth cranial nerve

THE COCHLEAR NERVE

The eighth cranial nerve has two components, the cochlear (auditory) and the vestibular.

The cochlear nerve arises from the end-organ in the internal ear called the organ of Corti, and the nerve fibres are gathered together as a single nerve from which arises a ganglion, the spiral ganglion. After a very short course within the internal ear, it is joined by the vestibular nerve to form a common eighth nerve which travels in the facial canal, exits through the internal auditory meatus, and then runs in the cerebello-pontine angle. The relationships of the eighth nerve in these sites have already been discussed.

In the cerebello-pontine angle, when it is near the brain stem the nerve again divides into its two components, the cochlear fibres going to the lower (caudal) part of the pons, where they terminate on each side in two nuclei, the dorsal (tuberculum acousticum) and ventral nuclei of the cochlea. The two dorsal nuclei are connected by fibres (striae acousticae) which run directly backwards, exit from the dorsal border of the lower part of the pons, and lie on the floor of the fourth ventricle. The two ventral nuclei are joined together within the substance of the central grey matter of the pons by a commissural tract, the trapezoid body (corpus trapezium) (*Figure 8*). By means of these commissural tracts, hearing from each ear passes to both sides of the brain.

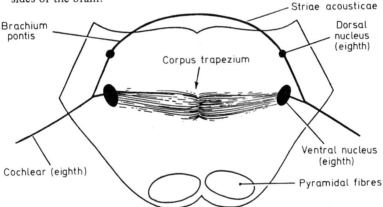

Figure 8. *Schematic diagram of the lower part of the pons showing the arrangement of the two ventral nuclei*

The relay arising from the dorsal and ventral nuclei on each side is known as the lateral lemniscus. This, after a short course through the pons, terminates in the medial geniculate body and the inferior corpora quadrigemina of the mid-brain. From these centres the final relay, the auditory radiation, goes through the posterior limb of the internal capsule to the temporal cortex.

Clinical aspects
Hearing can be tested adequately only in a quiet room. As a routine it is usually sufficient to note the patient's ability to hear conversation

in a quiet tone. Each side is tested separately and hearing on the opposite side is prevented as much as possible by the patient inserting a finger into that ear or by the physician rubbing the tragus of the ear not being tested in a rotatory manner, rustling a piece of paper close to that ear, or using a specially constructed noise box. For accurate quantitative assessment of hearing, especially to detect early nerve deafness, an audiometer is essential. Using a watch is not a good method because it tests only sounds of high frequency.

If a patient is deaf, the first procedure must be an attempt to differentiate between nerve (perceptive) deafness and middle ear (conduction) deafness. This is done with a tuning fork, which should be of a pitch C256, C512 or higher, because perceptive deafness is always more marked for higher pitch. Normally, air conduction is better than that of bone. With an eighth nerve lesion, air conduction remains better than that of bone, but the patient is also deaf; whereas if the deafness is of middle ear type, bone conduction becomes better than that of air. There are various ways of demonstrating this. One test (Rinne* test) is carried out by placing the tuning fork over the mastoid process for a few seconds and then in front of the ear and noting which is louder, or keeping the fork over the mastoid process until it cannot be heard and then putting it in front of the ear, or the order of placing may be reversed. Hearing the fork better over the mastoid process indicates a conduction deafness. Another test (Weber), useful in unilateral deafness, is performed by placing the tuning fork in the centre of the forehead, when if the deafness is of conduction type it will be heard better on the deaf side and not equally well on both sides as is normal. Unfortunately these tests, as done by the inexpert, frequently give equivocal results because of crude technique; for example, when doing the first test the hearing should be completely excluded from the ear not being tested.

It follows from anatomical considerations that unilateral nerve deafness must be due to a lesion of the nerve itself and not of the brain. In an elderly patient with nerve deafness, the possibility of Paget's disease of the skull should always be considered, whereas in young adults the possibility of congenital syphilis must be borne in mind.

THE VESTIBULAR NERVE

The vestibular nerve endings are in the labyrinth, which is part of the internal ear. It is situated in a tunnel in the petrous temporal bone and consists of the three semicircular canals, the saccule and the utricle.

The three semicircular canals are at right angles each to the others,

*Heinrich A. Rinne (1819–68), a German otologist.

representing the three planes of space, and are known as the horizontal (or external) and the anterior and posterior vertical canals. They are ring-shaped bony canals and within them is a membranous canal containing fluid, the endolymph. Part of the canal is dilated (the ampulla), and within this is situated the receptor organ, the crista acoustica, from which arise vestibular nerve endings. The crista is stimulated by movement of the endolymph.

In the saccule and the utricle there is a different mechanism. Their walls are lined by a gelatinous substance in which are concretions called otoliths, and also other vestibular nerve endings which are stimulated by movement of the otoliths. A simplification of the differences in action between the otolith and endolymph mechanisms is that the former indicates a patient's position in space, whether he is lying on his right side or left side, whether he is standing on his head or feet, whereas the latter mechanism comes into play on movement of the body. Stated differently, the otoliths record gravitational forces and the endolymph movement, especially rotation.

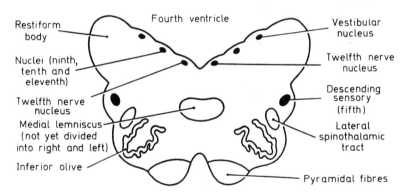

Figure 9. *Schematic diagram of the open medulla showing the pathway of the twelfth cranial nerve*

The vestibular nerve endings from both mechanisms form a single vestibular nerve within the labyrinth, which has on it a ganglion (vestibular) and which, after a very short course, is joined in the internal ear by the cochlear nerve. The combined nerve traverses the facial canal, exists through the internal auditory meatus and travels in the cerebello-pontine angle to the brain stem, near which the vestibular fibres separate from the cochlear nerve to terminate in a group of four nuclei situated in the lateral part of the dorsum of the open medulla (*Figure 9*). From these nuclei the next relay is mainly to the cerebellum via the restiform body but, in addition, there are the vestibulo-spinal tract (part of the extrapyramidal system) and fibres to the medial longitudinal bundle of the mid-brain, thereby making connections with the third, fourth, sixth and tenth nerves on both sides. The medial longitudinal bundle acts as a co-ordinating pathway for impulses from external ocular muscles, the neck muscles and the vestibular nuclei.

Vertigo

The principle manifestation of lesions of the vestibular pathway is vertigo. Vertigo is an hallucination of movement either of the patient himself or of objects around him resulting in a sensation of disturbed balance which varies in severity from a feeling of swaying to an inability to stand without support, the patient reeling and staggering if he attempts to walk and he may even fall. It is commonly accompanied by any or all of the following, and is usually accentuated by head movements.

1. A feeling of fear and apprehension.
2. Reflex bulbar phenomena, nausea, vomiting and sweating.

It is extremely important to realize that all these associated phenomena are common occurrences with vertigo from any cause, and that they should be considered as part of the vertigo and be included within the definition. Moreover, any one of them may dominate the clinical picture.

If this definition of vertigo is strictly adhered to then it becomes a very important localizing symptom indicating a lesion of the vestibular apparatus or the vestibular nerve or its central connections. Certainly if a patient spontaneously volunteers that he gets giddy spells and describes his symptoms in such terms as a sensation of whirling around, then the physician can have little doubt that the patient really has vertigo. Vertigo can be produced in a normal person if he turns round quickly around a vertical axis and then stops suddenly. This causes an overstimulation of the lateral canals and produces a sensation that everything is spinning round and the person himself actually becomes unsteady and may stagger or stumble. On the other hand motion in a ship, car or plane may produce vertigo in a normal person by overstimulation of centres in the cerebellum by stimuli from the vestibular end organs. The symptoms from this procedure are likely to differ from those produced by rotation, being mainly nausea and vomiting and sometimes without any feeling of disequilibrium as long as the motion continues, but they may develop when the person sets foot on firm ground. Motion sickness is a long-drawn-out and less severe form of vertigo but whether produced by rotation or by motion the symptoms can in each case correctly be called vertigo.

Attempts should be made to differentiate between vertigo, giddiness and dizziness, while appreciating that these terms are commonly used by lay people who regard them as synonyms. It is therefore imperative that the patient should attempt to describe his symptoms in simple language, explaining what he himself means by the terms he uses. But it is important that differences between these terms should not be suggested to the patient by the physician, who should also appreciate that it is difficult even for a trained observer to describe an attack which is transitory and often charged with emotion.

The physician in this context must never be guilty of the Procrustean offence of deciding whether or not the patient had vertigo after the physician has previously made up his mind that the patient has a lesion of the vestibular pathway.

Unfortunately attempts by neurologists to monopolize the word vertigo to its technical and restricted use described previously rarely has the support or understanding not only of lay people but also many doctors.

Vertigo may be (1) in brief paroxysms, (2) slight in degree but longer in duration with a continued sense of loss of balance, (3) only induced by certain movements or postures. These three types overlap and combinations of them may occur. Paroxysmal vertigo is most often due to lesions of the vestibular end organs. There is a considerable variety of the descriptions of the false sensations of movement which the patient may give. The sense of movement is usually in an horizontal plane but may occasionally be in a vertical or oblique plane. The vertigo may be subjective or objective and may last for minutes or hours; the longer it lasts the more likely is it to be followed by nausea and vomiting. When paroxysmal vertigo is due to a lesion of the brain stem, for example due to disseminated sclerosis or arterial occlusion, it often lasts for days.

The commonest complaint with the second type of vertigo, that is the more chronic forms, is a feeling of always being drunk and staggering and stumbling when walking. Often the peculiar sense of discomfort and anxiety which vertigo commonly implies is absent, but headache often described as 'a muzzy feeling in the head', is common. Chronic vertigo is most often due to progressive lesions of the vestibular pathway. A general rule is that vertigo from central lesions is likely to last longer and be more permanent than with peripheral lesions, and this is also true of the associated nystagmus.

Postural vertigo occurs only with changes of posture and is transient. It occurs especially when the vertigo is due to circulatory disturbance or closed head injuries. The patient usually exhibits symptoms as well as vertigo as long as the inducing posture is maintained.

Labyrinthine tests can be divided into those easily performed and those requiring special skills and apparatus. No investigation of labyrinthine function should ever be undertaken unless the patient's symptoms are characteristic of a disorder of the vestibular end organs or their connections.

The labyrinth may be stimulated by galvanic current applied to the mastoid, by rotation of the patient (but this stimulates both sides), or by caloric means, syringing the ear with either hot or ice-cold water. Stimulation of the labyrinth of a normal person will in 15–30 seconds produce (1) vertigo; (2) phasic nystagmus lasting one to two minutes (*see* section on nystagmus); (3) postural defects – for example, inability to maintain the position of the outstretched arms or a persistent falling in one particular direction on standing with the feet together and the eyes open; (4) hypermetria, which means that voluntary movements are excessive in range, producing overshooting of the mark on an attempt to touch an object (often referred to as 'past-pointing'). The rotation test has no localizing value within the vestibular pathway, but is of particular value in determining semicircular canal sensitivity. Further consideration of the details of the above phenomena as elicited by caloric tests, such as their precise direction, will depend upon whether hot or cold water is used and which semicircular canals are stimulated (this depends upon the position of the head), but all such details are beyond the scope of this elementary description and the non-specialist student is not advised to attempt to memorize them.

The standard procedure is for the patient to be lying down with his head raised about 30 degrees above the horizontal. This position brings the lateral semicircular canal into the vertical plane and is the position of maximal sensitivity to thermal stimuli. The labyrinths are stimulated by syringing the ear with water at 30°C and then at 44°C, each for 40 seconds. The cold water initiates nystagmus to the opposite side and the warm water to the same side. The patient fixes his gaze on a point straight ahead, and the physician records the time interval from the beginning of the syringing to the disappearance of the induced nystagmus.

The importance of the tests is that disease of the labyrinth will produce delayed, brief, diminished or absent responses and will be proof that the triad of symptoms (vertigo, tinnitus and deafness) is due to labyrinthine disease.

Apart from physiological stimulation, the common labyrinthine lesions are infection secondary to otitis media; toxic conditions due to quinine, salicylates, tobacco or streptomycin; haemorrhages, for example in blood disease such as leukaemia; and Ménière's* syndrome.

Minor epidemics, and occasionally sporadic cases, of severe vertigo of unknown aetiology occur. This condition has been given various appellations such as epidemic vertigo and vestibular neuronitis. The vertigo, which is often very severe, is of sudden onset and often associated with vomiting, but not with tinnitus or deafness. It usually lasts for several days, but may continue for weeks. It may simulate the ictus of a cerebral vascular lesion. It is of unknown pathology.

*Prosper Ménière (1799–1862), a French physician.

Ménière's syndrome

Ménière's syndrome is a condition characterized by paroxysmal labyrinthine disturbance in a patient with a previously healthy auditory apparatus. The aetiology of the disease is unknown and it is usually regarded as a degenerative lesion. Distension with endolymph of the whole of the labyrinthine system has been demonstrated. The syndrome is a disease of the middle and upper age groups, rarely occurring before the age of forty-five years. Headache, which may be severe, is a common accompaniment and may dominate the symptomatology. The tinnitus is described as a buzzing or ringing or whistling in the ear. The deafness is of the perceptive type, especially affecting low frequency sounds and later in the disease becomes bilateral although asymmetrical. It is usually most marked following each attack and improves quickly but not completely leaving ever increasing residual damage. An essential feature is that the symptoms are paroxysmal and not continuous. The severity, duration and frequency of the attacks are extremely variable. During the attacks nystagmus and ataxia of the limbs may occur but these clear up completely by the end of the attack leaving no residual signs. Between the attacks there must be no abnormal physical signs apart from some residual nerve deafness and reduced responses to caloric stimulation. If any other findings are present, such as ataxia, then the cause is an organic lesion of the vestibular nerve itself, for example, an acoustic neuroma.

Vestibular nerve lesions

The labyrinthine pathway must be affected along the course of the vestibular nerve itself, for example in the cerebello-pontine angle, and there is then likely to be involvement of the fifth, sixth and/or seventh cranial nerves and possibly of the cerebellum itself. But the vestibular nerve may be involved alone, and in the case of an acoustic neuroma, early diagnosis before other structures become affected is important.

Lesions of the vestibular nerve also give rise to the triad of vertigo, tinnitus and deafness because the cochlear nerve is running with it. In this case, if no other signs are present, the distinction between a labyrinthine and a vestibular nerve lesion may be difficult. Caloric tests used to be employed for this purpose because, whereas in lesions of the labyrinth itself depression of responses occurs, if the lesion is in the vestibular nerve qualitative rather than quantitative alterations will be present. However, no purpose is served by describing these subtleties because, for the purpose of this differentiation, caloric tests have been replaced by audiometric testing, the details of which the non-specialist should not attempt to memorize, especially if he cannot understand the technical jargon used.

Brain stem vertigo

The labyrinthine pathway may be involved in the lateral portion of the medulla because of a lesion of the vestibular nuclei, the restiform body, or both. In this case the vertigo will not be associated with tinnitus or deafness unless the pons is also involved, since the cochlear nerve travels independently to the pons. Usually there are other localizing signs indicating the medullary site of the lesion. The common lesions in this area are disseminated sclerosis, neoplasms, aneurysms and thrombosis of the posterior inferior cerebellar artery.

For details of the features of nystagmus associated with brain stem lesions, *see* the section on nystagmus.

Cerebellar giddiness

The labyrinthine pathway may also be involved by lesions of the cerebellum, especially those of the vermis. In this case the giddiness will not be associated with either tinnitus or deafness. An important point is that whereas any disease of the cerebellum may give rise to vertigo, in practice it is frequently found that extensive cerebellar lesions can occur without any vertigo whatsoever. That the vertigo is due to cerebellar disease will be proved by the finding of other cerebellar signs.

Cerebral giddiness

Under the heading of vertigo probably of cerebral origin are included raised intracranial tension (especially when due to a posterior fossa lesion), epilepsy and migraine. With raised intracranial tension, headache, vomiting and papilloedema are usually the dominant manifestations, but vertigo, which is not a localizing sign, is an extremely common association. Vertigo is a very frequent aura of epileptiform attacks, and in migraine it may dominate the symptomatology, being more distressing than the headache itself. The exact site of the lesion causing vertigo in these three instances is unknown, but there is presumed to be a transitory interference with cerebral function, probably affecting the temporal lobes.

Psychogenic giddiness

Giddiness of psychogenic origin is probably the commonest of all. It is usually objective rather than subjective, is rarely rotatory, and is often described as a 'light-headedness' or a 'swimming sensation' in the head. It is almost invariably associated with a feeling of uncertainty and paraesthesiae in the lower limbs, the patient complaining, for example, of numbness of the feet or that he feels he is walking on air.

Circulatory vertigo

Giddiness due to circulatory distrubance occurs in either hypertensive states or with the onset of an arrhythmia. It is always postural and transitory, lasting a few minutes only. When due to hypotension, it occurs when the patient suddenly assumes an erect posture, and when due to hypertension it is likely to come on with stooping.

The ninth, tenth and eleventh cranial nerves

Many of the anatomical details concerning these nerves are extremely complex and of no clinical importance. Moreover, during their course they have such ramifications and interconnections that it is sometimes controversial whether any particular sensation travels along the ninth or tenth or even the eleventh nerve, which is usually regarded as wholly motor.

The nuclei of all three nerves are situated in the dorsum of the open medulla in the floor of the fourth ventricle and are called the ventral (ambiguus), the dorsal and the solitarius. The details of the direct and indirect connections of these three nuclei individually with the ninth, tenth and eleventh cranial nerves are complex and controversial. The ventral nucleus is motor, the dorsal nucleus represents the autonomic outflow, and the nucleus solitarius is concerned with taste sensation.

THE NINTH CRANIAL NERVE

This nerve has a very short intracranial course, exiting through the jugular foramen together with the tenth and eleventh nerves. It has on it a ganglion (the dorsal) in the foramen and another (the petrosal) immediately below the foramen. Via these ganglia it forms connections directly and indirectly with the fifth, seventh, tenth and cervical sympathetic nerves. The nerve then passes between the jugular vein and the internal carotid artery, follows the posterior border of the stylo-pharyngeus, and passes beneath the hyoglossus muscle to the lateral wall of the pharynx. It supplies sensation to the back of the tongue (including taste), the fauces, the palate and the upper part of the pharynx, and secretory fibres to the parotid. Its motor supply is to the stylo-pharyngeus, the palato-pharyngeus and the palato-glossus, and partly to the pharyngeal constrictor.

THE TENTH CRANIAL NERVE

The vagus nerve also has two genglia on it — an upper in the jugular foramen (ganglion of root), and another about 1 centimetre below the foramen called the ganglion of the trunk.

In the neck the nerve passes down the carotid sheath, and has anastomotic branches to the ninth and possibly the twelfth nerve and also to the cervical sympathetic.

In the thorax and abdomen it has further connections with the sympathetic via the cardiac, pulmonary, oesophageal and gastric plexuses. The right vagus enters the thorax anteriorly to the subclavian artery and goes behind the root of the lung to take part in the right posterior pulmonary plexus. The left vagus in the thorax is between the right carotid and subclavian arteries and passes in front of the aortic arch. The nerve then goes downwards behind the root of the lung, taking part in the left posterior pulmonary plexus. It then unites with the right vagus to form the oesophageal plexus, and the combined vagi supply all the abdominal viscera. The vagi supply motor fibres to the palate, the larynx, the pharynx, and the thoracic and abdominal viscera, from which they also receive sensory impulses. The vagi also supply some sensation to a small part of the external ear.

THE ELEVENTH CRANIAL NERVE

This nerve is usually regarded as wholly motor. Some question whether it really is a cranial nerve, regarding its cranial portion as part of the tenth.

The cranial part arises from the ninth and tenth nuclei and passes through the jugular foramen, where it blends with the vagus.

The spinal part arises from the anterior horn cells of the fourth and fifth cervical segments. Ascending within the dura, it enters the skull via the foramen magnum and then turns laterally into the jugular foramen, where it joins the cranial part for a short distance. It then descends in the neck behind the digastric and stylohyoid and also the sternomastoid, which it supplies (together with branches from the second and third cervical nerve roots). It ends in the trapezius, which it supplies (together with branches from the third and fourth cervical nerve roots).

TESTING THE NINTH, TENTH AND ELEVENTH CRANIAL NERVES

The ninth and tenth cranial nerves are tested together by noting whether the patient has any dysphonia or dysphagia and observing palatal movement. Examination of movement of the pharynx on swallowing, and of the vocal cords on deep inspiration and phonation, is usually left to the specialist. It is important to have the vocal cords examined if it is suspected that the patient is hoarse, even though he himself denies it.

The spinal portion of the eleventh nerve is tested by examining the trapezius and the sterno-mastoids. The trapezius is tested by asking the patient to shrug his shoulders upwards against resistance and later to brace his shoulders back; in each case the muscle is observed and palpated. The sterno-mastoids are tested by asking the patient to rotate his head with his shoulders still so that his chin is turned towards each shoulder in turn, one of the observer's hands meanwhile pressing against the patient's chin to resist this movement and the other hand feeling the sterno-mastoid which is being brought into action. It is important to realize that gross weakness of the sterno-mastoid causes very little disability, the patient still being able to turn his head satisfactorily because this movement is taken over by other muscles such as the splenius. The observation as to whether or not the muscle is wasted is made on inspection and palpation of the muscle, particularly in the region of its sterno-clavicular attachment, and this is an important and extremely valuable diagnostic sign.

Localization of lesion

The ninth, tenth and eleventh cranial nerves have bilateral cerebral representation, and therefore the muscles which they supply will not be involved in any unilateral upper motor neurone lesion.

If there is a bilateral lower motor neurone lesion of these structures, then the lesion is likely to be either nuclear, forming part of a bulbar palsy (described later), or a muscle disease, such as dystrophia myotonica with its characteristic distribution of wasting and weakness affecting not only all the facial mucles but also the sterno-mastoids. The latter finding will be a clue to the diagnosis.

If the lesion is in the region of the jugular foramen, there will be unilateral involvement of various combinations of the structures supplied by these three nerve. Moreover, the twelfth nerve, passing through the anterior condylar foramen, is in very close proximity and may also be involved. Many syndromes are described which, in fact, merely represent different possible combinations of paralysed muscles, and the memorizing of these syndromes by eponym or otherwise is not profitable.

The commonest cause of a jugular foramen syndrome is a carcinoma of the pharynx. Other causes are lesions of the skull itself, such as a fractured base or Paget's disease; intracranial lesions, such as basal meningitis; or neoplasm or lesions in the foramen itself, such as jugular vein thrombosis. An isolated unilateral lower motor neurone lesion of the sterno-mastoid and/or trapezius is likely to be due to a lesion in the neck such as an injury.

Recurrent laryngeal nerve

The recurrent laryngeal nerves are clinically very important branches of the vagi. The right branch arises at the root of the neck anteriorly to the first part of the subclavian artery, passes around its inferior border and turns upwards behind it, and then passes behind the carotid sheath and the inferior thyroid artery to the groove between the trachea and the oesophagus. The left branch arises in the superior mediastinum and is anterior to the arch of the aorta, but then passes below its inferior border and turns upwards immediately behind it to pass between the trachea and the oesophagus. Both nerves are in close relationship with the inferior poles of the lateral lobes of the thyroid. At the level of the cricoid, each passes deeply beneath the inferior constrictor muscles to enter the larynx and supply its intrinsic muscles (except possibly the tensors). The sensory supply is from the superior laryngeal nerve, which arises from the inferior ganglion of the vagus and possibly contains fibres from the cranial root of the eleventh nerve.

Paralysis of the recurrent laryngeal nerve causes dysphonia, and bilateral lesions may also produce stridor. In any organic lesion of the vocal cords, the order of paralysis is always first the abductors, which move on inspiration; then the tensors of the cord; and finally the adductors, which move on phonation, with the end result that the affected cord is motionless in the cadaveric position. It follows from this law that an adductor paralysis without an abductor paralysis cannot occur in any organic lesion and always indicates hysteria.

A unilateral recurrent laryngeal paralysis does not cause complete loss of voice because the opposite cord crosses the midline to attempt glottic closure. The patient cannot talk loudly or shout but can produce a conversational volume. But if there is a combined recurrent and superior laryngeal paralysis then the paralysed cord remains further away from the normal cord and dysphonia becomes marked. A unilateral recurrent laryngeal nerve lesion may be due to lesions of the root of the neck or the superior mediastinum. The nerve is therefore likely to be involved by injuries (including surgery), by enlarged nodes in the neck or superior mediastinum, by enlargement of the thyroid or thymus, by aneurysms of the arch of the aorta and, rarely, by lesions, usually malignant, of the oesophagus or trachea.

Any of these lesions may compress other structures in this area such as the trachea or the superior vena cava. The manifestations of tracheal compression are stridor and a cough which is loud, explosive and metallic. The latter is often described as 'gander' or 'brassy', but most of us have never heard a gander cough or the noise of brass being turned on a lathe and such romantic terms have become meaningless. If a patient with such a cough later develops paralysis of the recurrent laryngeal nerve, then that cough must lose its previous characteristics and become husky (often referred to as a 'bovine cough').

The twelfth cranial nerve

ANATOMY

Part 1 of the course of the twelfth cranial nerve is the nucleus, which is situated in the dorsum of the medulla in the floor of the fourth ventricle, the two nuclei being close together near the midline (*see Figure 9*).

Part 2 of its course is within the substance of the medulla, the nerve coursing forward through the medulla to exit between the pyramidal fibres and the inferior olivary nucleus.

Part 3, which is very short, is within the cranium. The nerve leaves the skull via the anterior condylar foramen, which is immediately next to the jugular foramen, and therefore the nerve is in close proximity to the ninth, tenth and eleventh nerves.

Part 4 of its course is deep within the neck, the nerve descending vertically between the carotid artery and the jugular vein and being very near the vagus. At the level of the angle of the jaw, it turns directly forwards to supply the tongue muscles.

CLINICAL ASPECTS

In testing the twelfth cranial nerve, attention is confined to examination of the tongue, the patient being asked to protrude his tongue fully and straight. If there is any doubt as to weakness, the patient should be instructed to push his tongue hard against the inner aspect of each cheek in turn.

The usual mistake is to diagnose a non-existent paralysis. This error can be avoided if the following points are remembered:

1. The essential sign of a lower motor neurone lesion of the tongue is wasting. This is readily recognizable, and if it is not present, any apparent fibrillation or tongue deviation must be ignored.

2. A unilateral upper motor neurone lesion of the tongue does not occur except as part of an upper motor neurone hemiplegia, so that if the patient has not got a pyramidal lesion of the arm and leg he cannot have a pyramidal lesion of the tongue.

3. An apparent deviation of the tongue of no importance occurs in motor fifth and in seventh nerve lesions.

In any unilateral paralysis of the tongue of upper or lower motor neurone type, the tongue is always deviated towards the paralysed side. If the lesion is lower motor neurone, then in addition there will be wasting, and there may be fibrillation if the lesion is nuclear and is progressive. A bilateral lower motor neurone lesion of the tongue almost invariably forms part of a bulbar palsy (discussed below). A unilateral upper motor neurone lesion of the tongue will be characterized by slight difficulty of protrusion of the tongue, which is deviated to the paralysed side. However, as emphasized above, there is always an accompanying upper motor neurone hemiplegia and this usually also involves the face, the paralysis of which will accentuate the deviation of the tongue, making it more apparent than real. But in any patient with an upper motor neurone hemiplegia, whether the tongue is affected is of no clinical importance, because such a finding does not influence the anatomical diagnosis. A bilateral upper motor neurone lesion of the tongue forms part of a pseudo-bulbar palsy (discussed below).

If a patient has a lower motor neurone lesion of the tongue, an attempt must be made to localize the lesion more accurately. If it is an isolated unilateral lesion, it is likely to be in part 4 of its course, in the neck, usually as a result of injury. On the other hand, the nerve is unlikely to be affected alone at or near its passage through the anterior condylar foramen (part 3 of its course), but will be associated there with one of the jugular foramen syndromes (*see above*). In part 2 of its course, within the medulla, involvement will produce a crossed paralysis with an ipsilateral lower motor neurone lesion of the tongue and a contralateral upper motor neurone hemiplegia. The commonest cause of this rare syndrome is syringobulbia, but any other lesion in this area − for example, a neoplasm or aneurysm situated immediately outside the medulla and compressing the region of the groove between the pyramid and the olive − may give rise to it. A lesion of the nucleus is almost invariably a bilateral one because the two nuclei are so close together, and such involvement forms part of a bulbar palsy.

Bulbar palsies

Bulbar palsies are always labio-glosso-palato-pharyngeal palsies. Whether laryngeal and oesophageal involvement should be added is controversial, but most authorities do not include them, although no good explanation has been given why they do escape. The voice often lacks modulation, but this is ascribed to weakness of the muscles which fix the larynx and not to involvement of its intrinsic muscles. The involvement of the lip muscles, which are supplied by the seventh nerve, is explained by the fact that they are innervated by fibres which arise from the lowest part of the seventh nucleus, which extends right down to the twelfth nucleus. Involvement of other facial muscles is due to spread of the lesion to the pons, and then the fifth nerve nuclei may also be affected.

TYPES OF BULBAR PALSY

A bulbar palsy may be true, pseudo or myasthenic. A true bulbar palsy is a bilateral lower motor neurone labio-glosso-palato-pharyngeal palsy due to a lesion of the nuclei in the open medulla (the bulb). A pseudo-bulbar palsy is a bilateral upper motor neurone lesion of the same muscles. All muscles supplied by the cranial nerves are bilaterally innervated except those of the lower half of the face and probably the tongue, and therefore all except these muscles escape in a patient with an upper motor neurone hemiplegia due, for example, to a lesion of the opposite internal capsule. Moreover, all the trunk muscles and the diaphragm are bilaterally innervated. A myasthenic bulbar palsy is involvement of the myo-neural junctions of the same muscles by myasthenia gravis.

Whatever the type of bulbar palsy, the symptoms will be dysarthria and dysphagia. The dysarthria has been described in the section on speech defects. The dysphagia is a combined labial, glossal, buccal (mylohyoid and digastric muscles in the floor of the mouth), palatal, pharyngeal (including the muscles which raise and lower the thyroid and laryngeal cartilages, which all show early and marked involvement in bulbar palsies), and possibly oesophageal dysphagia as well. The greatest difficulty is with fluids, because these require a rapid and powerful action by the lips, tongue and buccal muscles and, moreover, due to the palatal palsy there will be regurgitation into the nose. The least difficulty will be with soft foods having the consistency of porridge.

True bulbar palsy
The signs of true bulbar palsy are bilateral wasting of the tongue with weakness and possibly fibrillation, together with paralysis of the palate and weakness of the orbicularis oris. The palsy may be acute, due to an inflammatory lesion such as poliomyelitis, acute ascending peripheral neuritis, encephalitis lethargica or botulism, or to injury. In these conditions the patients are critically ill because of respiratory muscle paralysis. The commonest cause of chronic bulbar palsy is motor neurone disease, but syphilis and lead poisoning may also give rise to the same signs.

Pseudo-bulbar palsy
A pseudo-bulbar palsy is characterized by paralysis of the tongue, which can scarcely be protruded at all. The tongue is spastic, but the only demonstrable manifestation of this apart from the dysarthria is that the tongue appears to be too small for that particular mouth, which is a difficult judgment. The palate is paralysed and there is often a pyramidal lesion of all four limbs, but frequently the limb signs on one side are extremely slight because of partial recovery. In addition there is jaw clonus due to a bilateral upper motor neurone lesion of the masseters. Spasticity of the facial muscles may cause a fixed facial expression. Gross emotional disturbance, the patient laughing and crying for no apparent reason, is frequently present and the cause of this is obscure.

The commonest cause of a pseudo-bulbar palsy is a bilateral lesion of the internal capsules due to bilateral cerebral thrombosis, the history of which is usually that, while the patient is recovering from the effects of one cerebral thrombosis, he suffers another. Sometimes the paralyses are not of dramatic onset but more gradual, suggesting that the capsular lesions are due to cerebral atherosclerosis *per se* without actual thrombosis. Pseudo-bulbar paralysis should be regarded as an anatomical rather than a pathological diagnosis, because although bilateral cerebral thrombosis is the commonest cause, diseases such as motor neurone disease and disseminated sclerosis can give rise to the same clinical picture.

The cervical sympathetic nerve

ANATOMY

The head ganglia of the autonomic nervous system are situated in the hypothalamus. From there, fibres pass through the pons and the medulla (probably not as a distinct bundle) to the lateral horns of the eighth cervical and first dorsal segments of the cord. From these cell stations, pre-ganglionic nerve fibres (rami communicantes) travel at first with the anterior nerve roots and later from the sympathetic chain, with cell stations in the superior cervical ganglion. The sympathetic fibres (post-ganglionic) then run in the carotid sheath with the internal carotid artery, enter the skull with it and, in the cavernous sinus, join the ophthalmic division of the fifth cranial nerve. They enter the orbit and, via the ciliary nerve, supply part of the levator palpebrae superioris, the dilator pupillae and Müller's muscle, and send vasomotor and sweat fibres to that side of the face.

CLINICAL ASPECTS

Paralysis of the cervical sympathetic system gives rise to a partial ptosis, a small pupil which fails to dilate in a dim light (or when shaded) or on emotion but is otherwise normal, enophthalmos, and lack of sweating on that side of the face. Partial involvement is much commoner than complete involvement, and the examiner must be prepared to make the diagnosis if, for example, only pupillary involvement is present. Enophthalmos is but rarely demonstrable.

Paralysis of the sympathetic may be due to a lesion of the brain stem, for example thrombosis of the posterior inferior cerebellar artery; to a lesion of the eighth cervical or first dorsal segments of the cord, for example syringomyelia; to a lesion in the superior mediastinum, such as aneurysm or a mass of enlarged glands from whatever cause; to a lesion of the neck, such as injury or a mass of glands; or to a lesion of the cavernous sinus, but then the ophthalmic fifth will also be involved. Stimulation of the cervical sympathetic by emotional disturbance or by drugs – for example, adrenaline (or its derivatives) or cocaine – will produce bilateral lid retraction, large but otherwise normal pupils, and sweating and flushing of the face. Theoretically, pressure on the sympathetic in the superior mediastinum or the neck may, prior to producing paralysis, produce signs of stimulation, but in actual fact this probably never occurs.

Involuntary movements

Having examined the cranial nerves, the examiner must then proceed in a methodical fashion to examine the limbs and the trunk. It is advisable to look first for any involuntary movements. All such movements should be regarded as being due to release of normal inhibitions rather than to focal irritative phenomena. With any involuntary movement, the physician must note (1) its type, (2) which parts of the body are involved, (3) whether it is present or not at rest, (4) effects of voluntary movement and alteration of posture and (5) the effects of emotion and sleep. Any of these may be an important clue to the localization of the lesion.

TREMOR

A tremor is an involuntary rhythmic movement of small amplitude. All tremors are by definition rhythmic, and therefore it is a tautology to talk of a 'rhythmic tremor' as is frequently done. Any tremor may be rapid or slow, fine or coarse, simple or compound. By 'simple' is meant that the tremor involves only one joint, while a 'compound' tremor involves many joints.

Extrapyramidal tremor

An extrapyramidal tremor is a coarse compound tremor, and its association with rigidity is known as Parkinsonism. Such a tremor, which may affect any limb, therefore indicates a lesion of the extrapyramidal system. It is sometimes stated that senility also produces such a tremor; however, distinction between this and Parkinsonism is often hair-splitting, although the distinction is sometimes said to be that rigidity does not occur in senility.

A coarse compound tremor disappears during sleep and is aggravated by emotion and on attempting fine movements (but it then must not be confused with the cerebellar intention tremor, which is not present at rest and occurs only on voluntary movement).

Passive movements, and strong movements such as gripping an object and sudden changes of posture will diminish the tremor. As Parkinson himself observed if the patient develops an acute pyramidal lesion (usually due to a middle cerebral artery thrombosis) the tremor will disappear, 'paralysis agitans sine agitantati' as he called it. He wrote of one of his patients who subsequently had a stroke: 'Neither the arm or the leg of the paralysed side was in the least affected by the tremulous agitation, but as the paralysed state was removed the shaking returned.' Involuntary movements necessitate the integrity of the pyramidal system.

In Parkinsonism other types of tremor may also be seen, involving the head, the lips, the jaws and the closed eyelids, but these are not pathognomonic, whereas the coarse compound tremor is. When the tremor is completely confined to the head it is very unlikely to be of extrapyramidal origin.

Cerebellar tremor
The characteristic cerebellar tremor is the intention tremor, an involuntary movement which is not present at rest, is brought out only on movement and, moreover, is accentuated as the range of movement is increased. It must be emphasized that other tremors and other involuntary movements may be accentuated by movement but, unlike the intention tremor, they are also present at rest.

Intention tremor is tested by asking the patient to touch with his index finger, repeatedly in rapid succession, his own nose and the observer's index finger. Since the tremor may be brought out only on full movement, it is important that the patient's arm be fully abducted, held above the horizontal, extended at the shoulder and elbow and not supported on pillows. In the lower limb, intention tremor may be sought by asking the patient to touch with his big toe the examiner's finger held about 2 feet away, and to keep his toe stationary in that position for a few seconds until the examiner moves his finger to a new position.

In cerebellar disorders, tremors of the head (titubation), may be present, but these are not diagnostic as they may also occur with extrapyramidal lesions and in elderly people without other evidence of Parkinsonism, and they may also be familial.

Tremor in general paralysis of the insane
The characteristic tremor is the backward and forward trombone tremor of the tongue, present especially at rest but also on attempted protrusion. Other tremors affecting the lips and the hands are frequent but are not diagnostic.

Fine rapid tremors
Fine rapid tremors of the limbs, especially of the outstretched hands, are seen in fatigue, cold (shivering), anxiety states, emotion, thyrotoxi-

cosis, and in poisoning by alcohol (notably in delirium tremens), tobacco, cocaine, opium (especially on withdrawal of the drug), tricyclic anti-depressants, mercury and amphetamine. Tremor of psychogenic origin usually takes the form of an aggravation and perpetuation of such fine rapid tremors, but sometimes a very coarse compound bizarre tremor, of variable severity is present and may be associated with an hysterically paralysed limb. Tremor of one or more limbs, unassociated with any other signs of neurological disease, may be hereditary and is then often confined to the hands and usually occurs only on attempting to maintain a posture and although the tremor continues with movements it is not exaggerated thereby. Titubation (head tremor) may also be genetic. All familial tremors are often greatly diminished by alcohol. In severe liver disease the outstretched upper limbs may show a 'flapping tremor', which consists of irregular bursts of flexion-extension movements at the wrists and the metacarpo-phalangeal joints and is often associated with abduction-adduction movements of the fingers. This type of tremor is grossly exaggerated by attempted voluntary movements and is called flapping because of its supposed resemblance to a bird flapping its wings. An identical tremor occasionally occurs in cardiac or respiratory or renal failure.

CHOREIFORM MOVEMENTS

Choreiform movements are involuntary, abrupt, jerky and of short duration. The same movement is never repeated twice in succession. The movements may be localized to any part of the body or may be very extensive, involving not only the limbs but also the neck and trunk muscles so that the patient is unable to keep still and walking becomes impossible. The face is nearly always involved, producing facial distortions and grimacings. In severe cases dysarthria and dysphagia occur. Choreiform movements flit from one part of the body to another in an unpredictable way. Severe unilateral choreiform movements affecting the upper and lower limbs of the same side are also known as hemiballismus and are most often seen in elderly people who have had a middle cerebral artery thrombosis with partial recovery.

Choreiform movements indicate a lesion of the extrapyramidal system. Such movements may be caused by any of the same drugs which may cause Parkinsonism; it may be a form of a toxaemia of pregnancy (chorea gravidarum); or as part of Huntington's* Chorea which is a genetically determined disease characterized by choreiform and athetoid movements, mental disturbance, dysarthria and dysphagia all of which start about the age of thirty and gradually

*George S. Huntingdon (1851–1916) of Long Island, New York, wrote his paper in 1872. All his patients were descended from British Quaker immigrants.

become worse. It is extremely doubtful whether rheumatic chorea has anything whatsoever to do with the extrapyramidal system, although the features of the involuntary movements are identical.

ATHETOID MOVEMENTS

Athetoid movements are involuntary, slow, sinuous, writhing, twisting, snake-like and purposeless, affecting principally the periphery of the limbs. The fingers are flexed at the metacarpo-phalangeal joints, with the thumb flexed and adducted into the palm and with flexion of the wrist. In severe bilateral cases the lips, jaw and tongue may exhibit involuntary movements.

Athetoid movements indicate a lesion of the extrapyramidal system. Similar movements, but affecting the trunk, shoulder girdle and hip muscles and occurring especially on attempted voluntary movement, are called dystonia musculorum or torsion spasm or torsion dystonia. Compared with choreiform movements they are much slower and longer sustained and are often regarded as a proximal variety of athetosis. The condition is most often seen as part of a cerebral palsy syndrome. These also indicate an extrapyramidal lesion.

Choreiform and athetoid movements are frequently seen in the same patient. Both are aggravated by either emotion or attempted voluntary movements, the latter being thereby always rendered clumsy.

TICS

A tic is a frequent explosive repetition of the same movement, which may have originated in some physical or psychological stimulus and may originally have been purposive, but is perpetuated as a compulsive, involuntary, stereotyped movement. Tics can be readily imitated. The person may be able voluntarily to control his tic but the effort causes anxiety and distress.

Tics are most commonly seen in the facial and neck muscles, causing blinking, raising of the eyebrows, grimacing, shrugging of the shoulders, twisting of the neck and nodding of the head. Tapping, rubbing and scratching of the hands, either individually or in any combination, are another common form of tic. Spasmodic toticollis consists of involuntary unilateral head turning associated with spasm of neck muscles and later with their hypertrophy. Though often regarded as psychogenic it may be due to a brain lesion, especially one involving the corpus striatum. A tic may take the form of repeated sniffing or grunting. Tics in their severest form may be associated with disorders of behaviour and explosive utterances which often consist of very foul language. The condition always starts in childhood. They are nearly always due to some psychological disturbance, but rarely may occur with lesions of the corpus striatum due to drugs which cause Parkinsonism.

MYOCLONIC MOVEMENTS

A myoclonic movement is a sudden brief shock-like contraction of a single large muscle or group of muscles, independent of their antagonists, as if stimulated by a faradic electric current. Such movements are most commonly seen in the limbs, usually the flexors of the upper and the extensors of the lower limbs, and are usually but not necessarily associated with displacement of the limb.

There is only one common cause of myoclonus, and that is epilepsy. An exception to this is hiccup (singultus), which is due to myoclonic movements of the diaphragm and has no relation to epilepsy.

Muscle power

The next procedure should be to assess the power of the limb and trunk muscles by attempting passive movements against the patient's resistance or the patient attempting active movements against the examiner's resistance and gravity. The possibility that any limitation of movement, difficulty in walking, or inability to use the limbs properly may be due to arthritis must first be excluded. A good plan is always to start at the periphery of the limbs — for example, testing power of movements first at the fingers, then at the wrists, elbows and shoulders, and finally at the scapulae. When testing power, the examiner should always demonstrate exactly what he wants the patient to do. The trunk muscles can be tested by the patient attempting to raise himself from the supine position without using his hands, and also by flexing his head fully against resistance while lying supine and also by noting his respiratory excursion. There is no satisfactory way of measuring strength in individual muscle groups and the use of numbers to record the results does not make their performance any more accurate.

If any weakness (paresis) is present, the examiner must next determine whether it is caused by a lower or upper motor neurone, extrapyramidal or cerebellar lesion, is hysterical, or is due to malingering or lack of co-operation. It is important to appreciate that any patient with sensory disturbance may describe such disability as weakness.

LOWER MOTOR NEURONE LESIONS

Lower motor neurone lesions are those caused by involvement of the motor pathway anywhere from the anterior horn cells to the muscles.

A quibble is whether muscle diseases should be included within this definition, and the author proposes to do so because the clinical manifestations are the same even though the electrical reactions and pathology are not. The exception to this statement is that in muscle diseases the reflexes are usually present until late in the disease.

The manifestations of a lower motor neurone lesion are (1) weakness with wasting, (2) flaccidity (hypotonicity), (3) diminished or absent reflexes, and (4) fasciculation.

Muscle wasting

The fundamental sign is wasting and without it, except in the initial acute phase, the physician should hesitate to diagnose a lower motor neurone lesion. Where such a lesion affects muscles which are not visible, for example iliopsoas, or muscles in which assessment is difficult such as those of the trunk, the diagnosis of a lower motor neurone lesion can be considered even in the absence of wasting, but only after other possibilities have been ruled out.

Wasting is probably the most frequently missed sign in neurology, and this is usually because, although it has been observed, it has been dismissed as due to either disuse or old age. The differentiation between wasting caused by a lower motor neurone lesion and that resulting from disuse is that the former involves comparatively few muscles and rarely the whole limb. If a patient had been in bed for a long time, disuse would not be a satisfactory explanation for wasting of the quadriceps or peroneal muscles with sparing of all other muscles. Or if a patient had an upper motor neurone lesion of an upper limb, this in itself would not cause focal wasting confined to the intrinsic muscles of the hand, however severe the degree of pyramidal paralysis.

In malnutrition from any cause, the limb muscles may lose their bulk but still retain their power except in extreme cases. It is advisable never to refer to wasting unless a neurological lesion is implied.

The most important technique for diagnosing muscle wasting is inspection. Palpation of muscles is a very minor and frequently misleading sign, and stroking them is a sheer waste of time. A common cause for wasting being missed is that it is sought for in the wrong place: for example, if a patient has foot drop — that is, plantar flexion of the foot with inability to dorsiflex and evert the ankle completely — then he must have weakness of the tibialis anterior and peroneal muscles. If this is due to a lower motor neurone lesion there will be wasting, but the correct place to look for this is the upper part of the outer aspect of the leg and not elsewhere. A pyramidal lesion of cortical origin, with lack of growth of the whole or part of a limb, should not be mistaken for a lower motor neurone lesion.

Hypotonicity

Hypotonicity is much more difficult to appreciate or demonstrate clinically than hypertonicity. It is recognized by the following signs:

1. A diminished resistance to passive displacement of the limb. This presumes full co-operation by the patient, who must keep his muscles completely relaxed.
2. An excessive range of active or passive movement at a joint without the presence of arthritis.
3. Difficulty in maintaining posture, for example of the outstretched limbs.
4. Palpation of the muscles, which is the least satisfactory method of all.

Hypotonicity due to a lower motor neurone lesion will never be recognizable clinically unless the wasting is very extensive, affecting the whole or the major part of a limb. It is not pathognomonic because it occurs also in cerebellar, posterior column, sensory nerve root and occasionally extrapyramidal lesions, and as a transitory phenomenon, lasting usually a few days but occasionally a few weeks, in acute lesions of the cerebral hemisphere or spinal cord.

Reflexes
All reflexes at the level of the lesion will be diminished or absent with a lower motor neurone lesion, but there may be no demonstrable reflex at the particular level. Between the second dorsal and the second lumbar segments inclusive, the only reflexes usually tested are the abdominal and cremasteric. The latter is at the level of the first lumbar segment and is occasionally a valuable localizing sign, but the abdominal reflexes are notoriously unreliable.

Fasciculation
Fasciculation is a visible fine rapid irregular flickering, rippling or twitching of bundles of muscle fibres which does not cause displacement of the part and which occurs spontaneously or on tapping the muscle. The patient himself is never aware of fasciculation, which is a purely visual objective phenomenon. Many seconds or minutes elapse between each twitch seen in the same part of the same muscle. Twitching of a muscle without wasting of that muscle is of no significance, and a diagnosis of a lower motor neurone lesion should never be based solely on apparent fasciculation. The term muscle fibrillation implies a spontaneous contraction of a single muscle fibre and is now no longer used except to denote an electromyographic phenomenon.

Fasciculation indicates a progressive lower motor neurone lesion (for example, motor neurone disease), but its diagnostic importance is often grossly exaggerated. It is not found in non-progressive lesions such as poliomyelitis or injury, and does not occur in the genetically determined muscular dystrophies.

Localization of lower motor neurone lesions
If a patient has a lower motor neurone lesion, the next task is to localize it to the anterior horn cells, nerve roots, plexus, peripheral

nerve or muscle. Such localization depends entirely upon testing all important individual muscles, finding out which are affected and then considering the problem as a purely anatomical exercise. *Aids to the Investigation of Peripheral Nerve Injuries* (London: H.M. Stationery Office, 1945) is an illustrated pamphlet describing how to test muscles and gives a detailed account of their supply in terms of peripheral nerve, plexus and cord. The best way of learning all this is by practising on patients with the above manual in front of you.

The distribution of the anterior nerve roots is as follows: Diaphragm C4; shoulder muscles and flexors of elbow C5 and 6; extensors of elbow, wrists and fingers C7; flexors of wrist and fingers C7 and 8; hand muscles T1; intercostal and abdominal muscles T2 to L3; quadriceps and thigh adductors L3 and 4; ileo-psoas L1 to L4; glutei L4 and 5; hamstrings L4 and 5 and S1; flexors of ankle L5; extensors of ankle S1; muscles of foot S1 and 2.

Some general rules may, however, be enumerated. If the lower motor neurone lesion is extensive and completely unilateral, the lesion is likely to be outside the cord. If there is a lower motor neurone lesion of all four limbs, then the likelihood is that peripheral neuritis, a muscle disease, poliomyelitis or, less likely, motor neurone disease is present. These conditions can usually be differentiated by the distribution of the wasting and by its mode of onset and progress.

The term 'myopathy' is used in two ways:
1. As a generic term to include all diseases in which the primary lesion is in the muscles.
2. As a more restricted term to describe a group of conditions, otherwise named the primary muscle diseases or muscular dystrophies, which are characterized by a progressive bilateral symmetrical wasting of muscles, which nearly always commence in childhood or adolescence, and which are familial and hereditary. Pathologically the changes are confined to the muscles themselves, but the urine usually contains creatine instead of the normal creatinine, and electromyographic tracings have a distinctive pattern, discussion of which is outside the scope of this volume.

MUSCULAR DYSTROPHY

The types of muscular dystrophy are as follows:
1. Facio-scapular-humeral, which begins in the facial muscles and later involves the scapular muscles, triceps and biceps, but may spread to other muscles of the shoulder and pelvic girdles.
2. A badly named 'juvenile' type which usually starts in adolescence but may be found much earlier or later. It affects the proximal limb muscles, especially of the pelvic and shoulder girdles, but spares the face.

3. A pseudo-hypertrophic form which is extremely rare in girls and in which wasting of proximal muscles is preceded by pseudo-hypertrophy (due to fatty infiltration) of the calves, glutei and infraspinati.
4. A rare distal form affecting the hands, forearms, feet and legs.

It must be emphasized that there is no sharp distinction between these four types.

PERONEAL MUSCULAR ATROPHY

This is characterized by a hereditary progressive wasting of all four limbs. However, unlike the true muscular dystrophies it shows, clinically often and *post mortem* always, evidence of peripheral nerve or cord damage, and therefore does not really belong to the same group. Moreover, the wasting is peripheral, always starting and maximal in the lower limbs. The early case may be difficult to diagnose because for a long time the wasting and consequent weakness are confined to the peronei and tibialis anticus, with bilateral foot drop and inversion deformity but comparatively little disability. Late in the disease the wasting spreads to involve all the muscles below the knee and the hand muscles, with resultant claw hands and feet. But the wasting never spreads further than the lower third of the thighs and forearms, giving, finally, the distinctive 'inverted champagne bottle' appearance to the limbs. The trunk and facial muscles are never affected. There may be sensory or pyramidal signs.

MYOTONIA ATROPHICA

Myotonia atrophica (dystrophia myotonica) is another condition characterized by hereditary, progressive, symmetrical, bilateral wasting and weakness of muscles, especially the facial muscles and the sternomastoids. Wasting may occur in the limb muscles, being then usually first seen in the forearms and later in the vasti and tibialis anterior. Peculiar features are baldness, gonadal atrophy and myotonia (muscle contraction being slow and prolonged, with difficulty in relaxation of the hand grip and persistent dimpling of the tongue on percussion with, for example, the handle of a tuning fork).

MYASTHENIA GRAVIS

Myasthenia gravis is another muscular disease characterized by bilateral symmetrical weakness of muscles, especially those supplied by the cranial nerves, but is not genetically determined. With the resultant weakness of all the facial muscles, the facies resembles that of facio-scapulo-humeral myopathy and also that of myotonia atrophica, and this similarity includes the fact that in all three conditions there is bilateral ptosis but no compensatory wrinkling of the forehead. In myasthenia gravis, however, because the muscles of the upper lip are often less affected than the other facial muscles, the upper teeth become much more visible than the lower when the patient smiles, producing the 'snarling facies'.

Undue fatigability is a feature of any type of paralysis, but myasthenia gravis is the only condition in which repetitive use of a muscle produces actual paralysis. It is also the only condition due to a lesion of the myoneural junctions not caused by drugs. The muscles histologically show whorls of lymphocytes known as 'lymphorrhages', an appearance not seen in muscular dystrophies. In myasthenia gravis, the first muscles in the limbs to show weakness and wasting are usually the deltoids. The tendon reflexes remain normal.

THYROTOXIC AND CARCINOMATOUS MYOPATHY

Occasionally muscle-wasting occurs in patients with thyrotoxicosis, and this is sometimes called thyrotoxic myopathy. It is bilateral and symmetrical and usually affects the proximal limb muscles. As in myasthenia gravis, the affected muscles exhibit lymphorrhages.

Localized wasting of muscles, often proximal, may occur in carcinomatosis, especially when the primary is bronchial. This is distinguishable from a carcinomatous peripheral neuritis only by electromyography.

The pyramidal system

ANATOMY

Any weakness of a limb may be due to a pyramidal (upper motor neurone) lesion.

The pyramidal fibres arise not only from the Betz cells, situated in the precentral convolution anterior to the Rolandic fissure, but also from a much more extensive area of the cortex especially of the postcentral gyrus. They pass through the internal capsule, immediately anterior and posterior to the genu (*see Figure 15*), through the middle part of the crus of the mid-brain and pons, where they form bundles of fibres in its anterior part, and so into the medulla where they decussate to form the pyramidal tracts (sometimes called the cortico-spinal tract) one on each side of the anterior median fissures. These pass down into the lateral column of the cord to enter the grey matter of the anterior horns, where they terminate by forming synapses with the anterior horn cells. In the brain stem, the pyramidal tracts give off fibres to the contralateral motor cranial nerve nuclei.

A few pyramidal fibres do not decussate in the medulla but go down the ipisilateral side of the cord as the ventral (direct) pyramidal tract.

CLINICAL SIGNS

A pyramidal lesion of the limb is characterized by (1) muscle weakness, (2) an extensor plantar response, (3) sustained clonus, (4) spasticity of clasp-knife type, and (5) increase of deep reflexes with diminution of superficial reflexes.

Extensor plantar response (Babinski*)

The plantar response is best elicited by stroking the outer aspect of the sole of the foot from the heel to the little toe and then across the sole to the hallux with a blunt instrument, the most popular being a key. A useful method is to use a tuning fork, the upper blade stroking the dorsum of the foot and the lower blade simultaneously stroking the sole from heel to toe. An extensor plantar response produces not only an extension of the hallux but also a fanning out of the other toes and a contraction of the hamstrings. It is essential that the limb be relaxed, the foot warm, and the stimulus applied firmly from heel to hallux. It is usually easier to elicit with the knee and hip slightly flexed and the hip externally rotated.

In those cases where the plantar response is equivocal, other techniques have been suggested for attempting to demonstrate it. These are as follows:

1. Stroking firmly around the external malleolus with a blunt instrument.
2. Tapping with a percussion hammer over the dorsal aspect of the metacarpo-phalangeal joint of the hallux, just internal to the extensor longus hallucis tendon.
3. Sudden sharp upward pressure on the sole of the foot just behind the ball of the hallux.
4. Firmly stroking the tibial border of the leg from above downwards.

One must beware of mistaking a withdrawal response for an extensor response, which is particularly likely to occur when the soles of the feet are very sensitive, for example in peripheral neuritis. With a withdrawal response the toes, other than the large toe, plantar flex and do not fan out. If there is complete paralysis of the extensor longus hallucis (due to a lesion at the level of L4 or L5), or gross loss of sensation on the sole of the foot, or a hallux rigidus, an extensor plantar response will be impossible to obtain even in the presence of a pyramidal lesion. It is advisable always as a routine to exclude a hallux rigidus before testing the plantar responses.

*J. F. F. Babinski (1857–1932), a French neurologist whose grandparents were Polish.

An extensor plantar response may be found in any deeply comatose patient and normally in the first year of life. But in anybody else, it is pathognomonic of a pyramidal lesion. Sometimes when the pyramidal lesion is minimal the plantar response is equivocal. Correct assessment is then probably the most difficult in the whole of neurology, and only an extensive clinical experience is the real guide.

In the upper limbs, equivalents to the extensor response have been described but are not satisfactory. For example, a tap on the palmar aspect of the semi-flexed fingers produces full flexion of all the fingers and the thumb if there is an upper motor neurone lesion of the upper limb.

Clonus

Clonus is a persistent rhythmical involuntary contraction of the calf muscles, quadriceps or pterygoids produced in response to maintenance of tension in these muscles by, respectively, forcible dorsiflexion of the ankle, pushing downwards of the patella, or percussion of the lower jaw with the mouth open. A sustained clonus, often called 'true clonus', is one which increases with pressure, while a 'pseudo-clonus' is abolished by increase of pressure. Sustained clonus is pathognomonic of a pyramidal lesion, but pseudo-clonus is not.

Spasticity

The spasticity of a pyramidal lesion has a clasp-knife character — that is, the resistance to a passive displacement is maximal initially. Spasticity is assessed by asking the patient to let his limbs 'go loose' so that the examiner can move them freely, and then noting any involuntary resistance to passive movement. Increased tone due to an extrapyramidal lesion is usually termed rigidity and not spasticity. Any apparent increase of muscle tone may be due to lack of relaxation. A localized increase of muscle tone can be felt in the abdominal muscles adjacent to an intra-abdominal lesion which causes peritoneal irritation, and also in the muscles around an active arthritis. Acute lesions of the pyramidal system are often followed by an initial transitory period during which the muscles are hypotonic and the tendon reflexes are diminished.

REFLEXES

The reflexes with which the physician is concerned in clinical neurology are (1) tendon; (2) cutaneous; (3) visceral — of which the only ones of clinical importance are the pharyngeal, vesical and rectal.

Tendon reflexes

Tendon reflexes (or jerks) are otherwise known as deep or muscle stretch reflexes (the latter term being perhaps the most accurate but pompous). Essential points in eliciting them are as follows:

1. Adequate relaxation. This is rarely obtained by merely asking the patient to 'let himself go loose'; a better plan is to attempt to distract his attention by engaging him in conversation.
2. The limb must be placed in the optional position for that particular reflex, so that there is adequate muscle tension (stretch), as too much or too little will interfere with the reflex.
3. There must be an adequate stimulus. The small light hammers which are so popular because of the ease with which they can be transported are almost useless. The hammer must be well balanced and fairly heavy, the main weight being in the head, and the handle should be long. The physician must flex his wrist as he strikes the blow.
4. Some technique of reinforcement must always be used before designating any tendon reflex as sluggish or absent. This consists in muscular effort of some other part of the body at the instant the hammer is used; for example, during the testing of the upper limb reflexes the patient clenches his teeth or presses his knees tightly together, and in testing the lower limbs the patient is asked to grip the observer's arm tightly or to attempt to separate forcibly his own interlocked fingers.

Tendon reflexes are diminished in any lower motor neurone lesion or any lesion of the first sensory neurone (posterior nerve root or posterior column). Stated differently, absent tendon reflexes without appropriate wasting — for example, absent ankle jerks without calf muscle wasting — are nearly always due to a posterior column or posterior nerve root lesion. In patients with myotonic pupils, some deep reflexes are often absent without known cause.

In myxoedema the tendon reflexes may be sustained, exhibiting a slowness of return to the starting stationary position. The importance of this as an aid to the diagnosis of myxoedema has been grossly exaggerated and some have even gone to the absurd length of devising a special construction to measure the tardiness of the reflexes. A similar response is sometimes found in rheumatic chorea.

Immediately after a severe cerebral or vascular lesion or traumatic lesion of the cord the tendon reflexes are absent and may remain so for several days and occasionally even for weeks.

Eliciting the reflexes
A method of testing each reflex is described below but it must be emphasized that there is no one correct way although there are certainly many poor ways. A distinguished German neurologist has described over a hundred ways of eliciting the plantar reflex.

Sluggish reflexes should never be dismissed as having no significance in any patient, however old, who has any other neurological signs or symptoms whatsoever.

Tendon reflexes are brisk with an upper motor neurone lesion, but this is not pathognomonic because it is a common finding in emotional people, in anxiety states, in hysteria, and in patients who have a tender or painful limb from any cause. With cerebellar lesions the tendon reflexes are pendular provided that there is no accompanying pyramidal or posterior column lesion.

Biceps reflex
All tendon reflexes in the upper limbs are best tested with the patient sitting up. The biceps reflex (C5 and 6) is elicited by flexing to a right angle and semi-pronating the patient's arm and then striking one's thumb or index finger placed on the biceps tendon. Flexion of the elbow and visible and palpable contraction of the biceps results.

Triceps reflex
The triceps reflex (C7 and 8) is obtained by a sharp blow on the triceps tendon in the region of the olecranon process, the elbow being flexed to a right angle and the forearm held loosely or supported by the observer. If the patient is sitting, it is often helpful to get him to rest his forearms on his thighs. Extension of the elbow and visible and palpable contraction of the triceps results. Sometimes with lesions at the level of C7 and 8, inversion of the reflex results — that is, actual flexion instead of the expected diminution of extension.

Radial reflex
The radial (*supinator*) reflex (C7 and 8) is not really a tendon reflex. It is obtained by tapping the lower end of the radius just above the styloid process while the elbow is flexed and semi-pronated. This normally produces flexion and supination and visible contraction of the brachio-radialis. If there is a lesion at C5 the sole response may be flexion of the fingers, referred to as inversion of the radial reflex. In these cases the radial reflex is brisk and the biceps reflex sluggish.

Knee jerk
The knee jerk (L3 and 4) is obtained by flexing the knees to about 120 degrees. The hammer blow must be a glancing one in a downward direction, because only in this way will the patella be drawn downwards and the quadriceps put on the stretch. It is better not to allow the patient to press his heels down as is usually done, but instead to press the anterior part of his soles against the observer's hand, or the floor or the bed. It is necessary not only to look for extension of the knee but also to observe and feel the contraction of the quadriceps.

Ankle jerk
The ankle jerk (S1) is best elicited if the patient is kneeling on a chair, gripping its back, with his feet just over the edge. If the patient

is lying down, the best procedure is with the hip externally rotated, the knees partly flexed, and the foot a little inverted and dorsiflexed to such an extent as to exert slight tension on the calf muscles. The physician's hand either presses lightly on the side of the foot or lightly grips the foot. Ankle jerks are often difficult to obtain in normal children and in elderly people, in patients with marked leg oedema, and in those who have had attacks of sciatica or lumbar disc displacement even though they appear to have made a complete recovery.

Hoffman reflex is done by flicking downwards the terminal part of the patient's middle finger placed between the examiner's thumb and index finger which results if the test is positive in an involuntary flexion of all the other fingers and thumb, and thumb adduction. A positive response suggests but is not proof of a pyramidal lesion affecting an upper limb and is more significant if the response and the lesion is unilateral. It is considered to be an equivalent to the extensor response of the lower limbs.

Superficial reflexes

Abdominal reflexes
The upper abdominal reflexes are at level T7–9, and the lower at T10–12. The patient must be lying flat with his head at the same level as his trunk. The appropriate abdominal segment is stroked, preferably with a blunt instrument such as a matchstick, after demonstrating to the patient exactly what you intend to do. A pin is not a suitable instrument for this purpose. The upper abdominal reflexes are best obtained if the stimulus is oblique from without inwards, roughly parallel to the costal margin. Such stroking usually produces a deviation of the umbilicus towards the stimulus. A response may be difficult to obtain in patients with poor abdominal musculature, in those who have had abdominal surgery and in the obese. The most significant observation is asymmetry of these reflexes.

The appropriate abdominal reflexes are lost with any lower motor neurone lesion at their level, but are also lost with pyramidal lesions. In most such lesions, but especially when they are due to disseminated sclerosis, this is a very early sign, but in motor neurone disease it is a late one, and in the cerebral palsies the abdominal reflexes often remain brisk. Abdominal reflexes are of no value in the localization of any brain lesion.

Cremasteric reflex
The cremasteric reflex (L1) is obtained by stroking the skin over the upper and inner aspect of the thigh, which produces retraction of the testicle on that side.

It is unnecessary to elicit all the above signs before a pyramidal lesion is diagnosed, an extensor plantar response by itself being sufficient. Moreover, any associated lesion, for example of the posterior columns or anterior horn cells, may alter these signs, especially if the involvement is greater than that of the pyramidal tracts, with the result that there may be absence of deep reflexes and hypotonicity even in the presence of a pyramidal lesion.

LOCALIZATION OF PYRAMIDAL LESIONS

A pyramidal lesion never affects a single muscle or muscle group apart from the face, but at the very least a whole limb. Commonly the muscles are not affected symmetrically, with the result that deformities often develop later. It is important to determine which limbs are involved, as this is the main clue to localization.

Hemiplegia

Hemiplegia is a paralysis of the arm, the leg and, sometimes, the face on one side. As indicated above, it does not necessarily imply a pyramidal lesion but may be lower motor neurone, extrapyramidal or hysterical. Therefore, the type of hemiplegia should always be stated.

A pyramidal lesion of the arm and leg on one side indicates a lesion of the opposite internal capsule unless some other sign such as aphasia is present, pointing to a cortical localization. An upper motor neurone hemiplegia of one side, with a lower motor neurone cranial nerve palsy on the other side (a crossed paralysis), indicates a brain stem lesion.

Monoplegia

Monoplegia is a paralysis of any type which is confined to one limb. An upper motor neurone monoplegia of an upper limb indicates a cerebral cortical lesion, but an upper motor neurone lesion of one lower limb may be due to either a spinal or a cerebral cortical lesion.

Paraplegia

Paraplegia is a paralysis confined to the lower limbs. It may be an upper or a lower motor neurone type of lesion. A pyramidal lesion of both lower limbs is nearly always due to a lesion of the cord. However, it may rarely result from a bilateral parasagittal cortical lesion affecting both leg areas of the cortex due, for example, to thrombosis of the superior longitudinal sinus, to fractures, or to developmental abnormalities of the skull such as craniostenosis or to a meningioma.

In a partial transection of the cord, the resultant spastic paraplegia is in flexion — that is, the lower limbs are involuntarily flexed at the hips and knees, because the extensors are always more paralysed than the flexors. But when the cord lesion becomes complete, paraplegia in extension results (reputedly because of coincidental involvement of the spinal extrapyramidal tracts), and then no voluntary movement of the lower limbs is possible and the tendon and plantar reflexes may be very difficult to obtain.

Quadriplegia
Quadriplegia is a paralysis of all four limbs, as is also diplegia. When it is of pyramidal type, the lesion may be in either the brain or the cord. The term diplegia, meaning a double hemiplegia, is often used as a synonym for a quadriplegia but some restrict the term to those cases, most commonly the cerebral palsies, where the lower limbs are affected much more than the upper and the site of the lesion is definitely cerebral.

A pyramidal lesion of all four limbs should never be considered as being due to a cord lesion unless there is a lower motor neurone lesion of the upper limbs as shown by wasting. However, in lesions of the upper three cervical segments it is usually extremely difficult to diagnose such wasting and, moreover, a brain lesion may be further simulated by the presence of sensory disturbances of the face and nystagmus. If the lesion is in the brain stem, then cranial nerve involvement will also be present. A bilateral internal capsule lesion is likely to be associated with a pseudo-bulbar palsy.

An extensive bilateral cortical lesion which causes an upper motor neurone quadriplegia is likely to be associated with intellectual impairment and possibly also with aphasia and/or epilepsy.

If an upper motor neurone lesion of any number of limbs is due to a cortical lesion which occurred before growth was completed, then it is frequently associated with lack of growth of the limb or limbs. This is often incorrectly interpreted as wasting due to a lower motor neurone lesion. However, it affects not only the musculature but the whole development including that of the bones, so that the limb may be shorter than its fellow or, even more striking, the hands or feet may be disparate. If both lower limbs are involved in such a process, then there may be dwarfism. Cases of pyramidal lesions with lack of growth due to cortical involvement must not be dismissed as due to birth injuries, because any lesion affecting the cortex before growth is completed may have a similar result – for example, congenital hydrocephalus, craniostenosis, or head injury in childhood. In all these cases the patient frequently states that he has got infantile paralysis, by which he means not poliomyelitis but paralysis which has been present since infancy.

The extrapyramidal system

ANATOMY
The extrapyramidal system is the old (evolutionary) motor pathway and consists of the following:
1. The corpus striatum, which consists of masses of grey matter deep in the cerebral hemispheres including the caudate and

lenticular nuclei. The caudate nucleus is an elongated curved mass lying in the floor of the anterior horn of the lateral ventricle and continues forward in the roof of the temporal horn of the ventricle ending in the amygdaloid nucleus deep in the temporal lobe. The internal capsule lies between the lenticular nucleus and the thalamus. The other parts of the lenticular nucleus are called the putamen and the globus pallidus.

2. The mid-brain structures – red nucleus, substantia nigra and the subthalamic nucleus, which is situated between the red nucleus below and the pulvinar of the optic thalamus above.

3. The spinal tracts – vestibulo-spinal, from the vestibular nuclei in the medulla; rubro-spinal, from the red nucleus in the mid-brain; and tecto-spinal (reticulo-spinal), from the reticular formation of the brain stem.

These various components should never be considered in isolation, because they are connected directly and indirectly with each other and also with the cerebellum and with areas of the cerebral cortex. Although, purely as a matter of descriptive convenience, the pyramidal and extrapyramidal systems are mentioned separately, they do in fact normally act in unison, and Sherrington's famous phrase, 'the integrative action of the nervous system', must always be remembered.

CLINICAL MANIFESTATIONS

Any lesion of the extrapyramidal system causes involuntary movements (described previously) and alteration of muscle tone. Either of these may dominate the clinical picture, but it is extremely unusual for there to be no involuntary movements at all. The involuntary movement is usually a coarse compound tremor and is then associated with increased tone. It may, however, be choreiform or athetoid and is then associated with diminished tone, but this is demonstrable only if the limbs are examined when no gross movements are present. The association of rigidity and tremor is called Parkinsonism. It is important to appreciate that the signs are often asymmetrical and may even be completely unilateral.

Exact localization within the extrapyramidal system is probably impossible, and the type of involuntary movement gives no certain clue. In paralysis agitans and encephalitis lethargica, lesions of the substantia nigra (with loss of its melanin pigment) and the globus pallidus are those most constantly found. Hemiballismus (severe choreiform movements affecting one side of the body but mainly the upper limbs, and always associated with rotary movements of the proximal joints) is regarded as indicating a lesion of the contralateral subthalamic nuclei and is often of vascular origin.

Extrapyramidal rigidity is always throughout the whole range of a passive displacement, and may be either jerky (cog-wheel) or uniform (lead pipe) throughout the movement. Lead pipe rigidity is more likely when the lesion is minimal and cog-wheel when it is more marked. It is unassociated with any alteration of any reflexes except when it is extremely marked, when the tendon reflexes may be sluggish. This rigidity gives rise to disturbances of facies, posture and movement.

Facies
The facies is often described as Parkinsonian or mask-like, although Parkinson himself did not include this as a feature of the condition. The latter description suggests that the expression is fixed and always the same, which is not true. Such patients can, for example, smile, although there is a slowness of initiation and relaxation of facial movements, and a better phrase is 'frozen face', with the implication of ability to thaw, albeit slowly. The patient often has difficulty in starting to walk and in turning.

Infrequency of blinking is a feature of Parkinsonism. Involuntary blinking whenever the base of the nose is tapped, no matter how often or how rapidly, is reputed to be a pathognomonic sign of Parkinsonism.

Posture
The abnormality of posture is one of 'universal flexion' of the head, spine, hips, elbows and wrists and adduction of the shoulders, the hands usually being held with the thumbs adducted, the metacarpophalangeal joints flexed and the interphalangeal joints extended or only slightly flexed.

Disorders of movement
The disorder of movement is a slowness of initiation and performance of emotional and voluntary movements which is sometimes described separately from the rigidity and designated bradykinesia but this is an unhelpful distinction. Parkinson himself wrote; 'There is difficulty in submission of the limbs to the direction of the will ... in the performance of the most ordinary offices of life.' The patient complains of weakness although there is no diminution of resistance to passive displacement. The speed and range of execution of active movements is lessened because of rigidity.

This poverty of all movements is well illustrated when the patient writes, walks or talks. Because of the rigidity of the hand muscles, writing is very slow and the letters produced are very small. Writing may also bring out a previously unobserved hand tremor. When walking, the patient maintains his attitude of universal flexion (if that is present at rest). There is a lack of associated movements (swing of the arms, and in females also of the pelvis). He walks with feet close together, scarcely raising them from the ground, and takes very small steps so that he shuffles along. As he walks, he goes more and more quickly as though 'chasing his own centre of gravity'; it is only the last phenomenon which is called 'festination'. If the patient is pushed, the festination will be so increased that he will fall unless he comes against an obstruction. This phenomenon is known as 'propulsion' or 'retropulsion' according to the direction of the impulse. Patients with Parkinsonism invariably find a walking stick a hindrance and not a help. Parkinsonism is often associated with emotional disturbance, seborrhoea, ptyalism and constipation.

CAUSES OF PARKINSONISM

Parkinsonism is always due to a lesion of the extrapyramidal system, and its manifestations are regarded as release phenomena. It may be degenerative, and is then called paralysis agitans or Parkinson's* disease. Parkinson's own description, published in *An Essay on the Shaking Palsy* in 1817, was brilliant. 'The condition produces involuntary tremulous motion with lessened muscular power in parts not in action and even when supported, with a propensity to bend the trunk forwards and to pass from walking to a running pace.' It may be inflammatory, as in encephalitis lethargica. It may be toxic, due to phenothiazine, rauwolfia (reserpine), butyrophenone or methyldopa derivatives, carbon monoxide or manganese. When the condition is drug induced it is reversible. It is sometimes secondary to arterial occlusion. It occasionally follows head injury, but is very unusual with neoplasms and extremely rare with syphilis. Cerebral atherosclerosis is often considered to be a common cause of Parkinsonism and a supposedly distinctive feature, differentiating it from the degenerative variety (paralysis agitans), is that the rigidity is marked and the tremor slight. Some neurologists consider that mental impairment and pyramidal signs are necessary accompaniments of arteriosclerotic Parkinsonism and indicating a more widespread involvement than the extrapyramidal system. An obvious aetiological difficulty is that most patients with paralysis agitans have coincidental arteriosclerosis because of their age.

The hypothalamus

ANATOMY

The hypothalamus is situated at the base of the brain and forms the floor and lower portions of the walls of the third ventricle. Anteriorly it begins at the lamina terminalis and the optic chiasma and just posterior to the chiasma is the infundibulum to which the pituitary

*James Parkinson (1755–1824), an English physician.

is attached and which contains blood vessels to the pituitary and to the hypothalmus. Behind the infundibulum the hypothalamus continues to the slight bulge in the region of the floor of the third ventricle called the tuber cinereum and then passes to the midbrain. There, in front of the interpeduncular space (fossa) are its two mamillary bodies one on each side of the median plane and with the optic tracts on either side of it. Many nuclei of the hypothalamus have been named but there is no agreement about their individual connections or precise individual functions.

The afferent fibres to it are from (1) the olfactory tracts; (2) the cerebral cortex, especially frontal; (3) the thalamus. The hypothalamus is closely linked with the limbic system, which comprises the hippocampus, the amygdalae and the septum lucidum. Clinical localization to any part of the hypothalamus is not justifiable. Moreover, the posterior lobe of the pituitary (pars nervosa), although it does not contain actual nerve cells, is traversed by many nerve fibres arising in the hypothalamus, and the pituitary and hypothalamus have a common blood supply. Because of this intimate association it is often virtually impossible to distinguish hypothalamic from pituitary signs, and they are often better designated by the term hypothalamic-pituitary or some similar phrase.

CLINICAL ASPECTS

The hypothalamus is a link between the central nervous system and the endocrines and exercises control over the internal milieu of the whole body. The hypothalamus activates, controls and integrates the peripheral autonomic nervous system and adjusts the balance to meet varying situations. It controls fluid and food intake, sexual impulses, rage, body temperature, and sleep. None of these activities depends solely on the hypothalamus. The anatomical and physiological relationships between the hypothalamus, the thalamus and the cerebral hemispheres cannot be summarized in a few sentences.

The manifestations of the hypothalamic-pituitary syndrome are as follows:
1. Obesity, especially of the trunk.
2. Hypogonadism, which, if it has occurred before puberty, may produce infantilism.
3. Diabetes insipidus.
4. Sleep changes, which may consists of prolonged episodes of diurnal sleepiness (hypersomnia), or inversion of sleep rhythm (the patient becoming restless at night and drowsy during the day), or narcolepsy.

Narcolepsy is characterized by an irresistible urge to sudden sleep produced by conditions usually conducive to sleep, such as boredom, or by emotional disturbance. The condition is frequently associated with cataplexy, but the two conditions may occur independently and should be regarded as separate entities. Cataplexy is a sudden momentary loss of power (associated with loss of tone) of the limbs produced by emotional disturbance, especially pleasurable. The severity varies from a transitory feeling of numbness of the limbs to a more widespread and severe weakness with lowering of the eyelids, drooping of the mouth and sagging of the limbs causing the patient to fall to the ground but without any loss of consciousness. The attacks last from a few seconds to a few minutes at most. Cataplexy must not be confused with catalepsy (catatonia), which is the maintenance for long periods of rigid statuesque attitudes of the limbs, frequently seen in schizophrenics and hysterics. Cataplexy must also be differentiated from another condition to which it has strong resemblance, namely sleep paralysis which occurs either at the moment of falling asleep or immediately on waking, the patient remaining fully conscious but unable to speak for about ten minutes and all the limbs remain paralysed. Sleep paralysis is often associated with hallucinations which although transitory are terrifying. Patients with narcolepsy or cataplexy or both may also suffer from sleep paralysis which is however a separate entity. No cause is usually found for any of these three conditions.

Other more unusual manifestations of hypothalamic damage are excessive salivation (ptyalism or sialorrhoea); greasy skin; high fever for no apparent cause and presumably associated with interference with the heat-regulating mechanism; and a liability to peptic ulceration and disorders of gastro-intestinal motility.

Causes of hypothalamic lesions
The commonest causes of hypothalamic damage are: (1) neoplastic, such as a third ventricle tumour, a suprasellar neoplasm or a chromophobe adenoma of the pituitary; (2) inflammatory, such as encephalitis lethargica or a tuberculous or syphilitic basal meningitis; (3) fractured base of skull. In some cases the aetiology is unknown.

The cerebellum

ANATOMY
For a proper understanding of the cerebellum it is important to know its anatomical connections, and these may most conveniently be described by listing the principal afferent and efferent tracts within each peduncle.

The inferior cerebellar peduncle (restiform body) connects the cerebellum and the medulla. The afferent tracts are (1) the dorsal (direct) spino-cerebellar tract, which arises at the roots of the posterior horns of the cord in a group of cells known as Clarke's column; (2) fibres from the vestibular nuclei; (3) fibres from the nuclei gracilis and cuneatus, which are the terminations of the posterior columns in the lower medulla. The efferent fibres are from the roof nuclei of the cerebellum, (emboliformis and fastigium) to the grey matter of the medulla and the vestibular nuclei.

The middle peduncle (brachium pontis) connects the pons and the cerebellum. Its afferent fibres arise from various parts of the cerebral cortex and pass through the posterior limb of the internal capsule, then the crura cerebri of the mid-brain, and so to cell stations in the pons (nuclei pontis). The efferent fibres are from the roof nuclei to the grey matter of the pons, and thence to the red nuclei and ventro-lateral nuclei of the thalamus.

The superior peduncle (brachium conjunctivum) connects the mid-brain and the cerebellum. Its afferent fibres are the indirect or ventral spino-cerebellar tract, situated in the lateral part of the spinal grey matter. The efferent fibres arise from the principal nucleus of the cerebellum, the dentate; from there they go via the peduncle to the grey matter of the mid-brain, and thus form associations with the third and fourth cranial nerves and the extrapyramidal system.

CLINICAL MANIFESTATIONS

The cerebellum has been described as the head ganglion of the proprioceptive system – that is, of the impulses arising from muscles, tendons, joints, bones and the labyrinth. Its main function is to control and co-ordinate all movements, probably by controlling muscle tone. The anatomical connections of the cerebellum indicate its integration with the motor and sensory parts of the cerebellum, and the extrapyramidal pathway, all of which control muscular activity. The cerebellum is not responsible for the design or initiation of movements but stabilizes, co-ordinates and smooths them out, ensuring their accuracy and precision.

Although it is generally agreed that the fundamental manifestation of cerebellar lesions is hypotonia and that all other signs derive from this, it is convenient for clinical purposes to subdivide the effects into (1) phasic nystagmus; (2) dysarthria; (3) intention tremor; (4) ataxia of the limbs, including gait; (5) hypotonicity of the limbs; (6) pendular reflexes. All cerebellar signs are ipsilateral. Precise localization to any part of the cerebellum or its connections is often impossible. When the physician refers to the patient as having a cerebellar lesion, he in fact means a lesion of the cerebellum or its connections.

Nystagmus

A nystagmus is an involuntary, more or less rhythmical movement of the eye, of small amplitude. It is essentially an ocular tremor.

When one is looking for nystagmus, the patient must be in a good light and preferably sitting. The examiner's moving finger must always be kept at least 10 inches away and never below the patient's eye level, and the patient should follow it to a point about 30 degrees to the left and right of the midline, which is roughly when the limbus and caruncle of the adducting eye meet. Nystagmus brought out only by extreme lateral gaze may be seen in normal people and patients on barbiturates and other anticonvulsive drugs and is of no significance. Such eye movements are sometimes called nystagmoid jerks to differentiate them from genuine nystagmus.

When due to a cerebellar lesion, nystagmus is phasic; that is, it has both a slow and a quick component, the quick component usually being towards and the slow component away from the fixing point. The direction of the nystagmus is labelled according to the direction of the quick component. Moreover, a phasic nystagmus is usually brought out only on full but not extreme conjugate deviation of the eyes, and therefore it is important to fix the head when looking for it. It can sometimes be best seen by careful observation of à scleral vessel, the movement of which may be easier to follow than that of the eyeball as a whole. Alternatively, looking at the fully conjugated eyes with a plus 15 lens is often useful.

Some irregular jerky movements of the eyeballs, of no significance, are sometimes seen either in normal people or in those with an ocular palsy. However, these movements lack the regular rhythm of a true nystagmus and cease when the patient keeps looking to the right or the left.

Regardless of which is the quick component, nystagmus on upward or downward gaze should always be regarded as significant, and is suggestive though not conclusive evidence of a brain stem lesion.

The description of a nystagmus as either fine or coarse is of little or no clinical value.

Type of nystagmus
Phasic nystagmus indicates a lesion of the vestibular pathway, the cerebellum or the cerebellar peduncles, but for some obscure reason it may also be seen with lesions of the upper cervical cord. Nystagmus of a phasic type occurs physiologically when the labyrinths are stimulated by rotation, or when a person watches a rapidly moving object (optokinetic nystagmus). The character of an optokinetic nystagmus is identical with that of a vestibular nystagmus. Labyrinthine (vestibular) nystagmus is horizontal and is more marked on looking in the direction of the quick component. It is influenced by alterations in the position of the head. Cerebellar nystagmus, which occurs even in the absence of vertigo, is usually of wider amplitude than the labyrinthine type and is accentuated when the patient looks towards the side of the lesion.

Phasic nystagmus occurring in only one eye is sometimes called a dissociated nystagmus. It may be due to local eye disease but is a common manifestation of a lesion, which is often vascular, of the brain stem, involving the longitudinal bundle connecting the third and sixth cranial nerves. A dissociated nystagmus is usually confined to, or much more prominent in, the abducted eye on lateral gaze to either right or left. If it is bilateral, that is, present in one eye on looking to the right and in the other eye on looking to the left, it is most often due to disseminated sclerosis.

Positional nystagmus occurs only when the patient's head is placed in certain positions. Whether or not the nystagmus alters when the position of the head is altered is immaterial. The patient, lying on a couch, is asked to fix his gaze on the examiner's forehead. The head is then turned to each side and the neck briskly hyperextended over the edge of the couch. If the patient has a lesion of the otolithic apparatus (utricle and saccule), this manoeuvre produces severe vertigo and a rotatory nystagmus (*see below*) directed towards the underneath ear and occurring only after a latent interval of a few seconds. The commonest cause of a lesion of the otolithic apparatus is head injury. Occasionally a positional nystagmus is found with posterior fossa neoplasms and also in disseminated sclerosis.

Phasic nystagmus is a common finding in barbiturate and also in alcohol habituation (especially in the presence of a peripheral neuritis). The nystagmus is not accompanied by any other signs of vestibular or cerebellar involvement, and its cause is obscure.

Contrasted with phasic nystagmus, which is linear along a horizontal or vertical line, is rotatory nystagmus, with a two-dimensional movement along a small (pendular) or large (oscillatory) arc of a circle. This form of nystagmus has not two components. It is often present even with forward gaze, and is due to a lesion of any part of the eye which has caused grossly defective vision. It may also be occupational — for example in miners, in whom, as a result of continually working in a dim light, there is interference with the development of visual purple. Albinos always have a gross oscillatory nystagmus.

Ataxia

Ataxia (inco-ordination), which literally means 'without order', is a clumsiness of movement. It is usual to restrict the term to inaccuracy of movement in the absence of obvious paralysis or involuntary movements of the limb. A patient with, for example, a pyramidal lesion or athetoid movement of a limb will have clumsy movements, but these should not be described as ataxia. Moreover, defective vision or a squint may interfere with the exact appreciation of the position of an object in space (erroneous projection), and such a patient's movements may appear clumsy.

Ataxia due to cerebellar lesions, unlike that due to involvement of the sensory pathway, is present even with the eyes open. It can be demonstrated in a large variety of ways. Although it can often be readily brought out by heel-to-knee and finger-to-nose tests, sometimes more delicate movements are necessary such as asking the patient to write quickly; to bring the tip of each finger rapidly in turn to touch the thumb of his own opposite hand; or to pat his knees first with the palmer aspect and then with the dorsum of both his own hands with increasing rapidity. Ataxia may be most obvious when the patient attempts to fasten his own clothes. Inability to perform a complex movement smoothly and rapidly is called dysdiadochokinesia, and is usually tested by asking the patient to pronate and supinate his forearms rapidly with his arms adducted to his sides. This is really another way of demonstrating ataxia. A good summary of cerebellar ataxia is 'In direction, range and force, movements err, even with the eyes open'.

Sometimes in cerebellar lesions, especially those involving its midline structure, the trunk muscles are more affected than the limbs, so that when the patient is examined lying down no ataxia of the limbs may be demonstrable, but the patient will have considerable difficulty in walking.

Gait
Often the best way of demonstrating ataxia of the lower limbs is by observing the patient's gait. With a cerebellar lesion the patient walks on a broad base in order to maintain his balance, and there is a lack of associated movement of the arms and pelvis (more noticeable in unilateral disease). In a mild case, unsteadiness is demonstrable only if the patient is asked to turn suddenly while walking. In a moderately severe case he will exhibit obvious unsteadiness, swaying, staggering or reeling to either side or backwards, the latter occurring especially if the lesion is in the vermis. 'They reel to and fro and stagger like a drunken man' (Psalm 107). Frequently the lower limbs are raised excessively and hyperabducted to compensate for the hypotonicity, and exhibit what is virtually an intention tremor during the replacement of the foot on to the ground. Moreover, this clumsiness is not corrected by vision and therefore, unlike a patient with a posterior column lesion, he does not look at the ground but straight ahead. In very severe cases, the loss of balance is of such a degree that the patient cannot even stand without falling.

Any abnormality of the gait due to a cerebellar lesion will, of course, be modified by the presence of other lesions, such as pyramidal or posterior column. Occasionally with cerebellar lesions, especially if acute, the patient adopts an abnormal posture of his head, which is flexed to the side of the lesion and turned to the opposite side (this is usually regarded as being due to interference with labyrinthine impulses).

Reflexes

Reflexes are not affected quantitatively in cerebellar disease because this pathway has nothing to do with the reflex arc, but the knee jerks may be altered qualitatively, becoming pendular. This must not be confused with increase of reflex.

CEREBELLAR DISEASES

Common examples of cerebellar lesions are as follows:

1. The hereditary and familial cerebellar ataxias. These constitute a group of conditions which have artificially been eponymously subdivided. They all commence in childhood or early adult life, with a gradual onset, and are gradually progressive. They are all characterized by cerebellar signs, which may be slight or marked. In addition they may show posterior column signs (which are gross in Friedreich's* type) and/or there may be pyramidal signs and occasionally primary optic atrophy. Skeletal abnormalities, such as pes cavus and scoliosis, are very common. Cardiac abnormalities may be present, usually taking the form of cardiac enlargement with or without arrhythmia.
2. The degenerative lesions of the cerebellum. These commence gradually in middle age or later and are gradually progressive but are not genetically determined. They also have eponymously described subdivisions. Probably the commonest is the primary cortico-cerebellar atrophy, in which signs are confined to the cerebellum. Olivo-pontocerebellar atrophy also belongs to this group.
3. Neoplasms. Because of their subtentorial position close to the ventricular system, these give rise early to signs of raised intracranial tension. In children, cerebellar tumours are nearly always highly malignant.
4. Inflammatory lesions of the cerebellum, such as abscess. These are usually secondary to middle ear disease. A tuberculous abscess of the cerebellum, sometimes referred to as a 'tuberculoma', is fairly common, especially in children. Disseminated sclerosis (often regarded as inflammatory) frequently affects the cerebellar pathway. It must be emphasized that it is extremely rare for syphilis to affect the cerebellum.
5. Toxic lesions of the cerebellum, due especially to alcohol and hydantoinates (Epanutin).
6. Thrombosis of the posterior inferior cerebellar artery. This is the commonest vascular lesion of the cerebellum. Because this artery also supplies part of the medulla, such lesions give rise to a distinctive picture (*see below*).

*Nikolaus Friedreich (1825–82), a German physician, wrote on this in 1863.

Sensory pathways

These are best considered by discussing separately the pathways for (1) joint, vibration, muscle and tendon sensations, and part of touch; (2) pain and temperature sensations. It is clinical judgment based largely on experience which should determine whether to do sensory testing in detail or minimally or not at all. Often the patient's history is a guide. When assessing the results the patient's intelligence, his power of concentration and suggestibility must always be taken into account.

Joint sense. Joint sense is the same as position sense. The patient should first be shown exactly what the examiner is doing and then, with his eyes closed, be instructed to reply 'up' or 'down' immediately the joint is moved passively. In testing joint sense at the toe or finger, care must be taken not to cause primarily a sensation of pressure instead of actual movement. This is done by holding one's finger and thumb on either side of the digit tested. The passive movements should always be done precisely and slowly at a uniform rate. Care must also be taken that there is no skin friction between the toes or fingers and that the patient does not attempt even the slightest active movement of the digit. Performed with care and with attention to all the details mentioned above, testing of joint sensation is a valuable diagnostic procedure, but as often performed it deteriorates into a meaningless ritual.

Vibration. Vibration sense is a test of bone conduction and is done with a tuning fork, preferably C128, with weighted ends, the heavier the better. A good plan is to place the oscillating fork first over the sternum, informing him that this is the guide and basis for assessment. Do not describe vibration sense to the patient in terms of sound or electricity as is often done. The fork after being struck by the physician is placed on a bony prominence always starting from the periphery of the limbs.

Muscle and tendon sense. Muscle sense and tendon sense are crudely tested by squeezing muscles or tendons, the sensation being normally only slightly painful. Such sensation is often referred to as 'deep pain'. An objection to this term is that within the cord, sensations are not divided into degrees, and terms such as 'superficial' and 'deep', 'epicritic' and 'protopathic', should be used only in reference to sensory peripheral nerve lesions. The best term, though not commonly used, is 'deep sensitivity'.

Pain. When testing sensation, it is important that the examiner should tell the patient exactly what he is going to do and exactly what type of reply is wanted. Pain sensation is tested with a pin and the examiner should show this to the patient, pointing out that one end is blunt and the other sharp, and that he should simply reply 'sharp' or 'blunt'. Ordinarily, the examiner does not wish the patient to attempt to analyse the degree of the sensation. The examiner must be very careful not to suggest an expected reply.

Pain and sensation to pin-prick are not really synonyms, pain being a much more complex and varied phenomenon, but response to pin-prick is the best simple way we have of testing pain.

Touch. Touch is best tested with a wisp of cotton wool, asking the patient simply to say 'yes' each time he is touched with it.

Temperature sensation. When testing thermal sensation, it is inadvisable to use very hot or very cold stimuli as they may cause a sensation of pain or discomfort rather than a thermal one. Tubes containing water at about 18°C and 40°C respectively are advised. It often helps to start by placing the tubes in turn on a part of the body which is not likely to be affected so that the patient knows exactly what is expected, and telling him 'This is warm' and 'This is cool' (or using two other related antonyms), and that a reply using exactly and solely the same words is expected.

ANATOMY

The pathway for joint, vibration, muscle and tendon sensations and part of the touch sensation is along the posterior nerve root with its root ganglion to cells in the posterior horn. The next relay is to the posterior columns (*Figure 10*). In the posterior columns the fibres from the lower parts of the cord lie most medially. These terminate

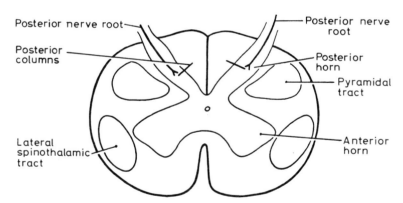

Figure 10. *Transverse section of the spinal cord showing the pathways for joint, vibration, muscle, tendon and part of touch sensations*

in the closed medulla in the nucleus gracilis (from leg and lower part of trunk) and nucleus ceneatus (from arm and upper part of trunk). From these nuclei are derived the internal arcuate fibres which cross the midline to form the sensory decussation (*Figure 11*). In the open medulla the sensory decussation is continued upwards as the medial lemniscus (fillet) which, at this level, is not yet split into its right and left components and is still separate from the lateral

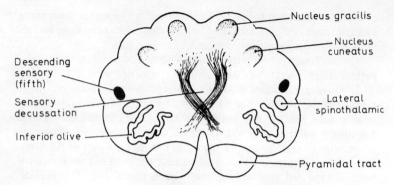

Figure 11. *Diagrammatic arrangement of the closed (lower) medulla*

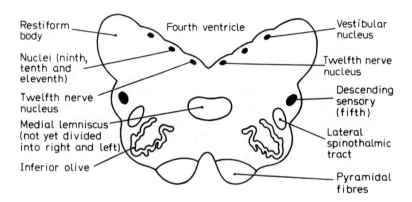

Figure 12. *Diagrammatic arrangement of the open medulla*

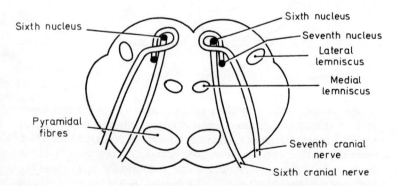

Figure 13. *Diagrammatic arrangement of the pons*

403

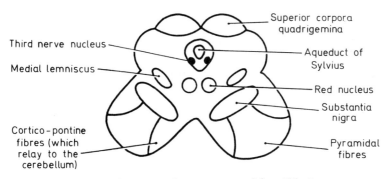

Figure 14. *Diagrammatic arrangement of the mid-brain*

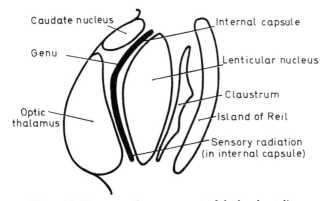

Figure 15. *Diagrammatic arrangement of the basal ganglia*

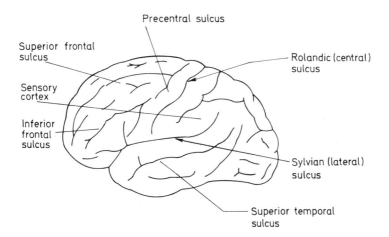

Figure 16. *Diagrammatic arrangement of the cerebral cortex*

spinothalamic tract (*Figure 12*). In the pons the lemniscus divides into right and left and is joined by the lateral spinothalamic tract (*Figure 13*). The medial fillet is continued through the mid-brain (*Figure 14*). The fibres (the sensory radiation) then go through the posterior limb of the internal capsule, terminating in the ventro-lateral nucleus of the thalamus (*Figure 15*), the reticular formation of the brain and the post-Rolandic area of the cortex (*Figure 16*).

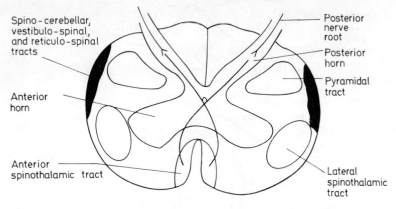

Figure 17. *Diagrammatic arrangement of the spinal cord showing pathway of half of the sensation of touch. The anterior spinothalamic tract joins the medial lemniscus in the medulla (see Figure 12)*

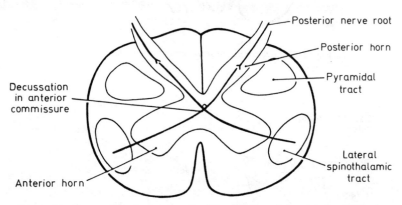

Figure 18. *Diagrammatic arrangement of the spinal cord showing the pain and thermal pathway. (For the rest of the pathway see Figures 11–16)*

The rest of touch travels along the posterior nerve root to the posterior horn and crosses over the midline of the cord to form the ventral spinothalamic tract (*Figure 17*), which joins the medial lemniscus in the open medulla, and from there onwards its pathway is the same as for the other sensations.

The pathway for pain and temperature sensation is along the posterior nerve root to the posterior horn and then across the midline in the anterior commissure to the lateral spinothalamic tract on the opposite side (*Figure 18*), which ascends the cord to the brain stem and, in the open medulla, is situated postero-laterally to the olivary nucleus, being still separate from the other group of sensations (*see Figure 12*) which are in the centrally situated medial fillet. In the medulla pain sensation from the face joins the lateral spino-thalamic tract, the fibres from the lowest segments of the cord being most lateral. In the pons the lateral spinothalamic tract joins the medial lemniscus, and from then onwards its pathway is the same as for touch and the proprioceptive impulses. In the thalamus sensations from the lower limbs are most laterally situated and in the cerebral cortex the most superiorly.

If any area of sensory impairment has both an upper and a lower limit, this indicates a lesion of the peripheral nerve, of the posterior nerve root, or of the sensory fibres within the cord before they have entered the long tracts. Either one's memory or reference to anatomical diagrams will show whether the distribution of the sensory loss conforms with the nerve root or the peripheral nerve pattern. If the area of impaired sensation has a well-defined upper limit but extends over the rest of the body below that level, not having a lower limit, then the lesion must affect the long sensory tracts of the cord. When localizing a cord lesion it is important to remember that the level of the various spinal segments do not coincide with the vertebral levels except in the upper cervical area. The C6 segment is opposite the centre of the body of the C7 vertebra, the upper thoracic segments are two above and the mid and lower thoracic are three above the corresponding vertebrae. The lumbar segments are opposite T12 and L1 vertebrae. The sacral and coccygeal segments are opposite L1 vertebra at which level the cord ends.

TERMINOLGY

It is important that terms used in regard to altered sensation should be precise and orthodox. No attempt is made to differentiate between complete loss and diminution of any particular sensation, for example between anaesthesia and hypo-aesthesia. 'Anaesthesia' in neurology means a diminution of touch unless it is preceded by an adjective such as 'total' (meaning loss of all forms of sensation), 'thermo-' (loss of temperature sensation), or 'dissociated' (*see below*). By analgesia is meant a diminution of pain sensation.

DISSOCIATED ANAESTHESIA

Dissociated anaesthesia is a diminution of pain and temperature sensations with a retention not only of touch but of all other sensations. The description of the sensory pathways explains how this comes about. Because the lateral spinothalamic tract joins the medial lemniscus in the pons, dissociated anaesthesia must always be due to a lesion below this level.

There are four causes, that is, four different anatomical localizations of dissociated anaesthesia. These are as follows:

1. With a lesion in the centre of the cord, the dissociated anaesthesia must always be bilateral and segmental (having an upper and lower limit, sometimes referred to as 'suspended'). It must be bilateral because it affects the fibres from both right and left posterior nerve roots which cross the centre of the cord. It must be segmental because it affects these crossing fibres at the level of the lesion and not the lateral spinothalamic tract. The dissociated anaesthesia and other signs produced by involvement of the nearby anterior horn cells and pyramidal tracts are frequently asymmetrical because the lesion, whatever its nature, is commonly not exactly central. The commonest pathologies at this site are syringomyelia, intramedullary neoplasm and spontaneous haematomyelia.

2. Dissociated anaesthesia will result from hemisection of the cord (Brown-Séquard* syndrome). This will be characterized by an ipsilateral lower motor neurone lesion at the level of the disease with posterior column and upper motor neurone lesions below that level, together with contralateral lateral-spinothalamic signs below the level of the lesion, giving rise to a dissociated anaesthesia of the opposite lower limb and possibly of the trunk. The only common causes of a Brown-Séquard syndrome are compression of the cord and intramedullary neoplasm, for example ependymoma.

3. Dissociated anaesthesia can be produced by a lesion confined to the anterior half of the cord, causing a lower motor neurone lesion at the site and bilateral upper motor neurone and lateral spinothalamic tract lesions below it. The only common cause of such a lesion is an anterior spinal artery thrombosis, and the dissociated anaesthesia produced is always a very transient phenomenon.

4. Dissociated anaesthesia will also be produced by lesions of the lateral medulla and in this case will affect the whole of the opposite side of the body, sometimes including the face. An important cause of such a lesion is a thrombosis of the posterior inferior cerebellar artery. A syringobulbia, because it is situated laterally, also typically gives rise to this distribution of dissociated anaesthesia.

---

*C. E. Brown-Séquard (1817–84), a French neurophysiologist, wrote his paper in 1850; born in Mauritius, he worked in Paris, London and Harvard.

The clinical picture of posterior inferior cerebellar artery thrombosis is as follows:

1. Dramatic onset of cerebellar signs, which are accentuated by the involvement of the restiform body.
2. Severe vertigo, usually unassociated with tinnitus or deafness.
3. Involvement of the sensory division of the fifth nerve, the sensory loss being ipsilateral and sometimes dissociated.
4. Dissociated anaesthesia of the whole of the opposite side of the body because of involvement of the lateral spinothalamic tract. This often clears up comparatively quickly.
5. Evidence of cervical sympathetic paralysis.
6. If the nearby pons is involved, ipsilateral fifth, sixth, seventh and occasionally cochlear eighth nerve lesions may occur.

POSTERIOR COLUMN LESIONS

A posterior column lesion will produce the following manifestations:

1. Diminution of joint, vibration, muscle and tendon sense. Touch is not affected because it has a dual pathway, crossed and uncrossed.
2. Diminution of deep reflexes.
3. Ataxia with the eyes closed, with the associated abnormalities of Rombergism and disturbance of gait.
4. Hypotonicity.

There is a great deal of needless and profitless quibbling about the reflexes in posterior column lesions. It is true that the reflex arc does not go through the posterior columns, and therefore theoretically the reflexes should not be diminished. But with any lesion of the posterior column, the intramedullary portion of the nerve root (including the posterior horns) and frequently the extramedullary portion also are affected, and it is because of such involvement that the deep reflexes are diminished. Which came first, the nerve root or the posterior column lesion, is a frequent but useless discussion, smacking of the hen-and-egg argument. Unfortunately, discussions of this type are great favourites with many clinicians. The position can be clarified by use of the term 'first sensory neurone', which includes the posterior nerve root, the posterior horn and the posterior column.

In the uncomplicated posterior column lesion, the patient walks on a broad base the better to maintain his centre of gravity and his limbs are lifted abnormally high. This is because such excessive range of movement is necessary before he can appreciate that the joints have moved at all, and the hypotonicity of the muscles necessitates an increased range of movement to 'pull in the slack', as it were. Due to lack of proper control of the legs, their movements are extremely clumsy and they are stamped back on to the ground. Moreover, when he walks he looks at his feet because vision may compensate in some degree for this ataxia and he can thereby control

o

his legs better. By Rombergism is meant that if a patient is completely steady when standing with his feet together and his eyes open, but becomes unsteady when he closes his eyes, he must have a lesion of the first sensory neurone. With involvement of an upper limb due to gross posterior column disease, the patient will not be able to appreciate the size or shape of objects held in his hand. Whether or not this should be designated astereognosis is a moot point (*see* section on cerebral cortex localization *below*).

Once again the sin of greed must not lead the student astray and he must be prepared to make a diagnosis of a posterior column lesion on very few of the above signs, sometimes even on only one sign such as diminution of some deep reflexes without wasting of the corresponding muscles.

PERIPHERAL NEURITIS

Peripheral neuritis is a condition caused by involvement of peripheral nerves anywhere from their nerve root to their termination. The term does not necessarily imply an inflammatory process, and the word neuropathy is pedantic. The involvement of the lower limbs is nearly always greater than that of the upper limbs, and sphincter disturbance is exceptional. Cranial nerve involvement may occur but is very unusual except in the severe forms, and is then often associated with paralysis rapidly ascending from the toes to the cranial nerve muscles.

Types of peripheral neuritis

Any peripheral neuritis may be wholly sensory, wholly motor or mixed, and recognition of this fact is extremely important. Thus, absence of subjective or objective sensory disturbance in one case, or absence of a lower motor neurone lesion in another, does not preclude this diagnosis. Most cases of peripheral neuritis are mixed.

Motor type

The best example of a purely motor peripheral neuritis is lead poisoning. While it is known that in this condition changes may occur in the muscles themselves, the orthodox viewpoint is to describe the condition as a peripheral neuritis.

Many cases of pure motor type were initially mixed — for example, that due to acute idiopathic polyneuritis, the sensory signs having cleared up.

A typical case of motor peripheral neuritis will be characterized by a lower motor neurone lesion of all four limbs, usually symmetrical and affecting mainly the peripheral muscles. The lower limbs are affected more than the upper, which may be spared.

The differential diagnosis from a myopathy has already been

discussed above and the sluggishness of deep reflexes excludes the likelihood of motor neurone disease.

Sensory type
The best example of a purely sensory peripheral neuritis is diabetic, and in such a case the differential diagnosis from a posterior column lesion may be extremely difficult. In peripheral neuritis there is pain on squeezing the muscles and tenderness of the soles, whereas in a posterior column lesion the squeezing of muscles causes no pain at all. However, such tenderness may be marked only in the acute phase and may disappear with improvement. In a peripheral neuritis all types of sensation may be lost, whereas in a posterior column lesion touch, temperature and pain are not affected. But often, for example in the diabetic, the sensory loss may be entirely of joint and vibration and a posterior column lesion will be very closely simulated, hence the term 'diabetic pseudotabes'. In a peripheral neuritis the distribution of sensory changes is of a 'glove and stocking' type, affecting the periphery of the limb without sharp demarcation from the normal, whereas in a posterior column lesion the sensory changes affect the whole limb. However, in a severe peripheral neuritis the sensory changes may even spread on to the trunk. This is often seen in acute idiopathic polyneuritis.

The difficulty of differentiation between a posterior column lesion and a sensory peripheral neuritis should always be borne in mind, and the points favouring one or the other should be carefully balanced and a verdict given according to the weight of the evidence observed.

Subacute combined degeneration of the cord
Rarer forms of diabetic peripheral neuritis are as follows:

1. A type affecting the motor and sensory supply of a few large peripheral nerves or even a single one such as the lateral popliteal or ulnar.
2. A purely motor variety, in which case the wasting frequently affects the proximal and not the distal muscles and is often asymmetrical. Some neurologists regard this variety not as a true peripheral neuritis but as being due to an anterior horn cell lesion. Other conditions causing peripheral neuritis which are often asymmetrical are polyarteritis and leprosy.

In subacute combined degeneration, the peripheral neuritis is the first manifestation of the condition. This may later be complicated by a cord lesion affecting the posterior columns and pyramidal tracts. But even in this condition it is important to attempt to differentiate between the relative degrees of cord involvement and peripheral neuritis, because the prognosis of the latter element is always good, whereas that of the cord lesion is equivocal, depending on whether or not irreversible changes have occurred.

The cerebral cortex

Cerebral cortical function is investigated by assessing (1) intelligence and memory and various aspects of speech all of which have been described previously, (2) special disturbances of sensation, and (3) the presence of apraxia or agnosia. If the patient has an upper motor neurone lesion of a limb or limbs associated with lack of growth of that limb this indicates not only that the lesion was present since infancy or childhood but also that it is localized to the motor cortex. Epileptiform attacks of any type are indicative of cortical dysfunction.

The sensory cortex is responsible for the following:

(a) Appreciation of fine differences in all types of sensation – for example, differentiation between the texture of silk and linen, velvet and wool, or wood and metal, and appreciation of minor degrees of differences in temperature, pin-prick and so on.

(b) One-dimensional localization (topognosis) – the patient not only appreicates that he has been touched or pricked, but can locate exactly where the stimulus was applied. An ability to recognize a number or letters traced out on the skin of the patient's limbs with a blunt instrument while his eyes are firmly closed is a special way of testing topognosis. This should be tested only if other sensations are normal.

(c) Two-dimensional appreciation – the ability to recognize two compass points as two and not one. The distance of minimal separation between two points which are still recognizable as two normally varies in different parts of the body, being about 1 centimetre on the palm and 3 centimetres on the sole. The compass or other points must be blunt.

(d) Three-dimensional appreciation (stereognosis) – the ability to recognize the size and shape of a readily identifiable object placed in the hand of a patient who has no obvious sensory disturbance, whilst his eyes are kept closed. If the hand is weak or arthritic then the object should be comparatively large. Astereognosis may be described as a tactile agnosia.

In the presence of gross intellectual impairment, it is useless to attempt the above sensory tests. Moreover, because of lack of complete attention, patients with cortical damage often give variable replies to identical stimuli.

PERSEVERATION

Perseveration is the continuation or repetition of movements which initially had a definite purpose but have become inappropriate, and which the patient is unable to control. For example, if a patient with perseveration is asked to close his eyes tightly and afterwards to protrude his tongue, he will obey the request perfectly, but either he will inappropriately continue to perform these movements or, if asked to repeat the performance, he will appear to be incapable of carrying it out although he had just demonstrated his ability to do so. This phenomenon is common in demented patients and in those with brain damage, whether due to injury, toxic agents, metabolic disturbances (including hypoglycaemic and gross electrolytic abnormalities, liver failure and hypoxia), or diffuse vascular lesions. It is not a localizing sign to any particular part of the brain.

The frontal lobes

ANATOMY

The frontal lobes are those parts of the cerebral hemispheres anterior to the sulcus of Rolando (coronal sulcus), and are for descriptive purposes divided into three parts as follows:

1. The prefrontal, which is anterior to the ascending frontal convolution and is devoid of any efferent motor impulses.
2. The post-frontal, which is continuous with the precentral convolution and includes the motor area and, on the left side, the motor speech area.
3. The orbital surface, which includes the olfactory bulb.

The motor cortex should not be considered as the highest hierarchial structure of the motor system or even the starting point of motor impulses but rather a link in a complex chain of impulses.

CLINICAL ASPECTS

Prefrontal lesions are common and are often neoplastic, and the signs of raised intracranial tension are often late and it is important to diagnose the lesion before such signs occur. The frontal lobes and their deeper connections give us our general sense of being alive, interest in living and ability to respond to the environment in a long-term and meaningful way, allowing for deliberation and consideration of possible actions, allowing us to plan intelligently and to adjust for future probabilities. These abilities allow us to stop and think, which animals do not do. Mental disturbance is common but far from inevitable with frontal lobe lesions. When present, it consists not only of emotional disturbance but also changes of personality and actual intellectual deterioration, which is usually subtle and rarely gross. Facetiousness, unwarranted jocularity, minor behaviour disorders and apathy are common manifestations. Epileptiform attacks are common.

If the lesion is in the upper and posterior portion of the lobe, especially if mesial, compulsive grasping and groping are often seen in the contralateral hand. Stroking the palm of the patient's hand close to the base of his finger causes an involuntary flexion of his finger, and may even produce marked tonic closure of his hand when the examiner slowly withdraws the stroking finger. This grasping may be present even if he is confused, but not if he is stuporose. Such contact, or the patient's seeing an object approaching his hand, may cause an involuntary groping towards the examiner's hand or the object. The grasping and groping reflex, to be significant, must be unilateral.

Post-frontal lesions give rise, at an early stage, to a contralateral upper motor neurone hemiplegia. Epilepsy is common and is often Jacksonian (*see below*). Acute involvement of the posterior part of the middle frontal gyrus causes impairment of voluntary eye movements to the contralateral side and in severe cases conjugate deviation of the head and eyes to the side of the lesion. Lesions of the posterior part of the inferior frontal gyrus of the dominant hemisphere if near a Broca area will cause a motor aphasia and may also cause apraxia. Lesions of the frontal lobe may also cause a distortion of the body image so that the patient cannot distinguish his right from left and he may neglect the side of his body opposite to the lesion and even deny that his paralysed limb is paralysed.

Lesions of the orbital surface of the frontal lobes may result in unilateral anosmia and sometimes unilateral exophthalmos, and if neoplastic may cause ipislateral optic atrophy and contralateral papilloedema.

The parietal lobes

Lesions of the parietal lobe affecting the area of the post-central convolution will cause sensory disturbance of a cortical type. If the dominant hemisphere is involved, visual aphasia is likely, and this may be associated with dyslexia and agraphia. Posteriorly situated lesions may cause a field effect, usually inferior homonymous quadrantic but occasionally a homonymous hemianopia. If there is an associated upper motor neurone lesion which occurred in early life, the affected limb or limbs will be small due to lack of growth.

APRAXIA

Apraxia may be a feature of parietal lobe lesions. This is an inability to perform familiar purposive complex acts, such as using a nail file or screwdriver or lighting a cigarette, in the absence of obvious mental disturbance, paralysis, ataxia, or sensory involvement of the limb. The disability is always confined to an upper limb and is independent of whether the attempted action is spontaneous, requested by the physician or imitative. Apraxia is difficult to test in a patient who has a disturbance of comprehension although it is probably present in a large number of patients with auditory or visual aphasia. It may be demonstrable by asking him to protrude his tongue which he may appear unable to do but later may be seen to do of his own volition. Or he may be asked to blow out a lighted match held by the physician. When testing limb apraxia each upper limb must be tested separately by such commands as asking the patient to salute or make a fist or use some instrument such as a screwdriver.

With parietal lobe lesions there may be a defect of spatial thought, and this can be demonstrated if the patient is asked to insert the numbers on a drawing of a clock face or surround a drawn circle with petals. In either case the patient may fail to fill in the side of the diagram opposite to the side of the parietal lesion. Allied to this there may be an apparent unawareness by the patient that a limb is paralysed, or he may even deny that one of his limbs is his. These abnormalities may be interpreted as a form of apraxia.

The occipital lobes

The main manifestation of an occipital lobe lesion is visual field defects. Cortical involvement of the dominant hemisphere may produce a visual aphasia. If epileptiform attacks occur, they are accompanied by visual hallucinations of a stereotyped pattern.

The temporal lobes

A temporal lobe lesion affecting the dominant hemisphere is likely to cause motor aphasia if anteriorly situated and auditory aphasia if posterior. Field defects usually take the form of a homonymous hemianopia, but a upper quadrantic defect may be produced if the lesion is superiorly placed. Bilateral lesions of the temporal lobes produce severe disturbances of emotion and behaviour, especially sexual and dietary. The emotional disturbances may include hallucinations, disordered recognition, disorders of memory and clouding of consciousness. Temporal lobe epilepsy is described below.

Hysterical anaesthesia

The features of hysterical anaesthesia are as follows:

1. All forms of sensation except joint sensation are usually affected.
2. The distribution usually does not conform with that produced by any known organic lesion. However, it may be a 'glove and stocking' distribution, simulating a peripheral neuritis, or it may be a total anaesthesia down the whole of one side of the body, such as can also occur in thalamic and occasionally with internal capsular lesions, but unlike with those lesions hysterical anaesthesia of the limbs is not always accompanied by severe disability.
3. The limits between normal and grossly abnormal are usually very sharply demarcated without any intervening zone of reduced sensation.
4. The extent of the anaesthesia varies at different examinations.
5. It can often be considerably modified by suggestion.

Epilepsy

It is impossible to give a pithy, precise definition of epilepsy. It might be regarded as paroxysmal cerebral dysfunction, a recurrent explosive disorder of consciousness. A difficulty of definition is that loss of consciousness is not an invariable accompaniment. The reason for the paroxysmal nature of epilepsy is obscure. Since the discovery of an abnormal electrical pattern (rhythm) recorded from the heads of epileptics, it has been fashionable to describe epilepsy as a cerebral dysrhythmia associated with the paroxysmal discharge in some part of the brain of an abnormal electrical rhythm.

Epilepsy is conveniently classified for descriptive purposes into four types: (1) grand mal; (2) petit mal; (3) Jacksonian; (4) psychomotor.

Grand mal is the occurrence of attacks of loss of consciousness together with convulsions. It is usually preceded by an aura, sensory, visceral or psychogenic.

Petit mal is the occurrence of attacks of clouding or actual loss of consciousness without convulsions. It is often accompanied by a fixed stare, a vacant expression and facial pallor, together with the sudden stopping of all motor activities. The loss of consciousness is very brief, lasting 10–45 seconds. Consciousness returns quickly and the patient resumes his discontinued activity, usually unaware that any attack has occurred.

Jacksonian attacks are those in which clonic movements occur. These always start at the same site, always exhibit the same order of spread (for example, from fingers to shoulder on that side), and are typically not followed by loss of consciousness. The pattern of the spread of the abnormal movements reflects the topographical relationship of the motor cells of the parietal cortex. Usually the trunk muscles escape. These movements are identical in every way with those obtained by electrical stimulation of the motor cortex. Jacksonian attacks may be followed by transient paralysis of the affected part which, following repeated attacks, may become permanent.

The above classification is, as stated above, purely descriptive, and any particular patient may at different times have any variety of epilepsy. The patient with grand mal often has petit mal attacks between the major paroxysms, and some Jacksonian attacks may be followed by loss of consciousness. Moreover, the causes of these types are not different. Jacksonian attacks are not necessarily associated with macroscopically identifiable lesions such as a neoplasm, although they are more likely to be so than the other types.

The causes of epileptiform attacks are as follows:

1. They may be caused by any organic disease of the brain, whatever its nature and wherever its site. Supratentorial lesions are much more likely than subtentorial ones to give rise to epilepsy, which is therefore unusual in lesions of the brain stem or cerebellum.
2. They may be due to known poisons such as lead and organic arsenic; to the unidentified poisons of uraemia, liver failure and toxaemias of pregnancy; or to any condition producing hypoglycaemic or gross electrolytic disturbance, especially of calcium or potassium.
3. They may be associated with cardiac arrhythmia, especially heart block (Stokes–Adams syndrome).
4. A large number of cases are idiopathic, but in these, genetic factors frequently play an important part.

Alternatively, the causes of epilepsy could be discussed as follows. Given an epileptogenic diathesis, which itself is often hereditary, any macroscopically recognizable lesion of the brain or disturbance of its function or biochemistry, by known or unknown poisons, will precipitate recurrent epileptiform attacks. The exact mechanism which causes such attacks in any given patient, or in any given pathology, is beyond the scope of this book, but it is important that the student understands the above basic principles before he gets immersed in any biochemical or biophysical discussions.

PSYCHOMOTOR (TEMPORAL LOBE) EPILEPSY

In any form of epilepsy, especially following petit mal, psychological disturbances such as compulsive behaviour and automatism sometimes occur after an attack, but paroxysmal pyschological disturbances may be the main or sole manifestation of epilepsy. In 1872 Morel* wrote:

> 'I have described a masked form of epilepsy in which there are no overt fits or convulsions but rather a great variety of other symptoms . . . periodic alternations of excitement and depression; unmotivated rage . . . amnesia for dangerous actions performed during these evanescent storms . . . true auditory and visual hallucinations . . .'

Since this masterly description, psychomotor epilepsy has been described under many names including temporal lobe epilepsy, epileptic equivalents, and uncinate fits (in which olfactory hallucinations are dominant). Its manifestations are many but are always paroxysmal and stereotyped (constantly having the same pattern). The patients usually have great difficulty in describing the attacks because they are outside normal experience. Hughlings Jackson† described the condition which may accompany these attacks as a dreamy state where dreams are mixed with present thoughts. The attacks are often accompanied by intense fear without there being any specific explainable reason for it. There may be hallucinations, and these are often very complex and may involve taste, smell, hearing or sight. The patient remains in touch with reality although his hallucinations appear very real to him. Illusions are also common, especially those in which objects appear to be grossly abnormal as regards their size or siting. Illusions may take the form of disorders of time perception, especially a *déjà vu* feeling (that is, of some familiar but previous environment) or the re-enactment of some previously experienced scene. Automatism may occur, the patient performing during an attack some complex co-ordinated activity of which later he has no memory. Other motor phenomena may occur during an attack, the commonest being twisting, writhing movements of the extremities, smacking of the lips and incoherent speech. Between the attacks, patients are often dreamy, hallucinated and agitated.

The lesion producing these attacks may not be localized to any particular part of the temporal lobe, although the mesial aspect is often incriminated. Indeed, the lesion may be beyond the anatomical limits of the temporal lobes, including the limbic lobe which surrounds the mid-brain, the hippocampus and the amygdaloid complex, the orbital aspect of the frontal lobes, and even the somatic sensory or visual areas of the occipital and frontal lobes. The cause of the lesion is often glial reaction, which may be secondary to injury or to inflammatory or vascular disease or, rarely, neoplastic.

---

*Benedict-Augustin Morel (1809–73), a French psychiatrist.
†John Hughlings Jackson (1835–1911), a London neurologist.

Autonomic nervous system

The nerve supply of involuntary muscles is from the autonomic nervous system with its two essentially antagonistic components, the sympathetic and the parasympathetic, both of which are integrated with the endocrines through the hypothalamus.

THE SYMPATHETIC SYSTEM

The cervical sympathetic has been described above. The rest of the sympathetic arises from the grey matter of the lateral part of the spinal cord, from the first dorsal to the second lumbar segment inclusive. The sympathetic fibres run with the anterior nerve roots and then leave the spinal nerves as white rami which terminate in the sympathetic ganglia. From these ganglia arise the two sympathetic chains lying on the antero-lateral aspects of the vertebral bodies. From them the fibres go to the various involuntary muscles, travelling either along the blood vessels supplying them or with the spinal nerves (grey rami). Efferent fibres go from the involuntary muscles via the posterior nerve roots and by white rami to the grey matter of the cord.

Sympathetic neuro-transmission is effected by the release of adrenaline at the post-ganglionic nerve endings. The exception is the fibres supplying the sweat glands, which release acetylcholine.

THE PARASYMPATHETIC SYSTEM

The cranial component is in association with the third (constrictor pupillae and ciliary muscles), the seventh (lacrymal and salivary glands), and the ninth and tenth nerves (to the viscera of the thorax and abdomen).

The cord component emerges with the sacral nerves and supplies the lower colon, rectum, bladder and genitalia.

All parasympathetic action is mediated by release of acetylcholine at the nerve endings.

PHYSIOLOGY OF MICTURITION

The bladder has a sympathetic and a parasympathetic innervation. The parasympathetic is the more important. The fibres of this are derived from the lower (pudendal) band of the sacral plexus which arises from the first, second and third sacral segments in the conus medullaris. The pudendal band is continued as the right and left pudendal nerves, the parasympathetic fibres of which are sometimes called the pelvic splanchnics or nervi erigentes. They supply the detrusor muscle and also carry efferent impulses from the bladder wall.

The lumbar sympathetic outflow forms the right and left aortic bands on either side of the aorta, being joined by splanchnic branches from the upper lumbar ganglia of the sympathetic chain. The main segments of the cord from which the sympathetic impulses to the bladder arise are the twelfth dorsal and first lumbar segments. The two aortic bands cross the iliac vessels and join together at the level of the fifth lumbar vertebral body to form the superior hypogastric plexus, which is sometimes badly named the presacral nerve. The superior hypogastric plexus divides to form the right and left pelvic (inferior hypogastric) plexuses.

A commonly held view is that the sympathetic conveys excitatory impulses to the internal bladder sphincter and inhibitory impulses to the detrusor. But most neurophysiologists consider that the internal sphincter is merely a part of the detrusor and, like the latter, is supplied by the parasympathetic, the sympathetic supplying only the relatively unimportant trigone musculature and possibly efferent impulses conveying the sensation of fullness and discomfort. This latter view, which ascribes a comparatively minor role to the sympathetic, is now generally accepted, although recently some experts have reverted to the view that the sympathetic plays the more dominant role in the control and performance of micturition.

In micturition not only the bladder musculature itself but also the muscles of the pelvic floor, especially the pubo-coccygeus and part of the levator ani (both of which are supplied by somatic fibres from the third and fourth sacral nerves), play a very important role. In addition, the posterior part of the male urethra has a ring of elastic tissue which is important in keeping the urethra normally closed.

A normal person has the ability to postpone or start micturition at will, emptying of the bladder depending on the initiation of stimuli from the cerebral cortex which are transmitted through the thalamus and the spinal tracts (probably pyramidal) to the cord. Moreover, the higher centres are capable of initiating bladder emptying in the absence of the stimulus of bladder distension by contracting the abdominal muscles and thus increasing the intra-abdominal pressure, or in response to emotion, cold, or certain sounds, any of which stimuli may cause small amounts of urine to be voided at frequent intervals.

With gradual bladder filling, there is increasing stretching of the bladder wall, which leads to involuntary contractions of the detrusor muscle developing in increasing strength. Fullness of the bladder produces a desire to micturate, but micturition does not normally occur until the voluntary release of impulses from the higher centres which allow forcible contracture of the detrusor muscle. As the intra-vesical pressure rises, the detrusor pulls open the neck of the bladder and shortens the urethra, while simultaneous contractions of the diaphragm and the abdominal muscles help to raise the intra-abdominal tension, although their action is probably not essential. In some complex way not fully understood, contraction of the detrusor is co-ordinated with relaxation of the muscles of the pelvic floor. Micturition is stopped by contraction of the external sphincter.

BLADDER INVOLVEMENT IN NEUROLOGICAL DISEASES

The type of bladder involvement which occurs in any neurological disease depends largely on (1) the completeness or otherwise of the spinal segmental lesion; (2) the acuteness of onset; and (3) whether or not the spinal reflex pathway in the conus medullaris is involved.

An acute complete segmental lesion is best exemplified by a cord injury. If the lesion is above the conus medullaris, then, during the phase of 'spinal shock', the detrusor is paralysed and retention results. If this is not treated properly, the bladder will subsequently become overstretched and lose its tone, resulting in retention with overflow incontinence and a consequent marked liability to infection. Otherwise, after a varying interval of days or of many months, the 'spinal shock' wears off and an 'automatic' bladder develops. In this condition, micturition can be initiated by sensory stimulation of the skin of the thighs or perineum but, because of lack of relaxation of the external sphincter, bladder emptying is never complete.

If the acute complete lesion involves the conus medullaris or the cauda equina, retention occurs, but after a while the patient learns that he is able to empty his bladder completely by the concerted action of his unparalysed abdominal muscles and his diaphragm aided by manual suprapubic pressure.

In chronic and incomplete lesion of the cord, due for example to cord compression, and in brain damage, voluntary control of micturition gradually diminishes and reflex hyperexcitability increases, resulting in frequency and urgency with occasional incontinence which later becomes permanent.

In tabes dorsalis, the bladder becomes insensitive to distension and the hypotonia results in incomplete emptying and, at a later stage, retention with overflow incontinence. The bladder may become huge, and cystitis is common.

In disseminated sclerosis, probably due to failure of cerebral inhibition allowing uncontrolled bladder contractions, urgency, frequency and precipitancy are early symptoms. However, sometimes difficulty in starting micturition is the first symptom. Retention occurs at a late stage of the illness, but the bladder never becomes as large as it often does in tabes dorsalis.

With any neurogenic disturbance of the bladder, a superimposed cystitis is likely and this increases the bladder reflexes, causing frequency. Bladder involvement is rare in the following neurological diseases: motor neurone disease, syringomyelia, subacute combined degeneration, peripheral neuritis and Parkinsonism.

In any male patient with disturbance of micturition due to neurological disease, more information can often be gathered by watching the patient attempting to pass urine than by complex pseudo-mathematical measurements of intravesical pressures and volumes.

Gait

Examination of the gait is an essential procedure in any case of definite or suspected neurological disease. An abnormality of gait may be the sole manifestation of even a serious neurological disorder. It is important to notice the patient's walk when he first enters the consulting room, because then his walking is likely to be more natural than when he is demonstrating it on request. But the gait must be carefully re-inspected at the conclusion of the examination.

EXAMINATION OF GAIT

Examination of gait must be in the following fixed sequence, with no omission of any detail.

1. Skeletal and cutaneous conditions which might interfere with the gait should have been recognized before the patient is finally asked to walk. Arthritis of the spine, of the sacro-iliac joints, or of any joints of the lower limbs more commonly causes difficulty in walking than do neurological lesions. The commonest reason for walking with a limp is undoubtedly some painful condition of the lower limbs, especially the feet, or of the trunk or abdomen. All these conditions must have first been excluded.
2. One must observe whether the patient can quickly and readily get out of his chair without any help.
3. Before the patient is asked to walk, he must stand as erect and still as possible and his posture and any involuntary movements must be observed. Involuntary movements often influence walking. If they are marked, and especially if they are of a choreiform or athetoid type, the gait may be rendered clumsy, but this must not be wrongly interpreted as evidence of a cerebellar or a posterior column lesion.
4. The patient is then asked to stand erect with his feet together and his eyes open. Any tendency to sway or lose balance should arouse suspicion of a cerebellar lesion.
5. Remaining in that position, the patient is next asked to close his eyes and is lightly pushed backwards, forwards and to each side in turn. If he was steady with his eyes open but becomes unsteady with his eyes closed, this is described as a positive

Rombergism and is indicative of a sensory peripheral neuritis, a posterior column lesion or, very rarely, a lesion of the sensory pathway in the brain.

6. The patient is then asked to walk straight with his arms swinging normally and without either hand in a pocket or holding anything. If he has become accustomed to using a stick, he should be persuaded to attempt to walk for at least a few steps without any aid and reassured that he will not be allowed to fall. He must be suddenly commanded to stop and turn quickly. This should not be done at any prearranged signal or when he has finished traversing the length of the room; the order must come unexpectedly, because only in this way will minor degrees of instability be brought out and recognized. If there is any suspicion of unsteadiness, it is often helpful to get the patient to walk quickly, first clockwise and then anti-clockwise, around a chair or table. This is a particularly useful manoeuvre in suspected unilateral cerebellar disease.

7. Sometimes it is helpful to get the patient to walk first on his heels and then on his toes, since these procedures accentuate any weakness of the appropriate muscle groups.

NORMAL GAIT

Very few normal people walk exactly alike. Sex, body build and race are important influencing factors. Females usually have smaller and quicker steps than males, swing their hips more and are more graceful. Apart from such factors there are subtle variations, perhaps distinctive for each individual, such as heaviness of tread, differences in pace and length of stride, carriage of the head and body as a whole, and range of associated movements of the upper limbs and pelvis. Some people claim to be able invariably to recognize familiar footsteps correctly, or to be able to identify people seen walking from behind by the individuality of their gait. Some also assert that they can assess a person's psychological make-up by his walk. While there may be some justification for such a claim, this ability must not be exaggerated.

A normal person while walking keeps his head erect and his dorsal spine fairly straight. The lower limbs, each in turn, are flexed slightly at the hip and knee and dorsiflexed at the ankle. The whole of the lower limb is then brought forward; the heel strikes the ground, and then the weight is thrust on to the ball of the foot while the other leg and arm are swung forward. Normally the arms are held adducted at the shoulders and slightly flexed at the elbows, and each upper limb in turn is swung rhythmically and freely over a roughly equal range. A normal person walks in a smooth and rhythmic manner, maintaining a perfect balance without any conscious effort.

ABNORMALITIES OF GAIT

Upper motor neurone hemiplegic gait

In cases of upper motor neurone hemiplegia, it may often be observed that when the patient is standing still he keeps the affected arm adducted and internally rotated at the shoulder and flexed and pronated at the elbow, with the fingers flexed. This posture will be maintained when he walks, with a proportionate loss of the arm swing. The hip on the affected side is often adducted, with the knee extended but the foot plantar-flexed. When the patient walks, the foot is dragged and the toes are scraped along the ground. With each step the affected lower limb is circumducted at the hip and swung out in a lateral arc, and the pelvis on the same side is tilted forward.

If the paralysis is mild, then the dragging and scraping of the toes may be observed only when the patient is fatigued, and the lack of swing of the arm is a more important but less obvious feature than in the severe case.

The upper motor neurone hemiplegic gait must not be mistaken for a unilateral Parkinsonism or vice versa.

Spastic paraplegia

The degree of interference with the gait in any patient with a spastic paraplegis depends on the severity of the lesion, so that in a mild case the patient may have a normal gait, and in a very severe case he may be unable to walk at all and may even be unable to stand unaided. In a moderately severe case the patient walks with stiff, jerky, slow paces, dragging and scraping his feet along the ground. In some cases bilateral adductor spasm causes a crossing of the legs with each attempted step (a scissors gait), and this makes progress very difficult. In any severe spastic paraplegia, when attempting to walk the patient often indulges in complicated movements of his upper limbs in an attempt to assist himself. In severe cases, walking is impossible without the aid of two sticks or other bilateral support.

Steppage gait

A steppage gait results from a bilateral or unilateral foot drop. This is a plantar flexion of the foot, with an inability to dorsiflex it completely, in the absence of arthritis of the ankle. It is often associated with an equino-varus deformity of the foot due to peroneal involvement.

Foot drop is due to weakness of the tibialis anticus and often of the peronei as well. Whether unilateral or bilateral, it may be due to an upper motor neurone lesion of these muscles, and then all the muscles of that lower limb will be affected. Alternatively, it may be caused by a lower motor neurone lesion, and then there will be wasting in the upper and outer compartment of the leg and possibly of other muscles as well. When foot drop is due to a muscle dystrophy (including peroneal muscular atrophy), the weakness, wasting and deformity are bilateral and symmetrical.

The steppage gait produced by foot drop is so called because the patient flexes the lower limb as a whole at the hip and knee, lifting it excessively so as to try and prevent the toes from catching on any ground object which might trip him, and then throwing the foot forward and slapping it on the ground. The patient with a bilateral foot drop walks as if traversing deep snow or dense ground vegetation. Especially when the peronei are involved (usually with a lower motor neurone lesion), he walks on the outer border of his foot.

Waddling gait

Patients with muscular dystrophy affecting the trunk and pelvic girdle muscles exhibit a duck-like waddling gait. Because of weakness of the trunk muscles and glutei, there is great difficulty in assuming and maintaining the erect posture. This difficulty is most apparent when the patient tries to stand from the supine position. He first turns on to his abdomen, pulls his knees under him and presses his hands on his knees to give leverage to his trunk muscles, meanwhile assuming a frog-like posture. He then gradually gets his trunk into the erect position by pressing his hands on his thighs at gradually progressively higher levels, pushing his trunk a little straighter with each movement. This manoeuvre has been described as climbing up his own thighs.

When the patient stands, he thrusts his trunk and shoulder girdles backwards to avoid strain on the weak erector spinae and other trunk muscles. This produces a marked lumbar lordosis and a protuberant abdomen. Such a patient walks with his feet wide apart and a marked swing of his body from side to side with each step, this being a compensatory movement of his trunk towards the alternating weight-bearing side because of inability to keep the pelvis at the correct angle relative to the side on which the weight is temporarily borne. A similar waddling gait is seen with bilateral congenital dislocation of the hips. Very fat people tend to waddle, but only to a minor degree.

Hysterical gait

An hysterical gait may mimic any type of abnormal walk. Its nature depends on which limbs are paralysed hysterically, walking being most affected when both lower limbs are involved. An extreme example of this is the condition of astasia-abasia, in which no gross weakness of the lower limbs is demonstrable when tested with the patient lying down but the patient cannot walk or even stand unaided.

In other cases, on attempted walking the striking features are bobbing, weaving, lurching or gyratory movements, which may be extremely bizarre. Frequently a prominent feature is that, in spite of these unusual movements when walking is attempted, the patient does not lose her balance but maintains it with the dexterity of an expert acrobat, which she could not possibly do if she had a lesion of the cerebellum or the sensory pathways. Often these patients are capable of expertly balancing on one foot as they slowly and hesitatingly transfer their weight from one side to the other. Such inconsistencies are a common and important feature of hysteria. Another important finding is that by coaxing and persuasion the physician can diminish the disability, albeit only temporarily.

The recognition of any walk as definitely hysterical requires skill, experience, and sometimes diagnostic courage. I have personally seen patients with hysterical paralysis diagnosed as organic disease, usually by those who have no diagnostic courage or suffer from the delusion that hysteria no longer occurs. On the other hand, I have often seen patients with organic neurological disease, especially disseminated sclerosis and myasthenia gravis, wrongly diagnosed as hysterical.

Abnormal gaits in lesions of the extrapyramidal system, the cerebellum and the sensory pathways have been described elsewhere in this chapter. Obviously any patients with combined lesions will have a gait more complicated than any described under the various anatomical headings. For example, disseminated sclerosis causes neither the typical gait of a cerebellar lesion nor that of a spastic paraplegia.

In order to learn and appreciate variations of gait, it is desirable first to study examples of localized lesions: for example, a unilateral cerebellar lesion due to a vascular episode; a bilateral cerebellar lesion due to a primary cortical cerebellar atrophy; a posterior column lesion due to tabes dorsalis; or a steppage gait due to a motor peripheral neuritis or a lesion of the lateral popliteal nerve. Too many doctors never correctly appreciate the diagnostic significance of the various abnormal gaits because their observations have been confined to patients with complex lesions. They fail to appreciate that there is no such thing as a typical gait of disseminated sclerosis, of subacute combined degeneration, or even of the hereditary spino-cerebellar ataxias. With few exceptions, it is not the specific disease itself but the anatomical site or sites which the disease affects that causes any recognizable alteration of gait.

Index